Outcomes in neurodevelopmental and genetic disorders

Edited by two leading authorities and written by a team of international experts in the field, this book describes the causes, course and treatment of a variety of developmental and genetic disorders, including attention deficit disorder, fragile X syndrome and autism. There is a particular focus on the course of disorders over time and prognosis in adulthood. Outcome is an area often overlooked in other books dealing with developmental disorders, but is an issue of great importance to parents and carers, and one that has important implications for education, health, social and employment services.

As well as offering succinct and up-to-date summaries of the most recent research, the authors provide clinicians with practical guidelines for intervention and management with children and young adults. This book is essential reading for clinicians and psychologists, and anyone working with or caring for individuals with neurodevelopmental disorders.

Patricia Howlin is Professor of Psychology at St George's Hospital Medical School in London. She is Editor of *Autism: International Journal of Research and Practice* and Annotations Editor of the *Journal of Child Psychology and Psychiatry*. Her book *Autism Preparing for Adulthood* won the NASEN Special Educational Needs prize.

Orlee Udwin is Consultant Clinical Psychologist at the Mary Sheridan Centre for Child Health, and Honorary Senior Lecturer in Clinical Psychology at the Institute of Psychiatry, King's College London. She is joint editor of the journal *Child and Adolescent Mental Health*.

Cambridge Child and Adolescent Psychiatry

Child and adolescent psychiatry is an important and growing area of clinical psychiatry. The last decade has seen a rapid expansion of scientific knowledge in this field and has provided a new understanding of the underlying pathology of mental disorders in these age groups. This series is aimed at practitioners and researchers both in child and adolescent mental health services and developmental and clinical neuroscience. Focusing on psychopathology, it highlights those topics where the growth of knowledge has had the greatest impact on clinical practice and on the treatment and understanding of mental illness. Individual volumes benefit both from the international expertise of their contributors and a coherence generated through a uniform style and structure for the series. Each volume provides firstly an historical overview and a clear descriptive account of the psychopathology of a specific disorder or group of related disorders. These features then form the basis for a thorough critical review of the etiology, natural history, management, prevention and impact on later adult adjustment. Whilst each volume is therefore complete in its own right, volumes also relate to each other to create a flexible and collectable series that should appeal to students as well as experienced scientists and practitioners.

Editorial board

Already published in this series:

Outcomes in neurodevelopmental and genetic disorders

Edited by

Patricia Howlin

and

Orlee Udwin

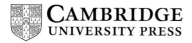

CAMBRIDGE
UNIVERSITY PRESS

PUBLISHED BY THE PRESS SYNDICATE OF THE UNIVERSITY OF CAMBRIDGE

The Pitt Building, Trumpington Street, Cambridge, United Kingdom

CAMBRIDGE UNIVERSITY PRESS

The Edinburgh Building, Cambridge CB2 2RU, UK

40 West 20th Street, New York, NY 10011-4211, USA

477 Williamstown Road, Port Melbourne, VIC 3207, Australia

Ruiz de Alarcón 13, 28014 Madrid, Spain

Dock House, The Waterfront, Cape Town 8001, South Africa

http://www.cambridge.org

First published 2002

Printed in the United Kingdom at the University Press, Cambridge

Typeface Dante MT 11/14pt   *System* Poltype® [v n]

A catalogue record for this book is available from the British Library

ISBN 0 521 79721 7 paperback

Every effort has been made in preparing this book to provide accurate and up-to-date information which is in accord with accepted standards and practice at the time of publication. Nevertheless, the authors, editors and publisher can make no warranties that the information contained herein is totally free from error, not least because clinical standards are constantly changing through research and regulation. The authors, editors and publisher therefore disclaim all liability for direct or consequential damages resulting from the use of material contained in this book. Readers are strongly advised to pay careful attention to information provided by the manufacturer of any drugs or equipment that they plan to use.

Contents

Contributors

Joseph H. Beitchman
Centre for Addiction and Mental Health
University of Toronto
250 College Street
Toronto
Ontario M5T 1RB
Canada

Patrick Bolton
University of Cambridge
Department of Psychiatry
2nd Floor, Douglas House
18B Trumpington Road
Cambridge CB2 2AH
UK

Jill Butler
University of Cambridge
Department of Psychiatry
2nd Floor, Douglas House
18B Trumpington Road
Cambridge CB2 2AH
UK

Janet Carr
2 Gaston Cottages
Little Bookham Street
Bookham
Surrey KT23 3BX
UK

Anupam Chakrapani
Birmingham Children's Hospital
Steelhouse Lane
Birmingham B5 6NH
UK

Nancy J. Cohen
The Hincks-Dellcrest Institute
Silverman Building
114 Maitland Street
Toronto
Ontario M4Y 1E1
Canada

Robert Goodman
Institute of Psychiatry
Department of Child and Adolescent
Psychiatry
De Crespigny Park
Denmark Hill
London SE5 8AF
UK

Paul J. Hagerman
University of California at Davis
Department of Biological Chemistry
School of Medicine
One Shields Ave
Davis CA 95616
USA

Randi J. Hagerman
MIND Institute
UC Davis Medical Center
4860 Y Street, Suite 3020
Sacramento
CA 95817
USA

A. J. Holland
University of Cambridge
Department of Psychiatry
2nd Floor, Douglas House
18B Trumpington Road
Cambridge CB2 2AH
UK

Patricia Howlin
St George's Hospital Medical School
Department of Psychology
Cranmer Terrace
London SW17 0RE
UK

Alison Kerr
University of Glasgow
Monitoring Unit, Academic Centre
Department of Psychological Medicine
Gartnavel Royal Hospital
1055 Great Western Road
Glasgow G12 0XH
UK

Orlee Udwin
Mary Sheridan Centre for Child Health
5 Dugard Way
off Renfrew Road
Kennington
London SE11 4TH
UK

Petrus J. de Vries
University of Cambridge
Section of Developmental Psychology
Douglas House
18B Trumpington Road
Cambridge CB2 2AH
UK

John Walter
Royal Manchester Children's Hospital
Willink Biochemical Genetics Unit
Pendlebury
Manchester M27 4HA
UK

Jody Warner-Rogers
Guy's Hospital
Newcome Centre
St Thomas Street
London SE1 9RT
UK

Joyce Whittington
University of Cambridge
Department of Psychiatry
2nd Floor, Douglas House
18B Trumpington Road
Cambridge CB2 2AH
UK

Arlene R. Young
Simon Fraser University
Department of Psychology, RCB 8307
8888 University Drive
Burnaby
British Columbia V5A 1S6
Canada

Preface

Much of the research and the majority of descriptive and clinical accounts related to developmental or early onset genetic disorders have an understandable focus on children. The parents of young children with such conditions have a pressing need to know why the disorder has occurred, whether it can be prevented, what are the genetic implications for other family members, what the long-term outcome is likely to be and perhaps most importantly what they can do to help their child. As time moves on, teachers and others responsible for educational provision need to know what problems these children are likely to face in gaining access to the regular school curriculum and what extra help will be needed in order to meet any special educational needs. And, at every stage, paediatricians, child psychologists and psychiatrists, health visitors, language therapists and many other professionals are likely to be called on for support and advice. It is clearly crucial therefore that those involved in the care, education or therapy of children with developmental and genetic disorders are fully apprised of the nature of the problems with which they have to deal, and of how they can help to minimize difficulties, enhance skills and prevent the development of secondary problems.

However, conditions such as Rett syndrome, fragile X or autism do not suddenly disappear around the age of 16 to 18 years. Neither do problems related to language, specific learning difficulties or attentional deficits cease at these ages. Unfortunately, all too often, the help and care that children and their families have received comes to an abrupt halt when these children reach adulthood. Teachers are no longer available to provide advice on education or other issues, and specialist clinical services are typically replaced by generic adult services for people with chronic physical or mental health problems, or intellectual impairments. Faced with an ever increasing clinical load, few practitioners working in these areas can be expected to spend much time also learning about children's disorders. And anyway, how relevant is such knowledge likely to be? Knowing about the early development of a young girl with

Rett syndrome, for example, is unlikely to be of great help when it comes to dealing with the physical and emotional problems sometimes experienced by older women with this condition. Similarly, the early *specific* problems of a child with language or reading difficulties may be replaced by a range of different social or emotional problems in adulthood.

Knowledge about the long-term outcome of childhood disorders is crucial if families and clinical and social services are to be able to plan adequately for adulthood. Thus, our aim in the present volume has been to examine some relatively well-known conditions with an onset in childhood but from a developmental perspective. What happens to these children as they grow up? Does the condition change with time, bringing new difficulties or a decline in severity? What problems are parents, carers and the individuals themselves likely to face, and how can these be effectively managed? Above all, what can be done to help individuals live lives that are as full and as satisfactory as possible?

As well as addressing such issues in the various chapters, we have sought to provide up-to-date and accessible summaries of what is currently known about the causes of these conditions (particularly those related to genetic factors) and the principal problems with which they are associated. And, because research into adult interventions remains limited, we highlight therapies and approaches that seem to be helpful for children, in the hope that knowledge about effective strategies may be adapted to work with adults.

The conditions themselves vary in severity, pervasiveness and prevalence. Some, such as attention deficit disorders, specific reading and other learning disorders, and language impairments are relatively common. These are conditions that most professionals working in adult education, medical, mental health or learning disability services are likely to encounter. Thus, knowledge of the adult sequelae of childhood difficulties, and the ways in which they may change over time, is particularly important.

Other disorders, including tuberous sclerosis, Rett syndrome, Prader-Willi, Angelman, Williams and Smith-Magenis syndromes and various metabolic disorders are relatively rare. However, their severity is such that it is crucial for those working in adult services to have at least some basic knowledge about what physical, behavioural, social and emotional problems may be manifest in adulthood. Even more important is access to information on how to manage these difficulties when they do occur.

Finally, there is a group of disorders that occur relatively frequently, but in which the presentation can be very variable. Fragile X and Down syndrome for example, are amongst the most common known chromosomal causes of intellectual disability, but levels of functioning can range from borderline/ average to profound mental retardation. Cerebral palsy – which is the single largest cause of severe physical handicaps in childhood – and autism are both spectrum disorders. Both can lead to profound and pervasive handicaps, or relatively mild impairments that with appropriate support can be greatly helped. However, this means that outcome can be significantly affected – for better or worse – by the degree of support that is available, not only in childhood but also in later adolescence and early adulthood. Even in the case of those whose disability is less severe, appropriate provision can make the difference between leading a rich and fulfilled life, or one that is dogged by continuing social problems and emotional turmoil.

It is our hope that by providing an accessible and up-to-date account of what happens to children with developmental disorders as they progress to adulthood – and what help they may need to see them safely along that path – the journey both for them, and those caring for them may be made a little easier.

Patricia Howlin and Orlee Udwin

1

Attention deficit hyperactivity disorder

Jody Warner-Rogers

Attention deficit hyperactivity disorder (ADHD) is one of the most prevalent psychiatric disorders of childhood. Although once a vigorously debated issue, it is now accepted that ADHD can be reliably distinguished from other behavioural problems in childhood and adolescence (Goldstein, 1999). The disorder is also recognized as existing beyond childhood (Tannock, 1998), resulting in the need for clinicians to increase their understanding of the various developmental outcomes and age-related changes in presentation and response to treatment.

This chapter begins by summarizing the research and clinic-based evidence regarding the nature of ADHD. The manner in which the disorder can affect individuals as they mature from childhood to adulthood is then discussed and various intervention strategies are presented.

Diagnostic classifications and prevalence

An important difference exists between simple hyperactivity, which describes a tendency to behave in an inattentive, overactive and impulsive way, and the psychiatric diagnostic category of ADHD. Most children are hyperactive in some situations. Indeed, hyperactivity is a trait, not unlike intelligence, that appears to be normally distributed in the general population (Taylor et al., 1991). However, in most children, their behaviour is regulated by environmental demands. This influence, and accompanying behavioural control, increases with age and maturity. Society expects increased behavioural control as children develop. At school, for example, a 5-year-old child might be expected to sit quietly listening to a 10-minute story, whereas a 15-year-old child would be required to sit and attend for a 45-minute lesson.

Some children consistently exhibit hyperactive behaviour across many situations and appear to have difficulty modifying their behaviour in response to their environment. These children exhibit levels of inattention, impulsiveness and overactivity that can actually impair their functioning in one or more areas (e.g. academic, social). When such difficulties are early in onset (before the age of 7 years), persistent over time (at least 6 months), pervasive across situations (evident in at least two different settings), and, importantly, out of keeping with their general developmental level (global intellectual functioning), a psychiatric diagnosis may be appropriate.

The two main current classification schemes, namely the fourth edition of the *Diagnostic and Statistical Manual* (DSM-IV), published by the American Psychiatric Association (APA, 1994), and the tenth edition of the *International Classification of Diseases* (ICD-10), published by the World Health Organization (WHO, 1994) both contain a disorder characterized by a cluster of three core behavioural symptoms: inattention; hyperactivity; and impulsivity. However, the two schemes differ in important ways and it is these differences that have contributed, in part, to the different ways in which the symptoms have been conceptualized and managed in Europe and North America. Both the DSM-IV and ICD-10 classification schemes are now used in the United Kingdom (UK).

Currently, the DSM-IV lists ADHD as a primary disorder. However, the scheme allows for the subtyping of the disorder based on the predominance of symptoms: ADHD Combined Type (all three core symptoms present); ADHD Predominantly Inattentive Type; and ADHD Predominantly Hyperactive–Impulsive Type. In contrast, all three symptoms must be present for a child to meet criteria for an ICD-10 diagnosis of Hyperkinetic Disorder (HKD). Thus, all children with a diagnosis of ADHD or HKD exhibit hyperactivity. More-over, all children with HKD would meet criteria for ADHD Combined Type but those with ADHD Predominantly Inattentive Type or Predominantly Hyperactive–Impulsive Type would not meet the more stringent criteria for HKD. Prevalence figures for disorders, therefore, will vary depending on which diagnostic scheme is being used and whether or not the subtypes in the DSM-IV are being applied.

Approximately 1.7% of children meet criteria for HKD (Taylor et al., 1991). In comparison, ADHD, a more broadly defined disorder, affects 3–5% of children (Szatmari, Offord & Boyle, 1989). The ratio of affected boys to girls is around 4:1 (Ross & Ross, 1982; James & Taylor, 1990). Hyperactivity is more common in urban than rural areas (Taylor et al., 1991). Links exist between hyperactivity and pervasive developmental disorder (PDD) in that children with autistic spectrum disorders can be very hyperactive. However, in the hierarchy of diagnoses, PDD is given priority in such cases. The treatment of hyperactive behaviour in a child with a pervasive developmental disorder may be quite different to that used in straight forward cases of ADHD.

The diagnosis of either ADHD or HKD, is based on patterns of behaviours, *not* aetiological factors, and involves the ruling out of alternative, differential diagnoses such as autism. The issue of comorbidity, however, is addressed differently in the DSM-IV and ICD-10. The DSM system allows for multiple diagnoses to be given (e.g. ADHD *and* Conduct Disorder; or ADHD *and* Generalized Anxiety Disorder), but the ICD system views HKD as a relatively rare condition that occurs in isolation. When other problems are also present to a significant degree, then other diagnoses may be given (e.g. Hyperkinetic–Conduct Disorder or Mixed Disorder of Conduct and Emotion).

This chapter will use the terms hyperactivity and ADHD interchangeably to imply the presence of developmentally inappropriate levels of inattention, overactivity and impulsiveness. However, it is important that readers appreciate the subtle differences in the way terms are used within professional and lay circles.

Nature of the disorder

Hyperactive behaviour can be relatively easy to operationalize and quantify. Rating scales or direct observations can provide reliable measures of the occurrence and frequency of selected behaviours (e.g. number of times a child is out of his/her seat during a lesson; percentage of a task completed; frequency of calling out in class without raising a hand). In contrast, it has proven considerably more difficult to identify the specific cognitive delays, deficits or dysfunctions that might underpin these behaviours. Indeed, much of the recent research in the field has focused on the identification of cognitive and genetic factors, as well as the identification of abnormalities in brain structure and function (see Tannock, 1998, for a review).

Despite the name attention *deficit* hyperactivity disorder, children with ADHD do not necessarily have a deficit in their cognitive attentional processes, even though they may exhibit behaviours that are suggestive of cognitive inattentiveness, such as frequently changing activity or being easily distracted. Experimental studies indicate that the primary problem in ADHD is not one of a poor level of attention, or inability to sustain it or a failure selectively to attend (Taylor, 1995). Rather, research evidence is converging to support the theory that the underlying deficit lies in a problem with behavioural inhibition and self-regulation (Taylor, 1994).

Behavioural inhibition has been seen as three inter-related processes: (1) the inhibition of a prepotent response; (2) the cessation of an on-going response such that a delay occurs which allows an individual to make a decision about the response; and (3) the ability to maintain this delay and prevent other events and responses from interfering with the self-directed responses that are happening within it (Barkley, 1997a). Those areas of the brain that control attention and the organization of responses, namely the frontostriatal areas, are being extensively investigated.

It is quite possible that children with ADHD Primarily Inattentive Type differ in terms of aetiology, prognosis and response to treatment from children with ADHD Primarily Hyperactive–Impulsive Type or those with ADHD-Combined subtype. Although the inattentive behaviours may be topographically similar across the subtypes, the nature of the cognitive attention deficit may be quite different. In particular, the inattentive subtype appears more closely linked to educational difficulties (Warner-Rogers et al., 2000) and socio-economic disadvantage (Taylor et al., 1991). These children tend to be described by their teachers as inattentive and dreamy, but not particularly overactive or impulsive (Taylor et al., 1991). Many researchers now argue that children with ADHD Primary Inattentive Type should not be included in the same study groups as ADHD Combined Type (Barkley, 1997a).

In a book written primarily for parents raising a child with ADHD, Barkley (1995) provides a useful summary of the cognitive nature of the disorder and the associated behavioural symptoms. In terms of their *attentional* functioning, Barkley (1995) notes that children with ADHD have: (1) difficulty sustaining attention; (2) get bored or lose interest in work faster than other children; and are (3) drawn to the most rewarding, stimulating or fun feature of any situation – a tendency that can make them appear easily distractible. With regards to *impulsive* behaviour, children with ADHD have difficulty controlling their impulses and deferring gratification. These tendencies can lead to: (1) more risk taking; (2) impulsive thinking; and (3) problems managing money. The *hyperactivity* aspect is described as 'a problem with too much behaviour' (Barkley, 1995: p. 36). Children with ADHD are both more physically active and respond to more aspects of their environment than non-ADHD children, making them seem 'hyper-responsive'. Finally, these children have difficulty with following instructions and working consistently. All of these behavioural symptoms are linked theoretically and reflect a disorder of self-control, and the ability to organize and direct behaviour towards a future goal (Barkley, 1995, 1997a).

Aetiology of the disorder

The development of ADHD in any given individual is likely to be multi-factorial (Taylor, 1998). Genetic contributions, neurobiological factors, illness or injury, psychological variables and environmental factors may all play a role.

Tannock (1998: p. 65) describes ADHD as 'a paradigm for a true bio-psychosocial disorder', reflecting the complex relations and interactions between genetic, biological and environmental factors.

Twin studies indicate that the tendency to behave in a hyperactive manner is highly heritable (e.g. Goodman & Stevenson, 1989a,b; Silberg et al., 1996). Pervasive hyperactivity is more concordant in monozygotic than in dizygotic twins. Goodman & Stevenson (1989a,b) found concordance rates of 51% in monozygotic twins compared to 30% in dizygotic twins. Several possible genetic mechanisms are currently being explored, including variations in the dopamine 4 receptor gene (LaHoste et al., 1996). Current consensus among genetic researchers suggests that inherited variants of those genes that function to modulate dopaminergic neurotransmission may contribute to changes in the structure and function of particular brain regions. These changes in function at the neurological level may give rise to the abnormalities in psychological functioning, characterized by difficulties in inhibiting inappropriate responses (Taylor, 1999a).

However, genetic research highlights the impact that other, non-genetic factors, particularly non-shared aspects of a child's environment, can have on the developmental course of the disorder. Epidemiological research indicates that ADHD is not associated with minor obstetric abnormalities at birth (Taylor et al., 1991); however, prenatal exposure to alcohol is linked with hyperactive behaviour (Taylor, 1991). Other factors, such as maternal smoking during pregnancy and pre-eclamptic toxaemia are also associated with hyperactivity, although the exact mechanisms of the effect have not been firmly established (see Taylor, 1999a). Very low birth weight, severe anoxia, and early lead poisoning are also risk factors for the later development of ADHD. Problems related to family function may not give rise to ADHD symptoms per se, but can affect the development of conduct problems in children with ADHD (Taylor, 1999a), which in turn has implications for outcome.

Findings from magnetic resonance imaging (MRI) studies indicate that ADHD is associated with changes in brain morphology. However, the results from different studies have been contradictory at times and the disparate findings across some studies are believed to reflect the true heterogeneity of aetiological routes to ADHD symptoms (see Eliez & Reiss, 2000, for a review). There is a tendency for total brain volume to be slightly lower in children with ADHD compared to controls (e.g. Castellanos et al., 1996), with particular reductions in the white matter of the right frontal region (Filipek et al., 1997). Abnormal morphologies of the basal ganglia, corpus callosum and cerebellum have also been suggested, but the results across studies remain conflicting with regards to the exact pathology (Eliez & Reiss, 2000).

ADHD in childhood

Although the diagnostic criteria state that at the minimum, the three core behavioural symptoms – inattention, hyperactivity and impulsivity – must be present by the age of 7 years, in many cases the behavioural disturbance is evident much earlier in the child's development. In the pre-school years, many children are inattentive and can exhibit behaviours that are difficult to manage. However, the demands for sustained attention on pre-schoolers are limited and certainly not all difficult-to-manage young children will go on to develop ADHD. None the less, Cohen and colleagues (1981) suggest that 60–70% of children who are later diagnosed as having ADHD exhibited the characteristic behavioural symptoms by their pre-school years. Parental reports of hyperactivity at the age of 3 years have also been associated with the later presence of conduct problems (e.g. Campbell, 1987).

Speech and language difficulties are very common in young children with ADHD (Baker & Cantwell, 1987; Taylor et al., 1991). Poor motor co-ordination and delayed reading skills are also frequent (e.g. Taylor et al., 1991). Young children with hyperactivity are likely to be more impersistent in their activity, change activities frequently, and explore their environments in an unsystematic and disinhibited manner (Luk, Thorley & Taylor, 1987).

By the time children enter formal education, around the age of 4–5 years, they are expected to have some capacity for concentration and behavioural control. Even in reception classes, children are required to sit quietly for periods of time listening to stories or instructions. At this early stage in education, although the day is clearly structured and organized for them, the children still need to learn to modify their behaviour in accordance with the demands of the environment – lessons and assembly necessitate settled behaviour, playtime allows for more boisterous activity. Children must learn to socialize with other children – to wait their turn and to share the attention of the adult. Children who have difficulties with attention, activity control and impulsiveness struggle with the limits placed on them in the early school environment. It is often at this point that the characteristic difficulties begin to be formally recognized.

As children progress though the primary school years, the lessons become more structured and children are expected to begin to acquire the basic foundations for literacy and numeracy. The demands for behavioural control within this environment steadily increase and unmodulated and inattentive behaviour will pose an increasing impediment on a child's ability to function effectively at age-level expectations (Taylor, 1995). The rapid and often chaotic style with which children with ADHD tend to process information can impair their ability to learn. This in turn means that they may not develop their knowledge base at the same rate as their peers. As other children are consolidating new skills and applying them in their classroom work, the children with ADHD may be unable to keep up. As tasks become increasingly difficult for them, rates of inattentive and disruptive behaviours may increase. Socially, their peers may begin actively to reject them as their behaviour becomes more intrusive and disruptive.

In secondary school, the demands on independent learning and self-organization are considerably higher than in primary school. Children with ADHD are at risk of becoming disaffected with education if they cannot cope with these demands. Problems with peer relationships or compliance may become exacerbated. Some children will, by this stage, already have had their ADHD diagnosed and be linked into appropriate treatment services. However, the needs of these children will change as they mature and their progress must be carefully monitored at regular intervals.

Other youngsters will reach adolescence with their difficulties as yet unrecognized and untreated. Their poor inhibition and attentional skills render them ill-equipped to master the developmental tasks of adolescence. Why had their problems not been identified earlier? Some children may have coped successfully, having benefited from other strengths and supports, such as high general intelligence, a good primary school, or a supportive, accepting family. In other cases, the children might have had such disrupted early lives (e.g. neglect, abuse, multiple foster placements) that the professionals involved in their care had focused on these factors as the most likely cause of any dysfunctional behaviour, and thus overlooked the possibility of a neuro-developmental problem.

Associated difficulties in childhood

Although the core behavioural symptoms in children with ADHD cause impairment in functioning, these are not the only aspects of their development that jeopardize educational attainment. Recent reviews suggest between 50 and 80% of children with ADHD will also exhibit another disorder (see Jensen, Martin & Cantwell, 1997). Oppositional Defiant Disorder and Conduct Disorder are the most frequently co-occurring problems, with estimates of comorbidity ranging from 40 to 90% (Jensen et al., 1997). Another common problem is academic underachievement, with reading difficulties occurring in about one-third of clinic-referred children with ADHD (August & Garfinkel, 1990).

Poor peer relationships are another frequently encountered area of difficulty

(Pelham & Milich 1984), though the actual deficits in social skills functioning can vary widely. Some children with ADHD are very good at making friends, but have difficulty keeping them. Other children struggle to make appropriate overtures to children and are actively rejected or neglected by their peers (Nixon, 2001). Children with ADHD have a tendency to be more dominating and aggressive in their social interactions (Guevremont, 1990) and their impulsiveness can affect their ability accurately to process social cues and information (Milich & Dodge, 1984).

As children with ADHD tend to be frequently in trouble with adults, be unpopular amongst their peers, and do poorly at school, they often develop a low self-image. Emotional disturbance, including mood disorders and anxiety problems, may affect 15–25% of children with ADHD (Jensen et al., 1997). Collectively, ADHD and the associated difficulties can pose a major risk to a child's potential to succeed in school, to view themselves as a valued member of the family, peer group or wider community, or to develop a positive sense of self-worth. Clearly, therefore, the assessment of ADHD must address symptoms beyond the three core problems.

Historically, it was believed that when conduct problems were comorbid with hyperactivity, it was the conduct difficulties and not the hyperactivity that posed the greatest risk to development. It is now recognized that hyperactivity itself is a risk for poor psychosocial adjustment in adolescence and adulthood (Taylor et al., 1996) although the presence of comorbid difficulties may play a critical role in later functioning (Goldstein, 1999). It is not clear yet whether or not cases of ADHD that present comorbidly with other disorders, particularly conduct problems or anxiety, should be conceptualized and treated substantially differently from cases in which ADHD occurs in isolation. Certainly, the outcome for comorbid cases appears more negative (Barkley et al., 1993). The presence of comorbid disorders may also alter the response to treatment. Longitudinal research, in which comorbidity has been identified and classified more systematically, will hopefully address these issues.

Transition into adolescence

Until recently, parents of a child with hyperactivity were often reassured that their child would 'outgrow it'. In some cases, this is true – in general, the level of ADHD symptoms, particularly overactive behaviour, does decrease with time (Hill & Schoener, 1996). However, longitudinal studies that were published in the late 1980s and early 1990s, dispelled the idea that *most* children would outgrow their hyperactivity problems. To some degree, the majority of children with ADHD will continue to experience the core symptoms of the disorder into early adolescence and they remain at risk of developing other behavioural and relationship difficulties (Hinshaw, 1994). Indeed, less than a third of children with hyperactivity will outgrow their difficulties by late adolescence (Barkley et al., 1990).

Although not all these children may meet diagnostic criteria, residual, subclinical symptoms of the disorder, such as poor organization or rapid decision-making may remain aspects of their personality. These may or may not impair functioning but professionals are now suggesting that ADHD should be seen as a chronic problem that requires specific support and treatment over many years (Goldman et al., 1998). Some have even implied that ADHD should be viewed as a lifelong condition (Fargason & Ford, 1994).

Associated difficulties in adolescence

The two-thirds of children whose ADHD symptoms continue into adolescence are at increased risk for developing other disruptive behaviour problems, particularly aggression, oppositionality, antisocial behaviour and delinquency (Gittelman, et al., 1985; Barkley et al., 1990; Taylor et al., 1996). Poor academic performance and educational underachievement are additional serious problems (Fischer et al., 1990). Social incompetence and emotional maladjustment are also characteristic of children whose ADHD is identified for the first time in adolescence (Barkley et al., 1991). Substance abuse problems appear to be more associated with the development of conduct difficulties in adolescence (Gittelman et al., 1985). Adolescents with a history of attentional and hyperactivity problems also have a higher rate of driving accidents and other traffic violations (Cox et al., 2000; Woodward, Fergusson & Horwood, 2000).

Of the three core symptoms of ADHD, hyperactivity is the most likely to decrease with time, whereas difficulties with impulsivity and inattention are more likely to persist. When considering the longitudinal course of the disorder and its impact on development, one must separate the actual continuity of the core behavioural symptoms from the disturbance in functioning that might arise in reaction or response to these symptoms. These secondary difficulties may persist even if the core ADHD problems eventually remit.

Longitudinal studies, in documenting the developmental course of ADHD, have firmly established that childhood hyperactivity is a risk factor for future adjustment and behavioural difficulties. However, the exact mechanism whereby hyperactivity functions as a risk factor remains less well understood and this is now an area of intensive research. It is possible, for example, that other factors, such as how people respond to the child and how behavioural difficulties are managed, play an important role in the development and maintenance of future problems (Barkley, 1998).

ADHD in adulthood

Although professionals in the UK are becoming increasingly aware of the importance of assessing and treating *children* with ADHD (see Sayal & Taylor, 1997), services dedicated to the mental health needs of adults may be less well-informed. Wender (1998a: p. 761) recently described ADHD as 'probably the most common chronic undiagnosed psychiatric disorder in adults'. Although its very existence in adulthood remains controversial amongst some professionals, reviews of the current literature indicate that the disorder can be reliably diagnosed in adults and that it has a definable course and response to treatment (Spencer et al., 1998). None the less, like other developmental disorders and psychiatric illnesses originating in childhood, the presence of ADHD can remain unnoticed by adult psychiatrists (Burger & Lang, 1998). A recent survey of adult psychiatrists in the Trent region in England suggests that few felt they were seeing cases of ADHD (Bramble, 2000). This implies that many adult mental health services may be ill-prepared to deal with the increasing number of young adults who will require assessment and treatment of ADHD. As ADHD becomes increasingly recognized as a chronic, possibly life-long, condition, more services will need to be developed to address the needs of this population.

The presence of hyperactivity in childhood is associated with hyperactivity and poor social and academic adjustment in early adulthood in both community, non-referred samples (Taylor et al., 1996) and clinic-based populations (Lambert, 1988). Mannuzza and colleagues (1991), in their follow-up of children diagnosed with ADHD, found that almost half (43%) of their sample continued to meet diagnostic criteria for ADHD as young adults. Moreover, one-third of their sample met diagnostic criteria for antisocial personality disorder and one-tenth were abusing drugs. A recent study, comparing a clinically referred sample of adults with ADHD to a clinic-referred control group, highlighted the increased psychiatric and social morbidity of the ADHD group. The adults with ADHD were more impaired on measures of academic achievement and both antisocial and criminal behaviour (Young, Toone & Tyson, unpub. data). Prospective studies (e.g. Satterfield & Schell, 1997) indicate that the risk of adult criminality is mediated predominantly by the presence of conduct problems which may also be associated with hyperactivity. Children with hyperactivity, but no conduct problems, are not at increased risk for criminality in adulthood.

Poor peer relationships and lack of participation in constructive activities are also common in young adults with ADHD (Taylor et al., 1996). Not surprisingly, occupational status may be affected. Compared to other family members, individuals with ADHD may have lower-status occupations and more job-related problems than non-affected individuals (Young, 2000).

The risk of ADHD appears to continue into an individual's early 20s and 30s, with one study suggesting that more than half of those adults with a history of childhood hyperactivity will continue to exhibit at least one 'disabling' symptom of hyperactivity (Weiss et al., 1985). These individuals tend to have a more immature and explosive personality type (Weiss & Hechtman, 1986). They may also have a history of self-medicating with stimulants, such as caffeine or amphetamines (Wender, Wood & Reimherr, 1985).

Assessment of ADHD

Children and adolescents

The frequent presence of comorbid difficulties highlights the need for a comprehensive and multidisciplinary approach to the assessment and treatment of ADHD. A multi-modal, multi-informant approach to assessment of hyperactivity is absolutely necessary. The purpose of assessment is to identify the presence of the behavioural symptoms, quantify the severity and impact of the symptoms, detect any comorbid difficulties, rule out alternative diagnoses and develop a formulation that will lead to a comprehensive treatment plan. Several current sources provide detailed guidelines on assessment and diagnosis (Barkley, 1998; Goldman et al., 1998; Taylor et al., 1998; Warner-Rogers, 1998).

For children and adolescents, a diagnostic assessment should include the following six components: (1) clinical interview including detailed developmental history and in-depth description of current problems and their development; (2) physical examination; (3) behavioural observation and interview of child; (4) psychological assessment, or at the minimum a screen for global learning delay or specific learning difficulty; (5) completion of rating scales and behavioural questionnaires by parents and at least one other informant who knows the child well (such as a health visitor, nursery worker, or teacher); and (6) review of school records from all schools attended, including nursery and reception where available.

The purpose of the detailed history is to establish if the developmental course of the symptoms would be consistent with ADHD. Information about family functioning and problems such as financial difficulties, marital strife, as well as details about existing sources of support, will also be important (Taylor et al., 1998). The physical assessment should involve a general physical examination, screen for congenital disorders or evidence of immaturity in motor function, and document height, weight and head circumference. More specific medical investigations are not always needed, but may be indicated if any problems are identified in the general physical examination (Taylor et al., 1998).

Behavioural observation of the child or adolescent allows one to ascertain how they modify their behaviour in relation to environmental demands. It is important to note, however, that novel situations, such as an appointment in an outpatient clinic, may often suppress symptoms of hyperactivity. A lack of hyperactive behaviour in new situations should not be construed as evidence of its non-existence in other environments. Likewise, the clinical interview with the child or adolescent is an important component of the assessment process. Children can present their views regarding their emotional and social functioning and give an impression of how other people seem to be reacting to their behaviour. Adolescents tend to be poor sources of information regarding ADHD symptoms. Teenagers tend to underreport difficulties in the areas of inattention, impulsivity and overactivity (Danckaerts et al., 1999), but can provide important, valid reports about the nature of social interactions (Smith et al., 2000).

As the diagnosis of ADHD requires the behavioural symptoms to be inconsistent with the developmental level of the individual, an accurate understanding of an individual's general level of functioning is required. A comprehensive cognitive assessment will serve to identify the level of development. Evaluation of a child's academic attainment allows one to consider the presence of any specific learning disorders. Specialized neuropsychological assessment can provide data on cognitive attention abilities and response inhibition. Other areas, such as memory and visuospatial skills can also be examined. In general, decisions about the necessity for detailed neuropsychological assessment should be made on an individual basis. There is no one neuropsychological profile that is characteristic of ADHD. Indeed, it is important to emphasize that the diagnosis is based on behavioural symptoms and not any pattern of cognitive deficit.

A number of rating scales can be useful as screening devices to supplement detailed interviews. The Strengths and Difficulties Questionnaire (SDQ) is a good general behaviour screening measure as it taps behavioural, emotional and social functioning and includes positive as well as negative attributes (Goodman, 1997). The SDQ has forms for parents, teachers and young people (age 11–16 years), so views across informants can be compared. The Conners Rating Scales (Conners, 1969) were designed specifically for hyperactivity and are very sensitive to medication effects, making them ideal for monitoring behaviour change during treatment. The Home Situations Questionnaire (HSQ) and School Situations Questionnaire (SSQ), developed by Barkley (1997b) are expressly for hyperactivity and focus on specific settings, such as mealtimes or travelling, that may be problematic. One must remember, however, that it is not uncommon for two respondents to provide disparate ratings for the same individual. This may reflect true variation in behaviour across settings or the different expectations of the raters from different settings.

The views of the school are essential for a complete ADHD assessment. The diagnosis requires pervasiveness of symptoms across situations, and teachers can provide critical information about how the child's attention and behavioural control skills compare to others within the same environment. Moreover, soliciting the input of teachers and educational professionals at the assessment phase may serve to enhance their willingness to support and collaborate with treatment later.

Adults

There are, at present, no separate diagnostic criteria for adult ADHD (Wender, 1998a). As such, the goals of assessments for adults who may have ADHD are almost identical to those that apply to children. The methods, however, vary slightly. The first National Health Service clinic in the UK dedicated to ADHD in adulthood attempts to gather information from four sources: (1) parent/ informant report; (2) self-report; (3) objective retrospective information (e.g. school reports, police records, educational statements); and (4) psychometric assessment (Young & Toone, 2001).

For adults, the assessment must show that the individual experienced the core symptoms as a child. There is a semi-structured interview available that focuses on contemporary ADHD features (Barkley & Murphy, 1998). However, the developmental history, which necessitates the accurate recall of childhood behaviour, is obviously critical. One might speculate that it could be very difficult to gather information about early childhood functioning retrospectively. At least one study (Murphy & Schachar, 2000) has examined this issue by comparing recall of childhood behaviour from three sources: adults referred for assessment of possible ADHD; their parents; and their partners. Good correlations across informants were found for inattentive, hyperactive-impulsive symptoms. Although this suggests that adults may be accurate reporters of childhood behaviour patterns, it does contrast with low validity of the contemporary reports of adolescents. Until more research is completed regarding accuracy of retrospective reports, it may still be useful to include the views of parents or partners when possible. Review of all available school reports provides another source of information.

Assessment of cognitive and neuropsychological functioning also has a role in the evaluation of adults (Young & Toone, 2001). Psychological assessment and neuropsychological evaluation may support the diagnosis, but will not confirm or disconfirm it (Fargason & Ford, 1994). Although adults with ADHD have been shown to perform more poorly than controls on tests of neuropsychological functioning, scores on such tests alone cannot discriminate adults with ADHD from those with other psychiatric disorders (Downey et al., 1997; Walker et al., 2000). As with children, there is no one neuropsychological profile that captures the functioning of adults with ADHD.

Rating scales, such as the Wender Utah Rating Scale (WURS), are known to be sensitive to ADHD, but not necessarily specific to the disorder and reliance on rating scales alone would lead to high rates of misclassification (e.g. McCann et al., 2000). The Minnesota Multiphasic Personality Inventory, second edition (MMPI-2), has also been shown to be useful in the assessment of ADHD (Downey et al., 1997; Coleman et al., 1998), though the device is not generally widely used in the UK.

Treatment of ADHD

Interventions must go beyond simple symptom reduction. Treatment strategies can be used effectively to decrease behavioural symptoms and increase adjustment, although this is clearly not the same as 'curing' the problems. Thus treatment for ADHD includes, but should not be limited to, the reduction of core behavioural symptoms. Ideally, intervention should also focus on any comorbid difficulties or disorders by promoting academic and social functioning, enhancing self-esteem, preventing the development of conduct difficulties and relieving family distress (Taylor, 1994; Warner-Rogers, 1998). Given the heterogeneity in groups of children with ADHD, it is not surprising that treatment packages must be highly individualized, and generally there will be multiple targets for treatment.

Historically there have been three main treatment approaches to ADHD: pharmacological; psychological; and nutritional. The actual treatment options selected will vary depending on the targets of intervention. Services should not rely solely on one approach to intervention (Taylor, 1999b). Research efforts have focused primarily on pharmacological and psychological interventions and therefore these two options are reviewed here in more detail. Evidence for the effectiveness of any particular dietary approach is so limited that no guidelines for dietary treatment yet exist (Taylor et al., 1998). However, parents are generally reliable reporters of whether or not their children are sensitive to particular foods (Young et al., 1987) and when such a food–behaviour link is suggested, a food diary approach is a non-intrusive way in which to explore the associations in more detail (Taylor et al., 1998).

Pharmacological intervention

In childhood and adolescence

Historically in the UK, medication has not been the treatment of choice, but there is now increasing consensus that it should be used to treat severe cases of hyperkinetic disorder and even some cases of ADHD (Sayal & Taylor, 1997). The main, first-line pharmacological treatment for ADHD is methylphenidate (Ritalin, Equasym), a stimulant medication (Taylor et al., 1998), and multiple treatment trials have demonstrated its efficacy in reducing the behavioural symptoms of ADHD (Swanson et al., 1993; MTA Cooperative Group, 1999b). However, children on medication must be monitored consistently and doses titrated carefully against behavioural response. In contrast to the UK, medication is the most common treatment in the United States (Safer & Krager, 1988), with estimates suggesting that approximately 88% of children with ADHD are prescribed methylphenidate (Wolraich et al., 1990). Current guidelines for European practice indicate that medication should be used in severe cases of ADHD, with milder cases being given home- and school-based treatments first, followed by medication if improvements are not forthcoming (Taylor et al., 1998).

In addition to treating the core symptoms, stimulant medication has been linked to decreases in general disruptive behaviour and increases in time spent on task (Pelham, et al., 1985). Increased attention during play activities (Pelham et al., 1990) and improvements in academic functioning have been observed with some children (Pelham et al., 1985; Evans & Pelham, 1991). The driving skills of older adolescents with ADHD may also be improved when taking methylphenidate (Cox et al., 2000). However, a small percentage of children experience adverse reactions to stimulant medication, including poor sleep, nervousness, sadness and appetite reduction (see Taylor et al., 1998, for review).

Methylphenidate is a very short-acting drug, which means that multiple doses are required during the day to achieve maximum benefit. This may pose difficulties as children must often take the medication during school hours. Some schools can be resistant to the notion of a medication approach to what they see as a behavioural problem, and be reluctant to co-operate with the medical regime. Adolescents can be especially sensitive to being stigmatized by having to regularly attend the office or school nurse for their medication.

This can lead to difficulties with adherence. A slow-release preparation of methylphenidate is now available which may circumvent some of these problems (Ford, Taylor & Warner-Rogers, 2000).

Taylor and colleagues (1998) provide a review of alternative stimulants and other types of medication that might also be effective. Briefly, dexamphetamine is a stimulant medication that is sometimes used, particularly for children who also have a seizure disorder. Desipramine, a tricyclic antidepressant, can also function as an anti-hyperactivity medication and is often considered when children have tic disorders as well as ADHD. Atypical antipsychotic drugs can also be used in special cases, but they are not first line choices and are generally less helpful than stimulants (Taylor et al., 1998).

In adulthood

As yet, there are no widely established or empirically validated protocols for the pharmacological treatment of ADHD in adults, though some general guidelines from the American Academy of Child and Adolescent Psychiatry (Dulcan, 1997) and other specialist clinics are available (e.g. Roy-Byrne et al., 1997). Treatment trials are underway, however, and preliminary evidence indicates that stimulant medications, including methylphenidate, dexamphetamine and Adderall (a mixture of amphetamine salts) can be effective with adults (e.g. Gualtieri, Ondrusek, & Finley, 1985; Wender, 1998b; Patterson et al., 1999; Horrigan & Barnhill, 2000) and should be considered first-line choices for pharmacological intervention.

Psychological approaches
In childhood and adolescence

There is a wide variety of 'psychological' approaches to treatment. The main focus of such interventions is to change the environment in order to alter the behaviour of the child. Some psychological techniques focus on the parent or teacher, others centre directly on the child. The techniques used might include: (1) educating parents, teachers and caregivers about the disorder in general and the child's needs in particular; (2) parent training in child management; (3) modifying educational provision; (4) consulting with teachers regarding cognitive–behavioural treatment for impulsiveness; and (5) direct intervention with children, e.g. attention training, anger management. Reviews of psychological approaches for children with ADHD can be found in MTA Cooperative Group (1999a), Goldstein (1997), Goldstein & Goldstein (1998) and Warner-Rogers (1998).

In adulthood

Education about the disorder, advice on coping strategies, individual counselling for improving self-esteem, organizational skills and anger control may also prove useful treatments for adults (Fargason & Ford, 1994), although the efficacy of these approaches has yet to be studied in detail. Young (1999) suggests that structured cognitive–behavioural therapy may be an extremely important component of work with adults with ADHD. This approach seeks to empower individuals to develop self-efficacy and the will to change and to teach self-management skills. Specific targets may include: impulse control; time-management and organizational skills; problem solving; anger control skills; and social awareness and interaction skills.

A comment on treatment effectiveness

The Multimodal Treatment Study of Children with Attention-Deficit Hyperactivity Disorder (MTA Study; MTA Cooperative Group, 1999a,b) summarizes the results from the most extensive randomized controlled treatment trial of ADHD in childhood to date. Subjects (children with ADHD aged 7–9.9 years) were assigned for 14 months to one of four treatment protocols: medication management; intensive behavioural treatment; the two combined; or standard community care. The behavioural treatment component of the MTA Study included parent training, child-focused treatment and a school-based intervention.

Children in all four groups of the MTA Study exhibited reductions in symptoms. However, the results indicate that closely monitored medication management was more effective than intensive behavioural treatment alone or standard community care in reducing core ADHD symptoms. The care, consistency and precision with which doses of methylphenidate were titrated against behavioural improvement for the children in the medication management treatment group of the study is worth highlighting. The combined treatment approach, including both medication management and behavioural treatment, provided no *greater* benefit for core ADHD symptoms than medication management alone. However, the combined approach was superior to intensive behavioural treatment alone as well as community care in other areas such as oppositionality, aggression, family relationships and academic functioning, whereas medication management was not. In addition, those children who received the combined treatment approach could be maintained on lower doses of medication than those in the medication alone group. It is also noteworthy that over 75% of those subjects in the behavioural treatment group were maintained without any medication throughout the study. In addition, treatment satisfaction scores for the combined treatment and the intensive behavioural treatment were significantly higher than the satisfaction scores from the medication alone group.

The MTA Group went on to examine the moderators and mediators of treatment response, and in so doing highlighted the relative importance of comorbidity (MTA Group, 1999b). Specifically, children with anxiety problems fared better in the behavioural treatment group than in the community care group with regards to their core ADHD symptoms. For children from families of lower socio-economic backgrounds, the combined treatment resulted in more improvements in teacher-reported social skills.

The MTA Study was undertaken in the United States and one must take care when generalizing the results to children in the UK or elsewhere, as the traditions of child mental health may be quite different (Taylor, 1999b). There is clearly more to the treatment of ADHD than the simple reduction of core symptoms. The MTA study results are also limited in their generalizability to adult populations. Although estimates suggest that around two-thirds of adults with ADHD will show good improvements when treated with stimulants and psychoeducational interventions (Wender,1998a), there are no random alloca-tion treatment trials that have systematically compared pharmacological to psychoeducational interventions. The issue of comorbidity will also have to be addressed in future treatment studies with adults, as it is likely – as in the case with children – that the presence of other difficulties may affect treatment efficacy (Hornig, 1998).

Conclusions

Attention Deficit Hyperactivity Disorder, once seen as a problem restricted to the school-age years, is now recognized as also occurring in adults. Although ADHD can often co-exist with other learning or behavioural difficulties, the disorder itself functions as a serious risk factor for development. It is hoped that as mental health services for children with ADHD are becoming better organ-ized, more individuals will be accurately identified and appropriately treated. Guidelines for the treatment of ADHD in childhood are available from various sources (Dulcan, 1997; Taylor et al., 1998). Professionals must now grapple with the evidence that ADHD may be a chronic condition. New services for the specific needs of older adolescents and adults with the disorder will need to be developed. For a summary of the clinical issues for practitioners see Table 1.1.

Although treatment of affected individuals can be construed as symptomatic rather than 'curative' in focus (Wender, 1998a), the combination of medication

Table 1.1. Summary of clinical issues of attention deficit hyperactivity disorder (ADHD) for practitioners

Assessment	Formulation	Treatment
Should be multi-informant, multi-modal and multidisciplinary. Should include a detailed developmental history, description of current problems and identification of clients' strengths and available resources Measures should include rating scales (parent, teachers), behavioural observation, school reports, and psychological assessment	Hyperkinetic Disorder (ICD-10)[a] or ADHD (DSM-IV)[b] should be specified (if ADHD, use subtypes) Comorbid difficulties and disorders should be included and alternative diagnoses ruled out Multi-axial diagnostic systems should be used to highlight all aspects of child's needs and functioning	Should be multi-modal and individualised for child and family Specific targets should be clearly identified to enable quantification of improvements Treatment plans should be regularly monitored and modified as needed and should capitalize on interpersonal strengths and existing resources (family, school, community)

[a] *ICD-10 Classification of Mental and Behavioural Disorders* (WHO, 1994).
[b] *Diagnostic and Statistical Manual of Mental Disorders*. 4th edition (APA, 1994).

and psychological approaches may be the best means of ensuring long-term improvements in general psychological functioning. When pharmacological approaches are used, it is imperative to monitor behavioural change closely and to be aware of side-effects. Issues of adherence must be considered, especially in adolescence. Psychological approaches may include provision of education to parents, individuals, schools and others regarding the individual's specific needs and treatment. It is important that the initial assessment also serves to identify the individual's strengths and available resources, as these can be valuable when planning and implementing interventions. Behavioural approaches will strive to teach new skills for managing behavioural problems and facilitating the development of more appropriate behaviour. Overall, the goal of all treatments will be to improve the adjustment and well-being of affected individuals by increasing self-control, enhancing understanding of the disorder, and ultimately minimizing its impact.

REFERENCES

American Psychiatric Association (1994). *Diagnostic and Statistical Manual of Mental Disorders*, 4th edn. Washington, DC: American Psychiatric Association.

August, G.J. & Garfinkel, B.D. (1990). Comorbidity of ADHD and reading disability among clinic-referred children. *Journal of Abnormal Child Psychology*, **18**: 29–45.

Baker, L. & Cantwell, D.P. (1987). A prospective psychiatric follow-up of children with speech/ language disorders. *Journal of the American Academy of Child and Adolescent Psychiatry*, **26**: 546–53.

Barkley, R.A. (1995). *Taking charge of ADHD: The Complete, Authoritative Guide for Parents*. New York: Guilford Press.

Barkley, R.A. (1997a). Behavioural inhibition, sustained attention, and executive functions: Constructing a unifying theory of ADHD. *Psychological Bulletin*, **121**: 65–94.

Barkley, R.A. (1997b). *Defiant Children: A clinicians' Manual for Assessment and Parent Training*, 2nd edn. New York: Guilford Press.

Barkley, R.A. (1998). *Attention-Deficit Hyperactivity Disorder: A Handbook for Diagnosis and Treatment*, 2nd edn. New York: Guilford Press.

Barkley, R.A., Anastopoulos, A.D., Guevremont, D.C. & Fletcher, K.E. (1991). Adolescents with ADHD: Patterns of behavioural adjustment, academic functioning and treatment utlization. *Journal of the American Academy of Child and Adolescent Psychiatry*, **30**, 546–57.

Barkley, R.A., Fischer, M., Edelbrock, C.S. & Smallish, L. (1990). The adolescent outcome of hyperactive children diagnosed by research criteria: I. An 8-year prospective follow-up study. *Journal of the American Academy of Child and Adolescent Psychiatry*, **29**: 546–57.

Barkley, R.A., Guevremont, D.C., Anastopoulos, A.D., DuPaul, G.J. & Shelton, T.J. (1993). Driving-related risks and outcomes of attention deficit hyperactivity disorder in adolescents and young adults: a 3- to 5-year follow-up survey. *Pediatrics*, **92**: 212–18.

Barkley, R.A. & Murphy, K.R. (1998). *ADHD: A Clinical Workbook*, 2nd edn. New York: Guilford Press.

Bramble, D. (2000). Psychostimulants and psychiatrists: the trent adult psychiatry psychostimulant survey. *Journal of Psychopharmacology*, **14**: 67–9.

Burger, F.L. & Lang, C.M. (1998). Diagnoses commonly missed in childhood: Long-term implications for treatment. *Psychiatric Clinics of North America*, **21**: 947–50.

Campbell, S. (1987). Parent-referred problem three-year-olds: developmental changes in symptoms. *Journal of Child Psychology and Psychiatry*, **28**: 835–45.

Castellanos, F.X., Giedd, J.N., Marsh, W.L., Hamburger, S.D., Vaituzius, A.C., Dickenstein, D.P., Sarfatti, S.E., Vauss, Y.C., Snell, J.W., Lange, N., Kaysen D., Krain, A.L., Ritchie, G.F., Rajapaske, J.C. & Rapoport, J.L. (1996). Quantitative brain magnetic resonance imaging in attention deficit hyperactivity disorder. *Archives of General Psychiatry*, **53**: 607–16.

Cohen, N.J., Sullivan, S., Minde, K.K., Novak, D. & Helwig, C. (1981). Evaluation of the relative effectiveness of methylphenidate and cognitive behavior modification in the treatment of kindergarten-aged hyperactive children. *Journal of Abnormal Child Psychology*, **9**: 43–54.

Coleman, A.R., Norstrand, J.A., Moberg, P.J., Kohler, C.G., Gur, R.C. & Gur, R.E. (1998).

MMPI–2 characteristics of adults diagnosed with attention deficit disorder. *International Journal of Neuroscience*, **96**: 161–75.

Conners, K. (1969). A teacher rating scales for use in drug studies with children. *American Journal of Psychiatry*, **126**: 884–8.

Cox, D.J., Merkel, R.L., Kovatchev, B. & Seward, R. (2000). Effect of stimulant medication on driving performance of young adults with attention deficit hyperactivity disorder: a preliminary double-blind placebo controlled trial. *Journal of Nervous and Mental Disease*, **188**: 230–4.

Danckaerts, M., Heptinstall, E., Chadwick, O. & Taylor, E. (1999). Self-report of attention deficit hyperactivity disorder in adolescents. *Psychopathology*, **32**: 81–92.

Downey, K.K., Stelson, F.W., Pomerleau, O.F. & Giordani, B. (1997). Adult attention deficit hyperactivity disorder: psychological test profiles in a clinical population. *Journal of Nervous and Mental Disease*, **185**: 32–8.

Dulcan, M. (1997). Practice parameters for assessment and treatment of children, adolescents and adults with attention deficit hyperactivity disorder. *Journal of the American Academy of Child and Adolescent Psychiatry*, **36**(Suppl): 85S–121S.

Eliez, S. & Reiss, A.L. (2000). Annotation: MRI neuroimaging of childhood psychiatric disorders: a selective review. *Journal of Child Psychology and Psychiatry*, **41**: 679–94.

Evans, S.W. & Pelham, W.E. (1991). Psychostimulant effects on academic and behavioural measures for ADHD junior high school students in a lecture format classroom. *Journal of Abnormal Child Psychology*, **19**: 537–52.

Fargason, R.E. & Ford, C.V. (1994). Attention deficit hyperactivity disorder in adults: diagnosis, treatment and prognosis. *Southern Medical Journal*, **87**: 302–9.

Filipek, P.A., Semrud-Clikeman, M., Steingard, R.J., Renshaw, P.F., Kennedy, D.N. & Biederman, J. (1997). Volumetric MRI analysis comparing subjects having attention-deficit hyperactivity disorder with normal controls. *Neurology*, **48**: 589–601.

Fischer, M., Barkley, R.A., Edelbrock, C.S. & Smallish, L. (1990). The adolescent outcome of hyperactive children diagnosed by research criteria. II. Academic, attentional and neuropsychological status. *Journal of Consulting and Clinical Psychology*, **58**: 580–8.

Ford, T., Taylor, E. & Warner-Rogers, J. (2000). Sustained release methylphenidate. *Child Psychology and Psychiatry Review*, **5**: 108–13.

Gittelman, R., Mannuzza, S., Shecnker, R. & Bonogura, N. (1985). Hyperactive boys almost grown up. I. Psychiatric status. *Archives of General Psychiatry*, **30**: 671–710.

Goldman, L.S., Genel, M., Bezman, R.J. & Slanetz, P.J. (1998). Diagnosis and treatment of attention deficit/hyperactivity disorder in children and adolescents. *Journal of the American Medical Association*, **279**: 1100–7.

Goldstein, S. (1997). *Managing Attention Disorders in Late Adolescence and Adulthood: A Guide for Practitioners*. New York: Wiley.

Goldstein, S. (1999). Attention deficit hyperactivity disorder. In *Handbook of Neurodevelopmental and Genetic Disorders in Children*, ed. S. Goldstein & C.R. Reynold, pp. 154–84. New York: Guilford Press.

Goldstein, S. & Goldstein, M. (1998). *Understanding and Managing Attention Deficit Disorder in Children: A guide for Practitioners*, 2nd edn. New York: Wiley.

Goodman, R. (1997). The strengths and difficulties questionnaire: a research note. *Journal of Child Psychology and Psychiatry*, **38**: 581–6.

Goodman, R. & Stevenson, J. (1989a). A twin study of hyperactivity. I. An examination of hyperactivity scores and categories derived from Rutter Teacher and Parent Questionnaires. *Journal of Child Psychology and Psychiatry*, **30**: 671–90.

Goodman, R. & Stevenson, J. (1989b). A twin study of hyperactivity. II. The aetiological role of genes, family relationships and perinatal adversity. *Journal of Child Psychology and Psychiatry*, **30**: 691–710.

Gualtieri, C.T., Ondrusek, M.G. & Finley, C. (1985). Attention deficit disorder in adults. *Clinical Neuropharmacology*, **8**: 343–56.

Guevremont, D. (1990). Social skills and peer relationship training. In *Attention Deficit Hyperactivity Disorder: A Handbook for Diagnosis and Treatment*, ed. R.A. Barkley, pp. 540–72. New York: Guilford Press.

Hill, J.C. & Schoener, E.P. (1996). Age-dependent decline of attention deficit hyperactivity disorder. *American Journal of Psychiatry*, **153**: 1143–6.

Hinshaw, S.P. (1994). Attention deficits and hyperactivity in children. *Developmental Clinical Psychology and Psychiatry*, vol. 29. London: Sage Publications.

Hornig, M. (1998). Addressing comorbidity in adults with attention deficit hyperactivity disorder. *Journal of Clinical Psychiatry*, **59**(Suppl): 69–75.

Horrigan, J.P. & Barnhill, L.J. (2000). Low-dose amphetamine salts and adult attention deficit hyperactivity disorder. *Journal of Clinical Psychiatry*, **61**: 414–17.

James, A. & Taylor, E. (1990). Sex differences in the hyperkinetic syndrome of childhood. *Journal of Child Psychology and Psychiatry*, **31**: 437–46.

Jensen, P.S., Martin, B.A. & Cantwell, D.P. (1997). Comorbidity in ADHD: implications for research, practice and DSM-IV. *Journal of the American Academy of Child and Adolescent Psychiatry*, **36**: 1065–79.

LaHoste, G.J., Swanson, J.M., Wigal, S.B., Glabe, C., Wigal, T., King, N. & Kennedy, J.L. (1996). Dopamine D4 receptor gene polymorphism is associated with attention deficit hyperactivity disorder. *Molecular Psychiatry*, **1**: 121–4.

Lambert, N.M. (1988). Adolescent outcomes for hyperactive children: perspectives on general and specific patterns of childhood risk for adolescent educational, social and mental health problems. *American Psychologist*, **43**: 786–99.

Luk, S., Thorley, G. & Taylor, E. (1987). Gross overactivity: a study by direct observation. *Journal of Psychopathology and Behavioural Assessment*, **9**: 173–82.

Mannuzza, S., Klein, R.G., Bonagura, N., Malloy, P., Giampino, T.L. & Addalli, K.A. (1991). Hyperactive boys almost grown up. V. Replication of psychiatric status. *Archives of General Psychiatry*, **48**: 77–83.

McCann, B.S., Steele, L., Ward, N. & Roy-Byrne, P. (2000). Discriminant validity of the Wender Utah Rating Scale for attention deficit hyperactivity disorder. *Journal of Neuropsychiatry and Clinical Neurosciences*, **12**: 240–5.

Milich, R. & Dodge, K. A. (1984). Social information processing in child psychiatry populations. *Journal of Abnormal Child Psychology*, **12**: 471–9.

Murphy, P. & Schachar, R. (2000). Use of self-ratings in the assessment of symptoms of attention deficit hyperactivity disorder in adults. *American Journal of Psychiatry*, **157**: 1156–9.

MTA Cooperative Group (1999a). A 14-month randomised clinical trial of treatment strategies for attention deficit/hyperactivity disorder. *Archives of General Psychiatry*, **56**: 1073–86.

MTA Cooperative Group (1999b). Moderators and mediators of treatment response for children with attention deficit/hyperactivity disorder. *Archives of General Psychiatry*, **56**: 1088–96.

Nixon, E. (2001). The social functioning of children with attention deficit hyperactivity disorder: a review of the literature. *The Child Psychology and Psychiatry Review*. (In press.)

Patterson, R., Douglas, C., Hallmayer, J., Hagan, M. & Krupenia, Z. (1999). A randomised, double-blind, placebo-controlled trial of dexamphetamine in adults with attention deficit hyperactivity disorder. *Australian and New Zealand Journal of Psychiatry*, **33**: 494–502.

Pelham, W.E., Bender, M.E., Caddell, J., Booth, S. & Moorer, S.H. (1985). Methylphenidate and children with attention deficit disorder. *Archives of General Psychiatry*, **42**: 948–52.

Pelham, W.E., McBurnett, K., Jarper, G.W., Milich, R., Murphy, D.A., Clinton, J. & Thiele, C. (1990). Methylphenidate and baseball playing in ADHD children: who's on first? *Journal of Consulting and Clinical Psychology*, **58**: 130–3.

Pelham, W.E. & Milich, R. (1984). Peer relations of children with hyperactivity/attention deficit disorder. *Journal of Learning Disabilities*, **17**: 560–8.

Ross, D.M. & Ross, S.A. (1982). *Hyperactivity: Current Issues, Research and Theory*. New York: Wiley.

Roy-Byrne, P., Scheele, L., Brinkley, J., Ward, N., Wiatrak, C., Russo, J., Townes, B. & Varley, C. (1997). Adult attention deficit hyperactivity disorder: assessment guidelines based on clinical presentation to a specialty clinic. *Comprehensive Psychiatry*, **38**: 133–40.

Safer D.J. & Krager, J.M. (1988). A survey of medication treatment for hyperactive-inattentive students. *Journal of the American Medical Association*, **260**: 2256–8.

Satterfield, J.H. & Schell, A. (1997). A prospective study of hyperactive boys with conduct problems and normal boys: adolescent and adult criminality. *Journal of the American Academy of Child and Adolescent Psychiatry*, **36**: 1726–35.

Sayal, K. & Taylor, E. (1997). Drug treatment in attention deficit disorder: a survey of professional consensus. *Psychiatric Bulletin*, **21**: 398–400.

Silberg, J., Rutter, M., Meyer, J., Maes, H., Hewitt, J., Simonoff, E., Pickles, A., Loeber, R. & Eaves, L. (1996). Genetic and environmental influences on the covariation between hyperactivity and conduct disturbance in juvenile twins. *Journal of Child Psychology and Psychiatry*, **37**: 803–16.

Smith, B.H., Pelham, W.E., Gnagy, E., Molina, B. & Evans, S. (2000). The reliability, validity, and unique contributions of self-report by adolescents receiving treatment for attention deficit hyperactivity disorder. *Journal of Consulting and Clinical Psychology*, **68**: 489–99.

Spencer, T., Biederman, J., Wilens, T.E. & Faraone, S.V. (1998). Adults with attention deficit hyperactivity disorder: a controversial diagnosis. *Journal of Clinical Psychiatry*, **59**(Suppl.): 59–68.

Swanson, J.M., McBurnett, K., Wigal, T., Pfiffner, L.J., Lerner, M.A., Williams, L., Christian, D.L., Tamm, L., Willcutt, E., Crowley, K., Clevenger, W., Khouzam, N., Woo, C., Crinella,

F.M. & Risher, T.D. (1993). Effect of stimulant medication on children with attention deficit disorder: a 'review of reviews.' *Exceptional Children*, **60**: 154–62.

Szatmari, P., Offord, D.R. & Boyle, M.H. (1989). Ontario Child Health Study: Prevalence of attention deficit disorder with hyperactivity. *Journal of Child Psychology and Psychiatry*, **30**: 219–30.

Tannock, R. (1998). Attention Deficit Hyperactivity Disorder: advances in cognitive, neuro-biological and genetic research. *Journal of Child Psychology and Psychiatry*, **39**: 65–99.

Taylor, E. (1991). Toxins and allergens. In *Biological Risk Factors for Psychosocial Disorders*, ed. M. Rutter & P. Casear, pp. 199–232. Cambridge: Cambridge University Press.

Taylor, E. (1994). Syndromes of attention deficit and overactivity. In *Child and Adolescent Psychiatry: Modern Approaches*, 3rd edn., ed. M. Rutter, E. Taylor & L. Hersov, pp. 285–307. Oxford: Blackwell Scientific Publications.

Taylor, E. (1995). Dysfunctions of attention. In *Developmental Psychopathology*, vol II, *Risk, Disorder and Adaptation*, ed. D. Cicchetti & D.J. Cohen, pp. 243–73. New York: Wiley.

Taylor, E. (1998). Clinical foundations of hyperactivity research. *Behavioural Brain Research*, **94**: 11–24.

Taylor, E. (1999a). Developmental neurpsychopathology of attention deficit and impulsiveness. *Development and Psychopathology*, **11**: 607–28.

Taylor, E. (1999b). Development of clinical services for attention-deficit/hyperactivity disorder. *Archives of General Psychiatry*, **56**: 1097–9.

Taylor, E., Chadwick, O., Heptinstall, E. & Danckaerts, M. (1996). Hyperactivity and conduct problems as risk factors for adolescent development. *Journal of the American Academy of Child and Adolescent Psychiatry*, **35**: 1213–26.

Taylor, E., Sandberg, S., Thorley, G. & Giles, S. (1991). *The Epidemiology of Childhood Hyperactivity. Maudsley Monographs* No. 33. Oxford: Oxford University Press.

Taylor, E., Sergeant, J., Doepfner, M., Gunning, B., Overmeyer, S., Mobius, H.-J. & Eisert, H.-G. (1998). Clinical guidelines for hyperkinetic disorder. *European Child and Adolescent Psychiatry*, **7**: 184–200.

Walker, A.J., Shores, E.A., Trollor, J.N., Lee, T. & Sachdev, P.S. (2000). Neuropsychological functioning of adults with attention deficit hyperactivity disorder. *Journal of Clinical and Experimental Neuropsychology*, **22**: 115–24.

Warner-Rogers, J. (1998). Attention deficit hyperactivity disorder. In *Behavioural Approaches to Problems in Childhood*, ed. P. Howlin, pp. 28–53. London: MacKeith Press.

Warner-Rogers, J., Taylor, E., Taylor, A. & Sandberg, S. (2000). Childhood inattentiveness: Epidemiology and implications for development. *Journal of Learning Disabilities*, **33**: 520–36.

Weiss, G. & Hechtman, L.T. (1986). *Hyperactive Children Grown Up*. New York: Guilford Press.

Weiss, G., Hechtman, L., Milroy, T. & Perlman, R. (1985). Psychiatric status of hyperactives as adults: a controlled prospective 15-year follow-up of 63 hyperactive children. *Journal of the American Academy of Child Psychiatry*, **24**: 211–20.

Wender, P.J. (1998a). Attention Deficit Hyperactivity Disorder in adults. *Psychiatric Clinics of North America*, **21**: 761–74.

Wender, P.J. (1998b). Pharmacotherapy of Attention Deficit Hyperactivity Disorder in adults. *Journal of Clinical Psychiatry*, **59**(Suppl): 76–9.

Wender, P.J., Wood, D.R. & Reimherr, F.W. (1985). Pharmacological treatment of attention deficit hyperactivity disorder residual type. *Psychopharmacology Bulletin*, **21**: 222–31.

Wolraich, M.L., Lindren, S., Stromquist, A., Milich, R., Davis, C. & Watson, D. (1990). Stimulant use by primary care physicians in the treatment of attention deficit hyperactivity disorder. *Pediatrics*, **86**: 95–101.

Woodward, L.J., Fergusson, D.M. & Horwood, L.J. (2000). Driving outcomes of young people with attentional difficulties in adolescence. *Journal of the American Academy of Child and Adolescent Psychiatry*, **39**: 627–34.

World Health Organization (1994). *The ICD-10 Classification of Mental and Behavioural Disorders.* Geneva: World Health Organization.

Young, S. (1999). Psychological therapy for adults with Attention Deficit Hyperactivity Disorder. *Counselling Psychology Quarterly*, **12**: 183–90.

Young, S. (2000). ADHD children grown up: an empirical review. *Counselling Psychology Quarterly*, **13**: 191–200.

Young, E., Patel, S., Stoneham, M., Rona, R. & Wilkeinson, J.D. (1987). The prevalence of reaction to food additives in a survey population. *Journal of the Royal College of Physicians of London*, **21**: 241–7.

Young, S. & Toone, B. (2001). Attention Deficit Hyperactivity Disorder in adults: clinical issues. A report from the first NHS clinic in the UK. *Counselling Psychology Quarterly*, **13**: 313–19.

2

Developmental language disorders

Nancy J. Cohen

Once a child develops the capacity to understand and use language then learning and social communication shift dramatically. When language development goes awry, children may suffer life-long consequences in terms of social, emotional, academic and vocational well-being. This chapter examines these long-term outcomes. Because relatively few studies have followed samples into adulthood, follow-up studies including adolescents will also be considered, on the assumption that the adolescent period is pivotal in establishing opportunities essential for full participation in the world of school, work and social relationships. The chapter will not only consider language impairment itself but the cognitive, achievement and social–emotional characteristics with which language impairment is associated.

Nature of language and communication impairments

The term 'specific language impairment' (SLI) is used to refer to problems in the acquisition and use of language, typically in the context of normal development (Bishop, 1997). Although the latter criterion is being debated, the term SLI will be used here to refer to individuals with normal overall cognitive development.

Speech/language pathologists and psychologists have broken language into broad categories of receptive and expressive language. These categories are divided further into phonology, morphology, syntax, semantics and pragmatics. Although interrelated, the latter aspects of language will be described separately. Individuals with SLI exhibit problems in combining and selecting the speech sounds of a language into meaningful units (phonological awareness) (Wagner & Torgeson, 1987; Bird, Bishop & Freeman, 1995). Phonological processing problems are distinct from speech impairments that arise from difficulties in co-ordination of oral–motor musculature and include difficulties in articulation, fluency (e.g. stuttering) or voice (e.g. too loud or too soft).

Individuals with SLI use shorter sentences and have difficulties producing and understanding syntactically complex sentences. Morphological deficits refer to omission of inflectional markers such as plurals, past tense, auxiliary verbs and possessives. Syntax refers to the rules for ordering and combining words to form sentences. Additionally, SLI is associated with an impoverished vocabulary, word finding problems and difficulty learning new words (semantics). Whereas the basic tasks for development of phonology and syntax are completed in childhood, vocabulary continues to grow into adulthood (Bishop, 1997).

Increasingly, the literature refers to pragmatics and to the broader term 'communication impairment' (Gallagher, 1996). Pragmatics includes the rules guiding appropriate communication and language use in different social contexts and requires online recognition of the demands of conversation and estimation of the listener's state of mind. Pragmatics also includes discourse, that is, the speaker's ability to integrate ideas and link successive sentences together coherently. For adolescents and adults, discourse involving figurative language (i.e. understanding and use of idioms, metaphor, humour, ambiguity) becomes increasingly important (Vallance & Wintre, 1997; Schwartz & Merten, 1967). Pragmatic skills are particularly important to highlight because, in some cases, symptoms that warrant a psychiatric diagnosis and those that warrant a diagnosis of SLI or communication impairment are interchangeable. For instance, behaviours such as 'interrupts others' and 'blurts out answers' are among the criteria for diagnosis of attention deficit hyperactivity disorder (ADHD) (American Psychiatric Association, 1994), but these same symptoms could be considered as symptoms of pragmatic language problems. There is also evidence that some individuals who are withdrawn and exhibit social anxieties are actually deficient in language and pragmatic skills necessary for competent social interaction (Windsor, 1994). Moreover, recently, Bishop (2000) has described a small distinctive group of children with pragmatic language impairment but normal language skills. Interest in pragmatic skills is also significant because improved communication is one of the major goals and outcomes of mental health interventions. Teasing apart maladaptive communications that are part of SLI and those that are symptoms of psychiatric disturbance has become an important and challenging task.

Causes of specific language impairment

Although there are some specific syndromes in which language impairment is typical, for the most part, the causes of SLI remain unknown, and outcomes are likely to be multidetermined. Thus, although the following discussion may make it appear that causative factors can be separated, there is rarely, if ever, a linear path from cause to outcome. Rather, there is a transactional chain of mutually influential biological and experiential processes that characterize development (Rutter et al., 1997).

Brain functioning

Historically, because acquired brain injury was associated with loss of language functions, it was assumed that SLI was caused by alterations in brain function. Earlier work suggested that the brain is plastic in the sense that among children with early injuries, unaffected parts of the brain were able to take over functions (Rapin, 1996). The more recent work on neurodevelopment postulates that plasticity is a basic property of the developing brain and not a response to injury (Johnson, 1999). Such a view opens the way for experience to exert an impact throughout development through alteration of brain structures, such as those responsible for language competence (Johnson, 1999; Nowakowski & Hayes, 1999). A corollary of this is that abnormalities can initially be subtle yet have an impact on future development.

Genetic factors

The past decade has witnessed a rapid growth in research on the genetic underpinnings of language impairment. First, there are genetic syndromes associated with language impairment, such as Down syndrome, which is characterized by deficits in phonology and pragmatics, and fragile X syndrome which is associated with deficits in expressive language, speech and pragmatics (Tager-Flusberg, 1999). Second, family and twin studies provide evidence of familial aggregation of speech and language impairment (Tallal, Ross & Curtiss, 1989; Beitchman, Hood & Inglis, 1992; Bishop, North & Donlan, 1995, 1996). Third, molecular genetic studies have begun to localize specific chromosomes responsible for aspects of language development (Grigorenko et al., 1997).

Peri- and postnatal factors

A number of factors has the potential for influencing fetal development and thereby to have an impact on language development. Examples of pathogenic processes include exposure to alcohol, as in Fetal Alcohol syndrome (Jung, 1987). Premature birth is probably the most commonly studied perinatal factor. Studies of premature infants of very low birth weight have shown that these children are at risk for speech/language impairments. However, outcome is determined by whether they are reared in an environment that provides adequate stimulation and psychosocial support (Siegel, 1982).

The most frequent postnatal factor cited as a possible contributor to SLI is otitis media (Whitehurst & Fischel, 1994). However, although a history of recurrent intermittent middle-ear infections and consequent hearing loss has been associated with problems in language development, this finding is inconsistent and many children with recurrent ear infections develop language normally (Bishop & Edmundson, 1986).

Neurodevelopmental immaturity

In view of the association of SLI with other developmental problems in motor, perceptual-motor, cognitive and social cognitive functioning, it has been suggested that this is a reflection of an overall neurodevelopmental immaturity (Beitchman, 1985). However, the fact that most children who exhibit these developmental problems do not catch up as they get older suggests that immaturity is not a sufficient explanation.

Mental retardation

Language impairment and general cognitive delay often occur together. Thus, there has been considerable controversy concerning the use of general developmental delay as an exclusion criterion for diagnosis of SLI (Shaywitz et al., 1992; Bishop, 1997). Children with low overall IQ scores may still show disparities in language relative to overall functioning, and children with SLI often exhibit non-verbal deficits (Bishop, 1997; Cohen et al., 1998a). Moreover, there is evidence from research on Williams syndrome that children with a general cognitive delay exhibit rather better vocabulary skills than might be expected, indicating that general developmental delay and language impairment do not necessarily parallel each other (Rossen et al., 1996).

Child temperament

Children with different temperamental traits may vary in their style of interaction which, in turn, may influence language development. Slomkowski et al. (1992) reported a significant correlation between receptive language and both the affect-extraversion and task orientation dimensions of temperament at the age of 2 years and receptive and expressive language at ages 3 and 7 years. Affect-extraversion made a unique contribution to individual differences in language abilities at the age of 7 years. These authors suggested that extraverted toddlers are not simply talking more but that they also have better receptive language skills than children who are less extraverted.

Socio-economic status

Children from a lower socio-economic background have poorer language skills than those from a middle class background (Hart & Risley, 1995). This association has been shown to be a result of parents in lower socio-economic class samples having less verbal interaction with their children (Hart & Risley, 1995). While the impact is primarily on vocabulary growth, there is evidence that children raised in low socio-economic environments also differ from middle class samples in the development of grammatic forms and narrative skills (Puckering & Rutter, 1987; Whitehurst, 1997). Nevertheless, the pattern of impairment does not appear to be congruent with that typically observed for children with SLI where syntax is most significantly affected (Whitehurst, 1997).

Parent–child interaction

Both language and socio-emotional development are promoted by a sensitive and contingently responsive style of caregiver interaction (Hart & Risley, 1995) Impairments in structural language, including vocabulary, syntax, functional communication, discourse and labels for internal states have been observed in maltreated toddlers and pre-schoolers (Blager & Martin, 1976; Coster et al., 1989). The impact on language development is greater amongst neglected infants than amongst those who are physically abused, most likely because neglecting mothers are unresponsive to their infants' signals whereas abusing mothers are controlling of infant and toddler behaviour (Christopoulos, Bonvillian & Crittenden, 1988).

Chronic maternal depression can also have a negative impact on child language and cognitive development (Murray et al., 1996). For instance, using a community sample, a large group of infants has been followed from birth (NICHD Early Child Care Research Network, 1999) with maternal report of depressive symptoms obtained at 1, 6, 15, 24 and 36 months after birth. Toddlers whose mothers reported feeling chronically depressed had poorer receptive language at 36 months than those whose mothers reported never or sometimes feeling depressed. However, there was a beneficial effect on language development among children whose depressed mothers were able to be sensitive during play. Although children of depressed mothers are at risk, their language scores often fall within the normal range and therefore it is questionable whether these children can be labelled as having SLI. However, one might expect that children of depressed mothers would have poor pragmatic skills, such as less optimal gaze, facial expressions and vocalization, associated with poor quality interactions.

Deprivation

There is no question that extreme deprivation in childhood is associated with language and cognitive impairments (Skuse, 1984). Moreover, although recovery can be rapid once children are placed in an adequate environment, if deprivation is sufficiently prolonged, damage to language development is severe and irreversible.

Processes underlying SLI

Understanding the specific processes underlying SLI has important implications for assessment and treatment. At this point in time, however, the exact nature of the processes is unknown. Moreover, it is uncertain whether there are different subgroups of children whose language impairments are caused by somewhat different underlying processes. SLI has been suggested as arising as a result of a variety of processing deficits (Fletcher, 1999). One set of investigators suggests that processing of grammatical information is critical, working under the assumption that the hallmark of SLI is disordered morphosyntax (Crago & Gopnick, 1994; Leonard, 1997). Others have suggested that SLI arises from an impairment in processing generally, although syntax may be particularly vulnerable (Bishop, 1994). Further, two aspects of processing have been hypothesized to account for problems of children with SLI. One is that children with SLI have difficulty processing (discriminating) brief transient auditory information (e.g. ba/da; Tallal & Piercy, 1974; Tallal, Stark & Mellits, 1985). This explanation has gained increasing interest because of rapid positive effects on language comprehension from focused training that involves daily exposure to acoustically modified speech (Merzenich et al., 1996; Tallal et al., 1996). Anecdotally, P. Tallal (pers. comm., 1999) has also observed changes in behaviour among some of the children receiving this treatment. Another specific processing deficit in individuals with SLI has been linked to problems in storing representations of verbal material in working memory (Gathercole & Baddeley, 1990). The results of this can be seen in the poorer performance of children with SLI on sentence repetition tasks and on measures of nonword repetition (Bishop et al., 1996), the latter of which has been suggested as a genetic marker for SLI.

Persistence of language impairment into adolescence and adulthood

Faith in research findings is always dictated by the quality of the methodology used to arrive at conclusions. Before continuing, therefore, it is important to highlight methodological problems that are common in the literature. First, most studies have relied on clinical samples that tend to be small, self-selecting and heterogeneous in type and severity of SLI. Moreover, there is inconsistency in the information available from the initial evaluation, including diagnostic criteria on which to base conclusions at follow-up and to decide whether the subjects are representative of the SLI population. Second, while epidemiological studies have addressed methodological shortfalls of clinical studies, they rarely provide information on the extent to which samples are functionally impaired, or what proportion required interventions/therapeutic services. Third, although it is well known that SLI is associated with a range of difficulties in cognition, visual–motor performance, social relationships, intelligence and achievement, these have not been consistently examined. Such information is essential to understand the impact of early SLI across the life span. Fourth, although pragmatic and discourse skills are important, these have rarely been examined in longitudinal studies. Fifth, few studies have made repeated measurements across the developmental span, which is essential because the nature of SLI changes with age (Bishop, 1997). Finally, although we know something about the factors that contribute to healthy development generally (Rutter, 1987), there are few data specific to samples with SLI that identify factors that contribute to a positive outcome. Rather, the emphasis has been placed on cumulative risks (e.g. Minskoff, 1994; L. Atkinson et al., unpub. data).

Longitudinal studies of both clinic and community samples show that for many children language problems are chronic. Looking first at studies of speech/language clinic samples, with outcome data obtained from interviews or questionnaires from parents, Hall & Tomblin (1978) found that 50–60% of children with SLI continued to have problems as adults. Tomblin, Freese & Records (1992) observed that adults with a history of SLI performed more poorly than controls on tests of receptive and expressive language. Poor performance on a sentence repetition task differentiated adults with and without a history of SLI. Aram et al. (1984) directly examined language, achievement and behavioural adjustment in 20 adolescents seen as pre-schoolers in a speech–language clinic 10 years earlier. Of those with normal IQ scores, most continued to have language impairments that required special attention at school. Moreover, five children had lower IQ scores at follow-up than when seen initially.

The largest speech–language clinical sample has been followed by Cantwell & Baker (1991). They examined 300 of 600 consecutive referrals of children initially assessed at 2 to 15 years of age and re-assessed 5 years later. While *speech* disorders decreased, approximately equal numbers of individuals exhibited changes from normal to abnormal language functioning and from abnormal to normal functioning (Baker & Cantwell, 1987). Moreover, there was an increase in the prevalence of disorders in language usage and auditory processing. As children with general developmental delays were not considered separately, it is not possible to say whether these children were more compromised. In addition, although some individuals were in their late adolescence and early adulthood at the time of follow-up, data were not analysed to indicate how the older subjects fared in comparison to the younger ones.

Mawhood, Howlin & Rutter (2000) followed 20 boys with severe language impairments but with normal non-verbal intelligence. In their mid-twenties, half had poor conversational skills, low vocabulary scores and articulation abnormalities. The same proportion showed prosodic oddities such as limited variations in pitch or tone, or problems in voice including speech that was flat, exaggerated, slow, fast, jerky and either too loud or too soft. In some cases language and communication deficits of individuals with language deficits actually worsened over time such that they were similar to a group who had been diagnosed as autistic (Mawhood et al., 2000). A further follow-up, conducted in their mid-thirties indicated that the story was much the same (Clegg, Hollis & Rutter, 1999). Along with residual receptive and expressive language deficits, there were also specific impairments in phonological processing.

The most comprehensive of the clinic follow-up studies was conducted by Bishop and Edmundson (1987a,b) who undertook a prospective study of 87 children, aged 4 years, with SLI and a non-impaired control group assessed at four important developmental transition points: early pre-school (4 year olds); just prior to school entry ($5\frac{1}{2}$ year olds); at a point where language skills are presumed to be consolidated (8 years); and in adolescence (15 years). When the sample initially seen at the age of 4 years was retested at $5\frac{1}{2}$ years, 44% of children with normal non-verbal intelligence and 11% of those with below average non-verbal intelligence continued to meet the criterion for SLI (Bishop & Edmundson, 1987a,b). The remaining children no longer differed from controls and thus their SLI was considered to have resolved (good outcome group). When re-assessed again at 8 years, the children with a good outcome at $5\frac{1}{2}$ years continued to make progress and were within the average range on measures of both vocabulary and grammar (Bishop & Adams, 1990). The children who had continued to exhibit SLI at $5\frac{1}{2}$ years remained impaired. The best outcome was for children who at 4 years had specific phonological impairments with a relatively narrow range of impaired language functions and a mild degree of disorder. The best predictor of language outcome was a measure of narrative discourse, the Bus Story. In adolescence (15 years old), those who had a good outcome at $5\frac{1}{2}$ years continued to make progress whereas those with a poor outcome at $5\frac{1}{2}$ years continued to exhibit a wide range of residual problems (Stothard et al., 1998). Nevertheless, while none of the good outcome group met criteria for SLI at the age of 15 years, they showed subtle but significant deficits compared to controls on tasks tapping verbal short-term memory and phonological skills. This is consistent with follow-up studies of children diagnosed as dyslexic, which showed that phonological (Bruck, 1992; Lewis & Freebairn, 1992) and morphological (Bruck, 1998) awareness deficits persist, even for those with adequate reading skills as adults.

While studies of clinic samples provide some useful information, to understand fully the outcomes for individuals with a childhood history of speech and language impairments, it is necessary to use an epidemiological sample. Two community epidemiological prospective studies have followed children into adolescence and early adulthood, one in Sweden and the second in Canada. A third study in New Zealand (Silva, 1980) examined language early on but only reading and behaviour in adolescence; this study will be discussed in the next section.

In the Swedish study, psychologists rated the amount of vocalization (non-crying) at 3, 6 and 9 months on a 5-point scale (Klackenberg, 1980; Stattin & Klackenberg-Larsson, 1993). Vocal communicativeness was rated again by different psychologists at 12 and 18 months and at 2 and 3 years on a similar scale. Despite some concerns regarding the reliability and validity of the assessments, infant ratings were associated with the length and complexity of children's sentence formation, vocabulary use and success in communicating ideas verbally at 3 and 5 years, and intelligence at 17 years. While socio-economic status was related to language, when this was controlled for the results were unchanged.

The Canadian study carried out by Beitchman and colleagues (1986) is the most comprehensive of the longitudinal epidemiological studies of children with SLI. It provides prospective data on language, cognition, achievement and psychiatric disorder at each of three ages: 5 years; 12 years; and 19 years. Sampling at the age of 5 years used a 3-stage epidemiological survey of 1655 children in Ontario. Those who failed a screening assessment were administered a more comprehensive diagnostic battery. Using a relatively liberal criterion (i.e. for some measures a score of one standard deviation below the mean was sufficient), this second stage screening yielded a prevalence of 6.4% speech-only impairments and a 12.6% prevalence of language impairments. In the third stage, the final sample of 284 children, along with 142 controls, completed additional measures to obtain data on demographic information, developmental and medical history, cognitive skills, psychiatric status and parent marital and psychiatric characteristics. Similar comprehensive assessments were done at the ages of 12 and 19 years using age-appropriate measures. When followed at the age of 12 years, 72% of children classified as SLI at the age of 5 years remained impaired, especially those with both receptive and expressive language impairments. Moreover, a small percentage of children not identified as SLI at the first assessment were so classified at 12 years (Beitchman et al., 1994). A further follow-up at the age of 19 years yielded similar results; 73% of children who were language impaired at 5 years still met criteria for language impairment (Johnson et al., 1999). The results did not change appreciably when a more stringent criterion for diagnosis of SLI was applied to the original sample. Further analyses indicated that 23% of controls were impaired at the age of 19, although half of these had only a speech impairment. While the possibility of measurement error must be acknowledged, these latter findings raise the possibility that young children with mild language impairments may not encounter problems until language demands on academic and social life increase in adolescence (Cohen, 1996). When children with general delays were examined separately, there was a similar rate of language impairment in both the SLI and general delay groups, even though children with secondary language impairment had comparatively poorer language skills. Prognosis was better for those who had initial speech impairments and for children with SLI, than for those with more general delays.

In summary, the evidence points toward the long-term persistence of language difficulties in adolescents and adults with SLI, even amongst those whose SLI appears to be resolved and those who had received treatment. Further, some children who early in development do not meet criteria for SLI do so later on. Although we do not know the long-term outcome for those with more subtle SLI, the availability of markers, such as non-word repetition, may permit more systematic longitudinal study of the range of outcomes for individuals with a history of SLI.

The impact of SLI in adulthood

Social relationships and psychiatric disorder

Language impairments rarely occur in isolation. Beyond the obvious function of language as a means of communication, from early childhood SLI is associated with cognitive deficits (e.g. memory, problem solving, concept development), poor academic achievement, immature social cognitive skills, problems in social relationships and psychiatric disorder (Cohen et al., 1998a,b).

Cognitive and academic deficits

Studies examining speech–language clinic samples report a range of cognitive and academic deficits among individuals with a history of SLI. Aram et al. (1984) found that, by adolescence, two-thirds of children with SLI with IQ scores in the normal range had either repeated one or more school grades or had received special help. Problems in mathematics were also observed. Hall & Tomblin (1978) reported that those children and adolescents diagnosed as SLI continued to achieve at a lower level as adults than children with articulation problems, although scores were still within the average range. When their sample was interviewed again at 17–25 years, adults with a history of SLI did more poorly in reading and spelling than controls (Tomblin et al., 1992). Records, Tomblin & Freese (1992) also reported that those with early SLI received less education and were in lower status jobs than non-language impaired controls.

When their speech–language clinic sample was followed after 5 years, Baker & Cantwell (1987) reported that 25% had developed learning disorders since the initial assessment, especially the children with receptive language impairments. Again, this suggests that relatively mild SLI may exert an effect when demands on language and academic performance increase. Consistent with other investigators, problems with mathematics as well as with reading and spelling, were observed.

Mawhood and colleagues (Howlin, Mawhood & Rutter, 2000; Mawhood et al., 2000) reported that by their mid-twenties, none of the 20 men with severe language impairments had passed any national school examinations and approximately half had reading comprehension and accuracy scores at or below a 10-year level. Poor performance on tests of spelling and mathematics was also observed. Moreover, on tests of reading and spelling, there were no group differences when compared with a non-verbal IQ matched group initially diagnosed as autistic. Clegg et al. (1999) reported poor performance on measures of literacy and of social cognition (i.e. Theory of Mind) in the same group when they were aged, on average, 36 years.

Bishop & Adams (1990) found that at 8 years, children with SLI persisting from the age of $5\frac{1}{2}$ years exhibited deficits in reading accuracy and comprehension, spelling and visual–motor performance. When followed-up at 15 years (Stothard et al., 1998), children who appeared to have a good outcome at $5\frac{1}{2}$ and 8 years did worse on measures of literacy than controls, although their scores still exceeded those of the children with persisting SLI and those with general delay. Fifty-two per cent of children with resolved SLI scored below the Grade 12 (Wechsler Objective Reading Dimensions test) level on reading accuracy, reading comprehension or spelling, whereas only 22% of controls did so, and approximately half were receiving some kind of special education. Of the children with persistent SLI and those with general delay, 93% and 80%, respectively were performing below the Grade 12 level.

Turning to the epidemiological studies, Klackenberg (1980) observed that psychologists' ratings of language ability at the age of 3 years were related both to intelligence and to teachers' assessments of reading ability and performance in basic subjects at 11 and 14 years, and to educational level at 20 years.

Silva and colleagues (Silva, 1980) sampled 1037 children born over a one-year period in one maternity hospital in New Zealand. They began to assess expressive and receptive language as well as intellectual and motor ability when the children reached the age of 3 years. Applying a stringent cutoff of two standard deviations below the mean, 3% of the sample was delayed in verbal comprehension only, 2.5% in verbal expression only and 3% in both. Those with low intelligence had a range of other problems in reading, motor ability and language in childhood. Children with normal IQ scores also experienced other language problems and reading delays, but these were less severe (Silva et al., 1984). Although language development was not followed past middle childhood, at 15, 18 and 21 years, adolescents and young adults continued to have reading problems, and examination results were poor (Williams & McGee, 1994, 1996).

Beitchman and colleagues (1996a,b) found that at the age of 12 years, children with a history of SLI at 5 years had lower intelligence and poorer achievement scores than controls. Moreover, cluster analysis indicated that children with the most pervasive language impairments were the most compromised in performance on measures of cognition and achievement, followed by children with poor comprehension and children with poor articulation. As would be expected, young adolescents with high scores on all language tests were least affected. Consistent with the work of others (e.g. Bruck, 1992; Stothard et al., 1998), phonological awareness was an important predictor of reading and spelling abilities. When followed at the age of 19 years, those children diagnosed as having SLI at 5 years still lagged behind non-language impaired controls in academic achievement, regardless of intelligence, and were more likely to be classified as learning disabled (A. Young et al., unpub. data). Of note is that the lowest scores among the young adults diagnosed as learning disabled were not on language tests but on a test of mathematics.

In summary, children with SLI are at risk for problems in learning and achievement that extend into the adult years. Although those with general developmental delay are at the highest risk, the pattern of difficulties also applies to children with normal intelligence. There is some evidence that reading difficulties are particularly salient and these of course also affect subsequent learning and continued vocabulary growth. It is also notable that language impairment is consistently associated with other areas of deficit, particularly mathematics. While on the surface, mathematics appears to be a non-verbal skill, it is reliant on verbal concepts and applications, and on processes such as working memory that are associated with adequate language functioning.

Social functioning and psychiatric disorder

There is now ample evidence from cross-sectional studies of the association between SLI and psychiatric disorder in speech–language clinics, mental health clinics and community samples, with estimates as high as 71% (Camarata, Hughes & Ruhl, 1988). Moreover, a relatively large proportion of children and adolescents referred solely for psychiatric assessment and treatment have unsuspected language impairments that are detected only when a formal evaluation is completed (Cohen et al., 1993, 1998a).

In their follow-up of a speech–language clinic sample, Aram et al. (1984) found that parents rated their adolescent children as less socially competent and as having more behavioural problems than their peers. A follow-up by Baker & Cantwell (1987) indicated that the prevalence of psychiatric disorders actually increased, with 60% of the sample receiving some psychiatric diagnosis at the 5-year follow-up in comparison to 44% when seen initially. The pattern of diagnosis also changed. Diagnosis of ADHD doubled in prevalence, and anxiety disorders more than doubled.

When the group of children with severe SLI was followed by Mawhood and colleagues (2000) into their mid-twenties, only one-quarter of the sample was living independently from their parents and approximately one-third were reported by family members to have difficulty appreciating other people's feelings. When followed again in their mid-thirties, the social, emotional and occupational functioning of the language impaired group continued to be poor in relation to that of both siblings and non-related controls. Moreover, there was greater overlap in social functioning of individuals in this group when compared to individuals who had been diagnosed as autistic and also followed into adulthood (Howlin et al., 2000). Although most did not meet the criteria for a psychiatric diagnosis, the adults in this sample were obviously socially impaired and 3 of the 20 men had developed schizo-affective disorders (Clegg et al., 1999).

The only speech–language clinic study providing more positive outcomes with regard to socio-emotional functioning was that of Records et al. (1992). Although adults with a history of mild to severe SLI had received less education and were employed in lower status jobs, they rated themselves as similar to controls on a measure of quality of life reflecting personal happiness and satisfaction in the domains of family, job, social life and living situation.

Turning to the epidemiological studies, in their follow-up of 212 infants, Stattin & Klackenburg-Larsson (1993) found that measures of language vocalization taken as early as 6 months were related to registered criminality at 15 years. Although the authors themselves raise questions regarding their methodology, these findings are still provocative given the current interest in prevention.

In the New Zealand study, behavioural outcomes began to be examined when children were 9 and 11 years of age. Although language outcomes were not measured in adolescence, reading problems were associated with psychopathology at the age of 18 years (Williams & McGee, 1994, 1996). Using structural equation modelling techniques, these investigators traced a developmental pathway whereby language impairment leads to psychiatric disorder via reading problems, low achievement, poor verbal self regulation and school failure, including poor literacy, with low socio-economic status and attention problems creating a greater risk (McGee et al., 1988; Fergusson & Lynskey, 1997). Transactional effects were such that early reading ability predicted later conduct disorder while, at the same time, antisocial behaviour exerted a detrimental influence on later reading (Williams & McGee, 1994). This finding suggests young adults who become alienated from the mainstream are less likely to be motivated to continue in their attempts to achieve given the unrewarding outcome. In this context, it is pertinent to note that there is strong evidence of a higher than expected prevalence of SLI and language related learning disabilities amongst incarcerated (Myers & Mutch, 1992), runaway and homeless youths (Barwick & Siegel, 1996), school refusing adolescents (Naylor et al., 1994) and adult female offenders (Wagner, Gray & Potter, 1983).

When their sample was followed into early adolescence, Beitchman and colleagues (Beitchman et al., 1999) reported not only a continuing association between SLI and psychiatric disorder at 12 years of age but also that some children without psychiatric disorder at 5 years were so diagnosed at the age of 12. Moreover, children with the most pervasive language impairments and those with auditory comprehension problems were at the greatest risk for psychiatric disorder (Beitchman et al., 1996a,b). At the age of 19 years, SLI status at 5 years was associated with an overall higher rate of psychiatric disorder and with anxiety disorder (Beitchman et al., 2001). The most common anxiety disorder observed was social phobia, which the investigators suggest may reflect the impact of persisting social difficulties and humiliations related to poor performance. Although young adults who had been diagnosed as having SLI at the age of 5 years were not at greater risk for substance abuse than controls, those with comorbid SLI and substance abuse disorders were functioning less well than substance abusers with normal language (Beitchman et al., 1999). Moreover, substance abusers with SLI had a higher rate of comorbid psychiatric disorders, particularly antisocial personality disorder and internalizing disorders, and exhibited more impaired functioning. SLI alone did not predict outcome. L. Atkinson and colleagues (unpub. data) found that factors at age 5 years that predicted psychiatric and cognitive outcomes at 19 years included low socio-economic status, young maternal age at birth of child, large family size, maternal depression, maternal marital situation, parent conviction for criminal offences, along with presence of a speech–language impairment. These factors also predicted more high school dropouts and history of arrests.

In summary, while there are relatively few studies examining the social and psychiatric outcomes of children with SLI, the evidence that does exist indicates that as adults they are at continuing risk for psychiatric disorder and poor overall social functioning. In addition, the risk for psychiatric disorder increases rather than decreases over time. Nevertheless, one study reporting subjective well being is a reminder that self-perceptions of life quality must be taken into account along with the perceptions of relatives, mental health professionals and researchers.

Approaches to intervention from childhood to adulthood

For some time it has been maintained that the bulk of normal language development occurs by the age of 5 years and by no later than the age of 8 years. Because of this, much of the literature describing and evaluating interventions for SLI has focused on the period from infancy through the early school years (McLean & Cripe, 1997; Wetherby, Warren & Reichle, 1998). Over the past 20 years there has been a striking change in the way that interventions are delivered to these children. Specifically, there has been a move away from one-to-one clinic-based therapy for specific phonological, semantic and syntactic deficits to a focus on functional language in naturalistic environments (McLean & Cripe, 1997), and the active inclusion of caregivers and family members (Andrews & Andrews, 1990). Although it is beyond the scope of this chapter to consider these in detail, examples of such procedures include using activities that are preferred by the child and require caregivers to follow their child's lead (Manolson, 1992); arranging the environment to increase the likelihood that the child will engage with materials related to language targets or initiate communication around them (Warren, 1992), and combining structured, focused, didactic approaches with naturalistic techniques (Cole & Dale, 1986). Given the increased emphasis on social language, there has also been a move to enhance pragmatic skills in naturalistic settings with peers (Gallagher, 1996; Hayden & Pukonen, 1996). The goal is to help children interact with peers and adults more successfully by appropriately initiating conversations, asking and responding to questions, taking into account listeners' needs and shaping information through narrative (Gallagher, 1993). The absence of these latter behaviours may account for at least some of the socio-emotional and psychiatric problems observed in children with SLI. From their review of intervention research on young children, McLean & Cripe (1997) concluded that early interventions are effective when administered under controlled conditions, although successful transfer to naturalistic settings is not always made. This is consistent with reports that treatment produced negligible effects in the studies of speech–language clinic samples reported earlier (Aram et al., 1984; Baker & Cantwell, 1987).

From middle childhood onward, interventions typically take two directions. One is a shift from treating oral language skills to improving functional language (Apel, 1999). Most reading remediation programmes do not target linguistic underpinnings (Lyons, 1998 cited by Apel & Swank, 1999: p. 228), although some language focused programmes are effective in increasing competence in phonological awareness skills that underpin most reading problems (Hatcher, Hulme & Ellis, 1994; Lovett & Steinbach, 1997). The second direction is to teach students metacognitive strategies to monitor their own learning, including activities such as talking aloud about the thought processes that contribute to competent learning, emphasizing the relation between targeted skills to daily reading and writing activities, practising active listening (Apel & Swank, 1999), using aids such as visual tools or graphics to depict the structure of discourse and practising self observation of ineffective verbal expression (Zimmerman, 1989). In a recent meta-analytic review of the outcomes of interventions for language learning disabilities, Swanson, Hoskyn & Lee (1999) argued that a focus on isolated skills may be inappropriate because processing components seldom act independently but are compounded by ongoing experiences. Moreover, there is not a unidirectional process leading from lower order skills, such as phonological awareness, to higher order skills such as reading and use of metacognitive strategies. The review by Swanson and colleagues (1999) suggests that a combination of remedial and metacognitive approaches enhances treatment outcomes over using either one alone. Given the range of difficulties faced by children, adolescents and adults with SLI, treatment also often includes environmental modifications, remedial help, classroom consultation and modification, career and vocational planning and psychotherapeutic treatment (Forness & Kavale, 1996). Although there is no strong evidence that psychopharmacological interventions have direct impact on SLI, they may help individuals with psychiatric disorders and SLI to participate more fully in the learning and therapy process by helping to control behaviour, attention, anxiety or mood (Tankersley & Balan, 1999).

In middle childhood, adolescence and adulthood, individuals with SLI have been shown to exhibit social cognitive immaturities in emotion recognition, theory of mind and social problem solving (Bishop, 1997; Cohen et al., 1998b; Clegg et al., 1999). Some interventions emphasize enhancing social cognitive skills such as perspective taking and social problem solving in dyads (Selman & Schultz, 1988). Group interventions have also been implemented using role play, group discussions to clarify goals, brainstorming about social and communication skills, feedback to other group members and devising scripts for social interaction (Donahue, Szymanski & Flores, 1999). In older children and adolescents, functional interventions that link social problem solving skills to personal experiences, goals and self-evaluation are emphasized (Donahue et al., 1999).

Psychotherapy has among its goals increasing the capacity to identify and label emotional cues in oneself and others, verbally interpret and describe behaviour and emotional states and, generally, to become more thoughtful and articulate about intra- and interpersonal processes. In psychotherapeutic interventions, individuals with SLI often encounter difficulties expressing themselves and understanding syntactically complex, lengthy and emotionally loaded discussions with their therapist or family members. Consequently, therapy, at least in part, may be oriented toward helping individuals with SLI to understand the type and breadth of problems encountered, and reflect on the impact of their behaviour on others. Improving self-esteem and encouraging the use of areas of strength, and helping with career and educational planning are other therapeutic goals. It is also necessary to consider how language-based therapies, including some behavioural interventions such as cognitive behaviour therapy, may be modified to compensate for potential communication deficits. For instance, formulating answers to 'how' and 'why' questions, which require procedural knowledge and inferential skills, are particularly difficult for individuals with SLI. An answer of 'I don't know' may not signal resistance but, rather, difficulty creating a narrative, a task that requires formulating on demand cohesive, coherent responses to specific questions on topics chosen by the therapist. Even simple strategies, such as allowing an individual with SLI more time to respond, can be effective.

Interestingly, there is some evidence that psychotherapy has a beneficial effect on language functioning, particularly for children who have peer relationship problems and low self-esteem. Moreover, psychotherapy was more effective when verbal interactions were spontaneous rather than structured (Russell, Greenwald & Shirk, 1991). Shirk & Russell (1996) cautiously suggested that increased language proficiency may be promoted in verbal psycho-therapies by the patient's participation in focused communicative interactions that clarify and expand on verbalizations. This is consistent with the literature on child psychotherapy suggesting a move from interpretation to an approach that sees therapist and patient as 'coauthors' of patients' narratives (Slade, 1994). There are also some broad parallels in components of interventions for SLI and for psychotherapy such as feedback, monitoring and repetition. Al-though, obviously, communication therapy and psychotherapy are different undertakings, these findings offer hypotheses for further exploration in adolescent and adult populations.

There is a paucity of literature on interventions directed specifically at adults with SLI. Most of the literature on intervention with adults focuses on individuals with acquired aphasias who often have selective impairments. In contrast, SLI is characterized by complex patterns of deficit from early childhood, which are compounded over development so that even mild impairments can have long-term sequelae (Bishop, 1997). For example, children with phonological processing problems have difficulty decoding individual words and this, in turn, affects reading comprehension and subsequent vocabulary growth and acquisition of general knowledge. While the functional approach to intervention used with children and adolescents also applies to adults, at the same time it must be recognized that adulthood marks a qualitatively different developmental period with an increasingly more specific set of functional goals, focused on education and career (Forness & Kavale, 1996). On the positive side, adults with relatively mild SLI, higher intelligence and good academic competence may succeed at university. For most students with SLI, options depend on relative strengths and interests and the ability to maintain motivation despite setbacks. Educational and vocational planning and services should be available from early adolescence in order to avert school drop-out and increased alienation from the educational system. For all individuals with SLI, outcomes in adult-hood are related to the extent to which they are able to select school and work environments suitable for themselves and to adapt to and compensate for learning, performance and organizational deficits. This is often done through being taught to use compensatory strategies or benefiting from environmental modifications such as using a tape recorder for note taking (Spekman, Goldberg & Herman, 1992). On the negative side, socio-emotional problems may set limits on the adaptability of individuals with SLI because of reduced tolerance for frustration, low self-esteem and inadequate social problem solving skills (Windsor, 1994). This is compounded by prejudices regarding the competence of individuals with SLI (Wood & Valdez-Menchaca, 1996) and potential biases in job opportunities (Spekman et al., 1992).

There are also individuals in adult psychiatric populations for whom SLI has not been identified or even suspected. The prevalence of unsuspected language impairments in this population is probably quite high, given the findings regarding the high prevalence of unsuspected language impairments in children and adolescents presenting to mental health clinics (Cohen, 1996). Behaviours that might alert therapists to the need for assessment of language and associated conditions are that the patient: has difficulty understanding oral directions; feels frustrated in expressing thoughts; has difficulties adapting language to the listener's needs; has difficulties in joining groups and introducing, maintaining and changing topic; misunderstands words, jokes, metaphors and lengthy sentences; has poor expressive grammar and word finding problems; has non-verbal communication problems such as poor eye contact; and reports problems with literacy skills. All of these symptoms are frequently misinterpreted and misattributed by family, peers, teachers and employers as maladaptive or provocative with labels such as 'lazy', 'bad attitude', and 'uncaring' being commonly applied.

Mental health professionals and communication specialists are not immune to misattributing the potential sources of symptoms. It has been this author's experience in reporting findings concerning the overlap between SLI and psychiatric disorder that some mental health professionals maintain that it is the affective variables, rather than language and cognitive processing variables, that have primacy in explaining these findings. The argument is that individuals who are referred for psychiatric service are emotionally distressed and preoccupied and that this impedes achievement and processing efficiency. Thus, struggles to communicate coherently are seen to be related to the same factors that are causing the psychiatric disorder. An alternative explanation is that, given the high prevalence of SLI among individuals with social adjustment problems and psychiatric disorder, communication difficulties are related to underlying structural language impairments, pragmatic deficits and associated cognitive problems. This is not to say that affect does not influence cognitive processing and the efficiency of processing auditory verbal information (Rothstein et al., 1988), but that the way in which this happens is qualitatively different for individuals with SLI and those with normal language. In order to disentangle discourse deficits associated with SLI and those associated with psychiatric disorders, Vallance, Im & Cohen (1999) examined four groups of 7- to 14-year-old children: children with SLI (including both those with psychiatric problems referred to a mental health centre and community controls); and children with and without psychiatric disorder with normally developing language. Results indicated that children with psychiatric disorder and normally developing language exhibited discourse deficits but these were not as severe or extensive as those of children and adolescents with SLI. Specifically, they used more fillers, repetitions and repairs, and exhibited less emotion-state language in favour of mental-state language. Thus, these children might be particularly vigilant about monitoring the effects of what they say on the listener. The discourse of children with SLI was characterized by severe deficits in language structure and flow of information, including greater use of simple short sentences and poor cohesion within and across sentences, which could have an impact on communicative competence by impeding the capacity to express and elaborate on the complexity of thoughts. Children with comorbid SLI and psychiatric disorder were at greatest disadvantage. They exhibited discourse deficits displayed by both children with SLI and psychiatric disorder and also some distinct discourse problems relating to pronominal reference and the ability to construct causal chains of meaning across events and relationships. Taken together, the results of this study reinforce an alternative explanation for some of the difficulties that individuals may have in therapy, such as problems expressing their thoughts concisely and logically or communicating meaning in emotionally loaded situations.

For mental health professionals working with adolescents and adults, an important first step is to tackle the complex task of understanding the relative contributions of communicative and socio-emotional functioning. Assessment of communicative impairments in adults should be functional and comprise a comprehensive examination not only of language but of cognitive, social cognitive and academic abilities along with social and emotional competence. Both mental health and communication professionals deal with individuals who are encountering problems in coping adaptively in their family, with friends, in the community, at school and at work. Although there is increased awareness of the overlap between SLI and socio-emotional disturbance, collaborative integrative assessment and treatment planning is rare. Moreover, the impact of accurate and sensitive feedback from an integrative assessment concerning the intimate connection between SLI and psychiatric disorder and social impairments that reach across school, work and social relationships should not be underestimated as it is an intervention in itself. Such feedback provides an individual with SLI and his or her family with a better understanding of the reasons for social and learning difficulties and an opportunity correctly to attribute some behaviours to genuine difficulties in communication rather than to an unwillingness to co-operate or a disinterest in relationships. Obviously, collaboration needs to go beyond sharing assessment reports during a feedback interview. Rather, professionals need to work together to arrive at a diagnosis, determine the resources and strategies and the capacity of the individual and their family to utilize these, and maintain communication about an individual's needs and responses to intervention over time.

With recognition of SLI as a lifelong condition, there is an urgent need for further longitudinal research and for systematic investigation of interventions for adults with SLI. Systematic research and documentation is also needed on the collaborative process between professionals and between professionals and individuals with SLI of all ages and their families as there is not, as yet, a solid body of work to suggest how these partners can work together most effectively. Finally, while this review has highlighted the adverse outcomes for individuals with a history of SLI, outcomes in adulthood are not always negative. However, far less is known about factors that lead to a salutary outcome than is known about risks. Likely candidates are probably similar to those predicting positive outcomes for adults with a history of reading disability, such as receipt of special services during schooling and support from parents and teachers (Maughan, 1995).

Summary and conclusion

This review of the literature on the long-term outcome for individuals with SLI leads to rather sobering conclusions. Considerable evidence now points to the persistence of even mild language impairments and their association with problems in cognition, learning, achievement and socio-emotional functioning into adolescence and adulthood. Although the outcome for children with language impairments secondary to general cognitive delay is poorer than for those with SLI, both groups are significantly compromised. Moreover, there is evidence that problems worsen over time, even when SLI appears to have resolved or improved (e.g. Stothard et al., 1998). Just as worrisome is the fact that psychiatric disorder has been shown to increase over time even in individuals whose language impairments improve (Cantwell & Baker, 1991; Williams

& McGee, 1996). The prognosis for those with receptive impairments is especially poor (Whitehurst & Fischel, 1994). Receptive language impairments are also more subtle and difficult to detect, which means that some children, adolescents and adults are not identified unless a routine examination is done (Cohen, 1996). Leaving language impairments unidentified can lead to mis-labelling the source of behaviour problems, which may set into motion a pattern of erroneous attributions, resulting into escalation rather than amelior-ation of problem behaviours (Barwick, Im & Cohen, 1995).

An inevitable problem with examining data from longitudinal studies is that the context and knowledge-base change over time. Thus, for instance, there are no systematic longitudinal studies of pragmatic functioning. This is particularly important because of the close association of pragmatic skills and many psychiatric disorders.

While many adults with SLI are compromised with respect to achievement and occupational level, there is some evidence that this does not apply to all such individuals, nor does it necessarily compromise their sense of their own quality of life (Tomblin et al., 1992). More needs to be known about factors that predict positive outcomes that can contribute to improve services offered to individuals with SLI across the life span.

The material reviewed in this chapter suggests that there are important overlaps between the work of mental health and communication professionals. Mental health professionals are often unfamiliar with the nature of communi-cation impairment, and communication specialists are often unfamiliar with the nature of psychiatric disorders. Although mutual education regarding terminology, symptoms, prognosis and treatment approaches is a necessary first step, it must be acknowledged that there is still often a grey area in differential diagnosis. Finally, there is as yet little written regarding how best to collaborate, and the difficulties of such collaborative partnerships must be recognized. A new body of systematic research is required that: acknowledges that SLI is a lifelong condition; examines how existing knowledge can best be integrated into the assessment and treatment process, and systematically evalu-ates treatments for adults with a history of SLI.

See Table 2.1 for a summary of the clinical implications of SLI.

Table 2.1. Clinical implications of 'specific language impairments' (SLI)

- Language impairments persist into adolescence and adulthood and are associated with problems in cognition, learning, achievement and socio-emotional functioning
- Those at greatest risk are those with receptive language impairments and language impairments secondary to general cognitive delay. Moreover, psychiatric disorder, which is diagnosed in approximately 50% of children with SLI, increases over time
- Language impairments in children, adolescents and adults presenting for mental health service are often not identified unless a systematic assessment is done. Mental health professionals should be alerted to the need for this when patients have difficulties in expression or comprehension (both verbal and non-verbal) or problems with literacy. These symptoms of what may be a SLI often are erroneously attributed to poor attitude, being uncaring or lack of motivation
- The most effective interventions for SLI appear to be those that focus on accomplishing specific tasks in naturalistic settings
- Support for educational and vocational planning should be available from early adolescence in order to avert school drop-out and alienation from the mainstream
- Most mental health interventions rely on language yet rarely is language or communication assessed. Comprehensive, collaborative, integrative assessment is needed in order to plan or adapt interventions. Moreover, providing accurate and sensitive feedback to individuals with SLI and their families can be an intervention in itself

REFERENCES

American Psychiatric Association (1994). *Diagnostic and Statistics Manual of Mental Disorders.* Washington, DC: American Psychiatric Association.

Andrews, J.R. & Andrews, M.A. (1990). *Family Based Treatment in Communication Disorders: A Systemic Approach.* Sandwich, IL: Janelle Publications.

Apel, K. (1999). An introduction to assessment and intervention with older students with language-learning impairments: bridges from research to clinical practice. *Language, Speech, and Hearing Services in the Schools*, **30**: 228–30.

Apel, K. & Swank, L.K. (1999). Second chances: improving decoding skills in the older student. *Language, Speech, and Hearing in Schools*, **30**: 231–42.

Aram, D., Ekelman, B. & Nation, J. (1984). Preschoolers with language disorders: 10 years later. *Journal of Speech and Hearing Disorders*, **27**: 232–44.

Baker, L. & Cantwell, D.P. (1987). A prospective psychiatric follow-up of children with speech/language disorders. *Journal of the American Academy of Child and Adolescent Psychiatry*, **26**: 546–53.

Barwick, M.A., Im, N. & Cohen, N.J. (1995). Parent and teacher attributions underlying psychiatric referral for children with unsuspected language and learning impairments. Poster presented at the Meeting of the Society for Research in Child Development, April, 1995, Indianapolis.

Barwick, M.A. & Siegel, L.S. (1996). Learning difficulties in adolescent clients of a shelter for runaway and homeless street youths. *Journal of Research on Adolescence*, **6**: 649–70.

Beitchman, J.H. (1985). Speech and language impairment and psychiatric risk: Toward a model of neurodevelopmental immaturity. In *The Psychiatric Clinics of North America*, ed. J. Beitchman, pp. 721–35. New York: W.B. Saunders

Beitchman, J.H., Brownlie, E.B., Inglis, A., Wild, J., Mathews, R., Schachter, D., Kroll, R., Martin, S., Ferguson, B. & Lancee, W. (1994). Seven year follow-up of speech/language impaired and control children: speech/language stability and outcome. *Journal of the American Academy of Child and Adolescent Psychiatry*, **33**: 1322–30.

Beitchman, J.H., Douglas, L., Wilson, B., Johnson, C., Young, A., Atkinson, L., Escobar, M. & Taback, N. (1999). Adolescent substance use disorder: findings from a 14-year follow-up of speech/language-impaired and control children. *Journal of Clinical Child Psychology*, **28**: 312–21.

Beitchman, J.H., Hood, J. & Inglis, A. (1992). Familial transmission of speech and language impairment: a preliminary investigation. *Canadian Journal of Psychiatry*, **37**: 151–6.

Beitchman, J.H., Nair, R., Clegg, M. & Patel, P.G. (1986). Prevalence of speech and language disorders in 5-year-old kindergarten children in the Ottawa-Carleton region. *Journal of Speech and Hearing Disorders*, **51**: 98–110.

Beitchman, J.H., Wilson, B., Brownlie, E.B., Walters, H., Inglis, A. & Lancee, W. (1996a). Long-term consistency in speech/language profiles. II. Behavioral, emotional, and social outcomes. *Journal of the American Academy of Child and Adolescent Psychiatry*, **35**: 815–25.

Beitchman, J.H., Wilson, B., Brownlie, E.B., Walters, H. & Lancee, W. (1996b). Long-term consistency in speech/language profiles. I. Developmental and academic outcomes. *Journal of the American Academy of Child and Adolescent Psychiatry*, **35**: 804–14.

Beitchman, J.H., Wilson, B., Johnson, C.J., Atkinson, L., Young, A., Escobar, M. & Douglas, L. (2001). Fourteen-year follow-up of speech/language impaired and control children: psychiatric outcome. *Journal of the American Academy of Child and Adolescent Psychiatry*, **40**: 75–82.

Bird, J., Bishop, D.V.M. & Freeman, N.H. (1995). Phonological awareness and literacy development in children with expressive phonological impairments. *Journal of Speech and Hearing Research*, **38**, 446–62.

Bishop, D.V.M. (1994). Grammatical errors in specific language impairment: Competence or performance limitations. *Applied Psycholinguistics*, **15**: 507–50.

Bishop, D.V.M. (1997). *Uncommon Understanding: Development and Disorders of Language Comprehension in Children*. Hove: Psychology Press.

Bishop, D.V.M. (2000). Pragmatic language impairment: a correlate of SLI, a distinct subgroup, or part of the autistic continuum? In *Speech and Language Impairments in Children: Causes, Characteristics, and Outcome*, ed. D.V.M. Bishop & L.B. Leonard, pp. 99–113. Hove: Psychology Press.

Bishop, D.V.M. & Adams C. (1990). A prospective study of the relationship between specific language impairment, phonological disorders, and reading retardation. *Journal of Child Psychology and Psychiatry*, **31**: 1027–50.

Bishop, D.V.M. & Edmundson, A. (1986). Is otitis media a major cause of specific developmental language disorder? *British Journal of Disorders of Communication*, **21**: 321–38.

Bishop, D.V.M. & Edmundson, A. (1987a). Language-impaired 4-year-olds: distinguishing transient from persistent impairment. *Journal of Speech and Hearing Disorders*, **52**: 156–73.

Bishop, D.V.M. & Edmundson, A. (1987b). Specific language impairment as a maturational lag: evidence from longitudinal data on language and motor development. *Developmental Medicine and Child Neurology*, **29**: 442–59.

Bishop, D.V.M., North, T. & Donlan, C. (1995). Genetic basis of specific language impairment: evidence from a twin study. *Developmental Medicine and Child Neurology*, **37**: 56–71.

Bishop, D.V.M., North, T. & Donlan, C. (1996). Nonword repetition as a behavioural marker for inherited language impairment: Evidence from a twin study. *Journal of Child Psychology and Psychiatry*, **37**: 391–403.

Blager, F. & Martin, H. (1976). Speech and language of abused children. In *The Abused Child*, ed. H.P. Martin, pp. 83–92. Cambridge, MA: Ballinger.

Bruck, M. (1992). Persistence of dyslexics' phonological awareness deficits. *Developmental Psychology*, **28**: 874–86.

Bruck, M. (1998). Outcomes of adults with childhood histories of dyslexia. In *Reading and Spelling: Development and Disorders*, ed. C. Hulme & R.M. Joshi, pp. 179–200. Mahwah, NJ: Erlbaum.

Camarata, S.M., Hughes, C.A. & Ruhl, K.L. (1988). Mild/moderate behaviorally disordered students: a population at risk for language disorders. *Language, Speech, and Hearing Services in Schools*, **19**: 191–200.

Cantwell, D.P. & Baker, L. (1991). *Psychiatric and Developmental Disorders in Children with Communication Disorder*. Washington DC: American Psychiatric Press.

Christopoulos, C., Bonvillian, J.D. & Crittenden, P.M. (1988). Maternal language input and child maltreatment. *Infant Mental Health Journal*, **9**: 272–87.

Clegg, J., Hollis, C. & Rutter, M. (1999). Developmental language disorders: A longitudinal study of cognitive, social and psychiatric functioning. Poster presented at the biennial meeting of the International Society for Research in Child and Adolescent Psychiatry, June, 1999. Barcelona, Spain.

Cohen, N.J. (1996). Psychiatrically disturbed children with unsuspected language impairments: developmental differences in language and behaviour. In *Language, Learning and Behaviour Disorders: Developmental, Biological and Clinical Perspectives*, ed. J.H. Beitchman, N.J. Cohen, M.M. Konstantareas & R. Tannock, pp. 105–27. New York: Cambridge University Press.

Cohen, N.J., Barwick, M.A., Horodezky, N.B., Vallance, D.D. & Im, N. (1998a). Language, achievement, and cognitive processing in psychiatrically disturbed children with previously identified and unsuspected language impairments. *Journal of Child Psychology and Psychiatry*, **39**: 865–77.

Cohen, N.J., Davine, M., Horodezky, N., Lipsett, L. & Isaacson, L. (1993). Unsuspected language impairment in psychiatrically disturbed children: prevalence and language and behavioural characteristics. *Journal of the American Academy of Child and Adolescent Psychiatry*, **32**: 595–603.

Cohen, N.J., Menna, R., Vallance, D., Barwick, M., Im, N. & Horodezky, N. (1998b). Language, social cognitive processing, and behavioral characteristics of psychiatrically disturbed children with previously identified and unsuspected language impairments. *Journal of Child Psychology and Psychiatry*, **39**: 853–64.

Cole, K.N. & Dale, P.S. (1986). Direct language instruction and interactive language instruction with language delayed preschool children: a comparison study. *Journal of Speech and Hearing Research*, **29**: 206–17.

Coster, W.J., Gersten, M.S., Beeghly, M. & Cicchetti, D. (1989). Communicative functioning in maltreated toddlers. *Developmental Psychology*, **25**: 1020–9.

Crago, M.B. & Gopnick, M. (1994). From families to phenotypes: theoretical and clinical implications of research into the genetic basis of specific language impairment. In *Communication and Language Intervention Series*, ed. R.V. Watkins & M.L. Rice, vol. 4. *Specific Language Impairments in Children*, pp. 35–51. Baltimore: Paul H. Brookes.

Donahue, M.L., Szymanski, C.M. & Flores, C. (1999). When "Emily Dickinson" met "Steven Spielberg": assessing social information processing in literacy contexts. *Language, Speech, and Hearing Services in Schools*, **30**: 274–84.

Fergusson, D.M. & Lynskey, M.T. (1997). Early reading difficulties and later conduct problems. *Journal of Child Psychology and Psychiatry*, **38**: 899–907.

Fletcher, P. (1999). Specific language impairment. In *The Development of Language*, ed. M. Barrett, pp. 349–71. Hove: Psychology Press Ltd.

Forness, S.R. & Kavale, K.A. (1996). Treating social skills deficits in children with learning disabilities: a meta-analysis of the research. *Learning Disabilities Quarterly*, **24**: 80–9.

Gallagher, T.M. (1993). Language skill and the development of social competence in school-age children. *Language, Speech, and Hearing Services in the Schools*, **24**: 199–205.

Gallagher, T. (1996). Social-interactional approaches to child language intervention. In *Language, Learning and Behavior Disorders: Developmental, Biological, and Clinical Perspectives*, ed. J.H. Beitchman, N.J. Cohen, M.M. Konstantareas & R. Tannock, pp. 418–36. New York: Cambridge University Press.

Gathercole, S. & Baddeley, A. (1990). Phonological memory deficits of language disordered children: is there a causal connection? *Journal of Memory and Language*, **29**: 336–69.

Grigorenko, E.L., Wood, F.B., Meyer, M.S., Hart, L, A., Speed, W.C., Shuster, A. & Pauls, D.L. (1997). Susceptibility loci for distinct components of developmental dyslexia on chromosome 6 and 16. *American Journal of Human Genetics*, **60**: 27–39.

Hall, P. K. & Tomblin, B.J. (1978). A follow-up study of children with articulation and language disorders. *Journal of Speech and Hearing Disorders*, **43**: 227–41.

Hart, B. & Risley, T.R. (1995). *Meaningful Differences in the Everyday Experience of Young American Children*. Baltimore: Paul H. Brookes.

Hatcher, P.J., Hulme, C. & Ellis, A.W. (1994). Ameliorating early reading failure by integrating the teaching of reading and phonological skills: the phonological linkage hypothesis. *Child Development*, **65**: 41–57.

Hayden, D.A. & Pukonen, M. (1996). Language intervention programming for preschool children with social and pragmatic disorder. In *Language, Learning and Behavior Disorders: Developmental, Biological, and Clinical Perspectives*, ed. J.H. Beitchman, N.J. Cohen, M.M. Konstantareas & R. Tannock, pp. 436–67. New York: Cambridge University Press.

Howlin, P., Mawhood, L. & Rutter, M. (2000). Autism and developmental receptive language disorders – a follow-up comparison in early adult life. II: social, behavioural, and psychiatric outcomes. *Journal of Child Psychology and Psychiatry*, **41**: 561–78.

Johnson, C.J., Beitchman, J.H., Young, A., Escobar, M., Atkinson, L., Wilson, B., Brownlie, E.B., Douglas, L., Taback, N., Lam, I. & Wang, M. (1999). Fourteen-year follow-up of children with and without speech/language stability and outcomes. *Journal of Speech, Language, and Hearing Research*, **42**: 744–60.

Johnson, M.H. (1999). Cortical plasticity in normal and abnormal cognitive development: evidence and working hypotheses. *Development and Psychopathology*, **11**: 419–38.

Jung, J. (1987). *Genetic Syndromes in Communication Disorder*. London, ON: College-Hill Press.

Klackenberg, G. (1980). What happens to children with retarded speech at 3? Longitudinal study of a sample of normal infants up to 20 years of age. *Acta Paediatrica Scandinavica*, **69**: 681–5.

Leonard L. (1997). *Children with Specific Language Impairment*. Cambridge, MA: MIT Press.

Lewis, B.A. & Freebairn, L. (1992). Residual effects of preschool phonology disorders in grade school, adolescence, and adulthood. *Journal of Speech and Hearing Research*, **35**: 819–31.

Lovett, M.W. & Steinbach, K.A. (1997). The effectiveness of remedial programs for reading disabled children of different ages: does the benefit decrease for older children? *Learning Disabilities Quarterly*, **20**: 189–210.

Manolson, A. (1992). *It Takes Two to Talk*, 2nd edn. Toronto: Hanen Early Language Resource Centre.

Maughan, B. (1995). Annotation: long-term outcomes of developmental reading problems. *Journal of Child Psychology and Psychiatry*, **36**: 357–71.

Mawhood, L., Howlin, P. & Rutter, M. (2000). Autism and developmental receptive language disorder – a comparison follow-up in early adult life. I: Cognitive and language outcomes. *Journal of Child Psychology and Psychiatry*, **41**: 547–59.

McGee, R., Share, D., Moffitt, T.E., Williams, S. & Silva, P.A. (1988). Reading disability, behaviour problems, and juvenile delinquency. In *Individual Differences in Children and Adolescents: International Perspective*, ed. D.H. Saklofske & S.B.G. Eysenck, pp. 158–72. London: Hodderd Stoughton.

McLean, L.K. & Cripe, J.W. (1997). The effectiveness of early intervention for children with communication disorders. In *The Effectiveness of Early Intervention*, ed. M.J. Guralnick, pp. 349–428. Baltimore: Paul H. Brookes.

Merzenich, M.M., Jenkins, W.A., Johnston, P., Schreiner, C.G., Miller, S.L. & Tallal, P. (1996). Temporal processing deficits of language-learning impaired children ameliorated by training. *Science*, **27**: 77–80.

Minskoff, E.H. (1994). Post-secondary education and vocational training. Keys to success for adults with learning disabilities. In *Learning Disabilities in Adulthood. Persisting Problems and Evolving Issues*, ed. P.J. Gerber & H.B. Reiff, pp. 111–20. Boston: Andover Medical Publishers.

Murray, L., Hipwell, A., Hooper, R., Stein, A. & Cooper, P. (1996). The cognitive development of 5-year-old children of postnatally depressed mothers. *Journal of Child Psychology and Psychiatry*, **37**: 927–35.

Myers, W.C. & Mutch, P.J. (1992). Language disorders in disruptive behavior disordered homicidal youth. *Journal of Forensic Sciences*, **37**: 919–22.

Naylor, M.W., Staskowski, M., Kenney, M.C. & King, C.A. (1994). Language disorders and learning disabilities in school-refusing adolescents. *Journal of the American Academy of Child and Adolescent Psychiatry*, **33**: 1331–7.

NICHD Early Child Care Research Network, (1999). Chronicity of maternal depressive symptoms, maternal sensitivity, and child functioning at 36 months. *Developmental Psychology*, **35**: 1297–310.

Nowakowski, R.S. & Hayes, N.L. (1999). CNS development: an overview. *Development and Psychopathology*, **11**: 395–417.

Prizant, B.M. (1999). Early intervention: young children with communication and emotional behavioral problems. In *Communication Disorders and Children with Psychiatric and Behavioral Disorders*, ed. D. Rogers-Adkinson & P. Griffith, pp. 295–342. San Diego, CA: Singular Publishing Group.

Puckering, C. & Rutter, M. (1987). Environmental influences on language development. In *Language Development and Disorders*, ed. W. Yule & M. Rutter, pp. 102–28. London: MacKeith Press.

Rapin, I. (1996). Practitioner review: developmental language disorders. A clinical update. *Journal of Child Psychology and Psychiatry*, **37**: 643–55.

Records, N.L., Tomblin, J.B. & Freese, P.R. (1992). The quality of life of young adults with histories of specific language impairment. *American Journal of Speech and Language Pathology*, **1**: 44–53.

Rossen, M., Klima, E.S., Bellugi, U., Bihrle, A. & Jones, W. (1996). Interaction between language and cognition: evidence from Williams syndrome. In *Language, Learning, and Behavior Disorders: Developmental, Biological, and Clinical Perspectives*, ed. J.H. Beitchman, N.J. Cohen, M.M. Konstantareas & R. Tannock, pp. 367–94. New York: Cambridge University Press.

Rothstein, A., Benjamin, L., Crosby, M. & Eisenstadt, K. (1988). *Learning disorders: An Integration of Neuropsychological and Psychoanalytic Considerations*. Madison, CT: International Universities Press.

Russell, R.L., Greenwald, S. & Shirk, S.R. (1991). Language change in child psychotherapy: a meta-analytic review. *Journal of Consulting and Clinical Psychology*, **59**: 916–19.

Rutter, M. (1987). Psychosocial resilience and protective mechanisms. *American Journal of Orthopsychiatry*, **57**: 316–31.

Rutter, M., Dunn, J., Plomin, R., Simonoff, E., Pickles, A., Maughan, B., Ormel, J., Meyer, J. & Eaves, L. (1997). Integrating nature and nurture: implications of person-environment correlations and interactions for developmental psychopathology. *Development and Psychopathology*, **9**: 335–64.

Rutter, M. & Mawhood, L. (1991). The long-term sequelae of specific developmental disorders of speech and language. In *Biological Risk Factors in Childhood and Psychopathology*, ed. M. Rutter & P. Casaer, pp. 233–59. Cambridge: Cambridge University Press.

Schwartz, G. & Merten, D. (1967). The language of adolescence: an anthropological approach to the youth culture. *American Journal of Sociology*, **72**: 453–68.

Selman, R.L. & Schultz, L.H. (1988). Interpersonal thought and action in the case of a troubled early adolescent: toward a developmental model of the gap. In *Cognitive Development and Child Psychotherapy: Perspectives in Developmental Psychology*, ed. S.R. Shirk, pp. 207–46. New York: Plenum

Shaywitz, S.E., Escobar, M.D., Shaywitz, B.A., Fletcher, J.M. & Makuch, R. (1992). Evidence that dyslexia may represent the lower tail of a normal distribution of reading ability. *New England Journal of Medicine*, **326**: 145–50.

Shirk, S.R. & Russell, R.L. (1996). *Change Processes in Child Psychotherapy*. New York: Guilford Press.

Siegel, L.S. (1982). Reproductive, perinatal, and environmental factors as predictors of the cognitive and language development of preterm and full-term infants. *Child Development*, **53**: 963–73.

Silva, P.A. (1980). The prevalence, stability, and significance of developmental language delay in preschool children. *Developmental Medicine and Child Neurology*, **22**: 768–77.

Silva, P.A., Justin, C., McGee, R. & Williams, S.M. (1984). Some developmental and behavioural characteristics of seven-year-old children with delayed speech development. *British Journal of Disorders of Communication*, **19**: 147–54.

Skuse, D., (1984). Extreme deprivation in early childhood. II Theoretical issues and a comparative review. *Journal of Child Psychology and Psychiatry*, **25**: 543–72.

Slade, A. (1994). Making meaning and making believe: Their role in the clinical process. In *Children at Play: Clinical and Developmental Approaches to Meaning and Representation*, ed. A. Slade & D.P. Wolf, pp. 81–107. New York: Oxford University Press.

Slomkowski, C.L., Nelson, K., Dunn, J. & Plomin, R. (1992). Temperament and language: Relations from toddlerhood to middle childhood. *Developmental Psychology*, **28**: 1090–5.

Spekman, N.J., Goldberg, R.J. & Herman, K.L. (1992). Learning disabled children grow up: a search for factors related to success in the young adult years. *Learning Disabilities, Research and Practice*, **7**: 161–70.

Stattin, H. & Klackenberg-Larsson, J. (1993). Early language and intelligence development and their relationship to future criminal behaviour. *Journal of Abnormal Psychology*, **102**: 369–78.

Stothard, S.E., Snowling, M.J., Bishop, D.V.M., Chipchase, B. & Kaplan, C.A. (1998). Language-impaired preschoolers: a follow-up into adolescence. *Journal of Speech, Language and Hearing Research*, **41**: 407–18.

Swanson, H.L., Hoskyn, M. & Lee, C. (1999). *Interventions for Students with Learning Disabilities: A meta-analysis of treatment outcomes*. New York: Guilford Press.

Tager-Flusberg, H. (1999). Language development in atypical children. In *The Development of Language*, ed. M. Barrett, pp. 311–48. Hove: Psychology Press Ltd.

Tallal, P., Miller, S., Bedi, G., Byma, G., Wang, X., Nagarjan, S., Schreiner, C., Jenkins, W. & Merzenick, M. (1996). Language comprehension in language-learning impaired children improved with acoustically modified speech. *Science*, **271**: 81–4.

Tallal, P. & Piercy, M. (1974). Developmental aphasia: the perception of brief vowels and extended stop consonants. *Neuropsychologia*, **13**: 69–74.

Tallal, P., Ross, R. & Curtiss, S. (1989). Familial aggregation in specific language impairment. *Journal of Speech and Hearing Disorders*, **54**: 167–73.

Tallal, P., Stark, V.R. & Mellits, D. (1985). The relationship between auditory temporal analysis and receptive language development: evidence from studies of developmental language disorder. *Neuropsychologia*, **23**: 527–34.

Tankersley, M. & Balan, C. (1999). An overview of psychotropic drugs used in the treatment of behavior and language disorders. In *Communication Disorders and Children with Psychiatric and Behavioral Disorders*, ed. D. Rogers-Adkinson & P. Griffith, pp. 141–76. San Diego: Singular Publishing Group.

Tomblin J.B., Freese, P. & Records, N. (1992). Diagnosing specific language impairment in adults for purpose of pedigree analysis. *Journal of Speech and Hearing Research*, **35**: 832–43.

Vallance, D.D., Im, N. & Cohen, N.J. (1999). Discourse deficits associated with psychiatric disorder and with language impairments in children. *Journal of Child Psychology and Psychiatry*, **40**: 693–704.

Vallance, D.D. & Wintre, G. M. (1997). Discourse processes underlying social competence in children with language learning disabilities. *Development and Psychopathology*, **9**: 95–108.

Wagner, C.D., Gray, L.L. & Potter, R.E. (1983). Communicative disorders in a group of adult female offenders. *Journal of Communication Disorders*, **16**: 269–77.

Wagner, R.K. & Torgeson, J.K. (1987). The nature of phonological processing and its causal role in the acquisition of reading skills. *Psychological Bulletin*, **101**: 191–212.

Warren, S.F. (1992). Facilitating basic vocabulary acquisition with milieu teaching procedures. *Journal of Early Intervention*, **16**: 235–51.

Wetherby, A.M., Warren, S.F. & Reichle, J. (Eds) (1998). *Transitions in Prelinguistic Communication*. Baltimore, MD: Paul H. Brookes.

Whitehurst, G.J. (1997). Language process in context. In *Communication and Language Acquisition: Discoveries from Atypical Development*, ed. L.B. Adamson & M.A. Romski, pp. 233–65. Baltimore: Paul H. Brookes.

Whitehurst, G.J. & Fischel, J.E. (1994). Practitioner review: early developmental language delay. What, if anything, should the clinician do about it? *Journal of Child Psychology and Psychiatry*, **35**: 613–48.

Williams, S. & McGee, R. (1994). Reading attainment and juvenile delinquency. *Journal of Child Psychology and Psychiatry*, **35**: 441–59.

Williams, S. & McGee, R. (1996). Reading in childhood and mental health in early adulthood. In *Language, Learning, and Behavior Disorders: Developmental, Biological, and Clinical Perspectives*, ed. J.H. Beitchman, N.J. Cohen, M.M. Konstantareas & R. Tannock, pp. 530–54. New York: Cambridge University Press.

Windsor, J. (1994). Language impairment and social competence. In *Language Intervention: Preschool Through the Elementary Years*, ed. M.E. Fey, J. Windsor & S.F. Warren, pp. 213–40. Baltimore, MD: Paul H. Brookes.

Wood, M. & Valdez-Menchaca, M. (1996). The effect of a diagnostic label of language delay on adults' perception of preschool children. *Journal of Learning Disabilities*, **29**: 582–8.

Zimmerman, B.J. (1989). A social cognitive view of self regulated academic learning. *Journal of Educational Psychology*, **81**: 329–39.

3

Reading and other specific learning difficulties

Arlene R. Young and Joseph H. Beitchman

Background

Interest in following children with specific learning difficulties (SLD) into adulthood has increased considerably over the past decade (e.g. Patton & Polloway, 1992). Researchers are increasingly asking how children with SLD perform in secondary school, whether they enter and/or graduate from post secondary programmes and how they fare in the adult working and social worlds. An important consideration when examining the characteristics of adults with SLD concerns the unique demands and problems that arise in adulthood because of increased vocational, relationship and independence demands that were not as prominent during childhood.

In addition to differences between childhood and adult environments, the population with SLD is itself extremely diverse. For example, adults with SLD vary greatly in severity and types of processing deficits, reflecting both individual strengths and weaknesses as well as the underlying aetiology of their various forms of SLD. Additionally, wide variation in cognitive ability, language skills, cultural backgrounds and personality characteristics will effect outcome in adulthood. Given this variability, it would be a mistake to assume that outcome within any domain can be uniformly predicted. This variability has implications for interpreting the findings of most studies examining outcomes in adults with SLD. Many studies combine different subgroups of individuals together, regardless of the specific type of SLD they show (e.g. Sitlington & Frank, 1990; Levine & Edgar, 1995; Blackorby & Wagner 1996). This is to ensure sample sizes large enough to make meaningful comparisons. The cost of such comparisons, however, is the loss of information regarding outcome within SLD subtypes, which may have both theoretical and practical applications. While combined SLD samples are likely to contain mostly reading disabled (RD) individuals, failure specifically to identify the type of disability often makes definitive conclusions impossible. Thus, throughout this chapter the term RD is used when the sample is specifically reported to have reading disabilities, while the more general term SLD is used when the study sample is not restricted to individuals with RD. Furthermore, we will describe outcomes in SLD only and will not report on outcomes of individuals with mental retardation, who are referred to as learning disabled (LD) in some diagnostic systems (e.g. in the United Kingdom – UK). The term learning disability is used differently in the United States (US) and UK. In the UK it tends to be used as an alternative to 'mental retardation' to indicate individuals with an IQ below 70. In the US, however, it refers to individuals with *specific* difficulties related to reading, spelling, mathematics, etc. and it is in this sense the term is used here.

Keeping these provisos in mind, this chapter focuses on the characteristics of adults with reading and other specific learning disabilities. Outcomes will be described in the following areas: (1) cognitive characteristics; (2) educational attainments; (3) vocational outcomes; (4) self-perceptions and aspirations; and (5) mental health. We begin with a brief overview of the nature and purported causes of SLD, followed by a summary of recent research on outcomes in the domains listed.

The nature of reading and other specific learning disabilities

The definition of learning disabilities adopted into federal law in the US in the Education for All Handicapped Children Act (Public Law 94–142) has achieved wide acceptance for identifying individuals with SLD for educational and research purposes. This definition (Federal Register, August, 1977: p. 65083) reads as follows:

Specific learning disabilities means a disorder in one or more of the basic psychological processes involved in understanding or using language, spoken or written, which may manifest itself in an imperfect ability to listen, think, speak, read, write, spell, or to do mathematical calculations. The term includes such conditions as perceptual handicaps, brain injury, minimal brain dysfunction, dyslexia, and developmental aphasia. The term does not include children who have learning problems which are primarily the result of visual, hearing, or motor handicaps, of mental retardation, of emotional disturbance, or of environmental, cultural, or economic disadvantage.

DSM-IV (American Psychiatric Association, 1994) criteria for SLD (referred to as Learning Disorders) include three subtypes: reading disorder; mathematics disorder; and disorder of written expression. The diagnostic criteria require that achievement in a specific academic area is substantially below that expected given the age, grade and intellectual ability of the individual. A fourth subtype, learning disorder not otherwise specified, is used to reflect poor academic performance that cannot be attributed to any SLD. The diagnosis also requires that other factors that may be primary contributors to the learning problems (e.g. lack of educational opportunity, poor teaching, impaired vision or hearing, and mental retardation) be ruled out.

An important area of contention among researchers and clinicians is the requirement for a significant discrepancy between ability (as measured by a standardized intelligence measure) and academic achievement. Some (e.g. Siegel, 1992; Fletcher et al., 1993) argue that a significant discrepancy is unnecessary and actually excludes some of the most severely learning disabled individuals (i.e. those whose processing deficits impair performance on intelligence testing as well as acquisition of academic skills). The need for an ability–achievement discrepancy may be particularly unwarranted when assessing SLD in an adult population, as compensation and accommodation for areas of deficiency may serve to blur the boundaries between achievement and ability. The cumulative effect of deficits associated with SLD (e.g. limited exposure to reading materials in disabled readers) can also affect areas such as general knowledge and vocabulary acquisition which, in turn, negatively affect IQ (Stanovich, 1986).

Deficits underlying reading disability

Reading disabilities and the brain

Neuroanatomical and neurofunctional studies of individuals with RD have found evidence in support of a left hemisphere deficit. Using magnetic resonance imaging (MRI) scans the planum temporale has been shown to lack the normal left greater than right asymmetry, and the right planum temporale has been found to be greater than the left (Hynd & Semrud-Clikeman, 1989; Jernigan et al., 1991). On positron emission tomography (PET) studies, differences have also been shown in the left hemisphere of individuals with and without RD while performing language tasks (Flowers, 1993). Regional cerebral blood flow studies show that on language-related tasks there is a significant relationship between left temporal and parietal blood flow in childhood diagnosed dyslexia (Flowers, 1993).

In addition, the brains of individuals with RD compared to those of non-reading disabled individuals tend to have significantly more focal dysplasias, particularly in the language regions bordering the Sylvian fissure (Galaburda et al., 1985; Kaufman & Galaburda, 1989). Given the view that RD falls along a continuum and does not constitute a discrete entity (Shaywitz et al., 1992), the positive neuroanatomical results may represent findings at the extreme end of the spectrum; among individuals with less severe impairment, neuroanatomical and neurofunctional differences may be less evident. Until the results of more definitive studies are known, these findings should be considered tentative.

Biological factors

Between 35% and 40% of first degree relatives of children with RD have similar problems (Shepherd & Uhry, 1993), but because the condition is aetiologically heterogeneous, no single major locus is likely to be implicated. Evidence for a quantitative trait locus (QTL) in the HLA region of chromosome 6 that influences reading ability has been reported by Cardon et al. (1994). A recent study by Grigorenko et al. (1997) has shown linkage between RD and chromosomes 6 and 15. The specific genes have not yet been identified nor has the possible underlying mechanism of action. However, Grigorenko et al. (1997) reported that the link to the site on chromosome 6 is related to phonological awareness, and the link to the site on chromosome 15 is related to single word reading, each being a separable phenotype of reading ability and disability. Further study is needed to confirm and amplify the findings.

Core cognitive deficits

There is consensus among researchers that the central deficit underlying developmental reading disability is a very specific aspect of language processing referred to as 'phonological awareness' (e.g. Lovett, 1992; Torgesen, Wagner & Rashotte, 1994; Brady, 1997). This term refers to the awareness of and ability to manipulate individual speech sounds in words. Children with this type of deficit may, for example, have difficulty recognizing and producing rhymes for words or identifying the individual syllables in compound words at the same age as other children. They may also show persistent difficulty in performing certain tasks such as when they are required to substitute one phoneme for another (say 'brake' but substitute 'd' for 'b') or to omit a single phoneme within a word (say 'brake' without the 'b'). This core phonological awareness deficit has been associated with an array of problems often apparent in disabled readers. These include difficulties in working memory skills (e.g. Brady & Shankweiler, 1991; Stanovich, 1991, 1994) and in acquiring and remembering spelling-to-sound relationships, which are necessary for both reading and spelling skills (Torgesen, Wagner & Rashotte, 1997).

Longitudinal studies have confirmed that early occurring deficits in phonological awareness predict later reading difficulties (Bishop & Adams, 1990; Wagner, Torgesen & Rashotte, 1994; Snowling, Goulandris & Defty, 1996; Young et al., in press). Given the importance of phonological skills, interventions directed at preventing reading problems in at-risk children (e.g. Olson et al., 1997; Scanlon & Vellutino, 1997; Foorman et al., 1998) and treating reading problems in disabled readers (Lovett & Steinbach, 1997; Wise et al., 1997) typically focus on improving phonological reading skills.

Outcomes in adults with reading disabilities

Cognitive and academic outcomes

Studies of adults with a history of reading problems point to the persistent nature of these difficulties. Follow-up studies of children identified as having RD, for example, consistently report adult reading levels considerably below those of controls (e.g. Michelsson, Byring & Bjoerkgren, 1985; LaBuda & DeFries, 1989; Spreen, 1989; Maughan et al., 1994). Yet reading achievement outcomes are not uniformly negative. Naylor, Felton & Wood (1990) for example, reported that while 50% of a clinical sample of children with RD still met criterion for RD in adulthood, the reading levels of approximately one-third were within normal limits. Thus, while adults with RD as a group continue to perform below their peers in reading, there is considerable individual variability in outcome. In a review of long-term outcomes of RD in childhood, Maughan (1995) noted that reading comprehension and word recognition skills continue to improve into adulthood, and that this improvement results from continued practice and education rather than from maturity alone. However, a slower reading rate is often typical, even when reading identification and comprehension skills have improved (Denckla, 1993). According to Maughan (1995), the best predictors of later reading levels are IQ and initial severity of the reading disability.

As far as phonological processing deficits are concerned, both cross-sectional and follow-up studies indicate that these are stable throughout childhood and adolescence (Fawcett & Nicolson, 1995; MacDonald & Cornwall, 1995) and into adulthood (Pratt & Brady, 1988; Bell & Perfetti, 1994; Elbro, Nielsen & Petersen, 1994). Pennington et al. (1990) compared phonological processing skills in adults with RD with both reading age and chronological age controls. The adults with RD included a group of familial dyslexics (recruited from a genetic linkage study) and a group from a RD treatment programme. A clear deficit in phoneme awareness was evident in both these groups. The importance of phonological awareness was underscored in a prospective longitudinal study of adult outcomes in children first identified in a community sample as speech/language impaired at age 5 years (Beitchman et al., 1986a,b; 1996). At age 19, 36.8% (26.7% when an IQ cutoff is employed) of the early language impaired group met criterion for RD, compared to only 6.4% (5.8% with IQ cutoff) of matched controls (Young et al., in press). While these findings demonstrate the importance of language functioning generally to reading outcomes, examination of individual factors related to prognosis revealed that phonological awareness made a substantial contribution to reading skills in adulthood, regardless of initial language status.

Bruck (1992) reported that children and adults with RD show little if any increase in phonological awareness as their reading skills improve, regardless of age or reading level. In normal readers phonological awareness and reading are bidirectionally linked such that gains in reading skills facilitate gains in phonological awareness skills (e.g. Morais, 1987). The finding that, in the case of RD, improvement in word recognition is not reflected in improved phoneme awareness suggests that the pattern of development is different than in normal readers. Taken together, these results show that a core deficit (or related deficits) in phonological awareness persists in RD and that this underlying deficit is most apparent when the reader encounters unfamiliar words or difficult text. Thus, while adults with a history of reading problems often learn to compensate for weak phonological processing skills and show improved word identification and reading comprehension skills, they may still encounter difficulty when phonological skills are required.

Not unexpectedly, fewer youngsters with SLD compared with typically developing peers, complete secondary school and go on to further education. Maughan et al. (1994) reported that 40% of a sample of poor readers followed from 10 to 16 years of age left school early without any qualifications, and only 10% achieved the minimum school-leaving qualifications for entry into higher education. Nevertheless, some students with SLD do enter higher education and a few studies report positively on their outcome and adjustment.

Having entered post-secondary education, proportionately fewer students with SLD remain until graduation. Sitlington & Frank (1990), for example, reported that while 50% of a sample of high school graduates with SLD entered college, only 6.5% of these students were still in school one year later.

Vogel & Adelman (1990, 1992) reported on the educational attainments of college students with SLD compared with a sample of students matched for gender, and college aptitude test results. Results showed that students with SLD tended to take less intensive courses and graduated one year later than the matched sample. They also had significantly poorer essay writing skills. Nevertheless, the academic failure rate in the aptitude matched sample was three times greater than in the sample with SLD. This was because students with SLD in this study were all enrolled in a support services programme within the college. Thus, continued academic support appears to be beneficial to students with SLD, even within post-secondary settings.

Vocational outcomes

The majority of studies of vocational outcome in adults with SLD suggest that, on average, they do not fare well (Gajar, 1992; White, 1992). Higher rates of unemployment are frequently reported (e.g. Kavale & Forness, 1996), and individuals are often under-employed, in that they are more likely than their peers to work part-time and to have relatively unskilled jobs (Faas & D'Alonzo, 1990; Sitlington & Frank, 1990; Fairweather & Shaver, 1991; Fourqurean et al., 1991). While the effects of SLD are often most noticeable during formal schooling, adults often report continuing problems after leaving school. Greenbaum, Graham & Scales (1996), for example, reported that 80% of a sample of adults with SLD indicated that their difficulties significantly affected them at work and in other aspects of their lives. According to White (1992), only about 50% of adults with a prior history of SLD were able to live independently and the majority were not self-supporting. This finding should be viewed with caution since there is little information about the characteristics of the subjects in White's study, and the type and severity of their learning disabilities is unknown. Psychosocial difficulties (Ryan & Price, 1992), social competence deficits and poor self-advocacy skills (Hoffman et al., 1987) are additional areas of difficulty that are likely to have an impact on vocational success.

Outcomes in gifted students with SLD

Holliday, Koller & Thomas (1999) examined outcomes in a sample of gifted adults with SLD. Their mean age was 23 years (age range 18–45 years), and their Performance or Verbal IQ was at least 120. The mean academic grade level completed was 12.7 years, with only 21% of the sample completing more than four semesters at college. Most (76%) of the subjects earned only the minimum wage and 52% worked in unskilled jobs; 36% worked in skilled jobs and 9% in professional jobs. A clear discrepancy was also evident between the participants' expressed educational and vocational aspirations and their actual educational and vocational attainments.

These results highlight the struggle that many adults with SLD face in both academic and vocational arenas, even when intellectual abilities are significantly above average. When interpreting these results, however, it is important to note that for 85% of the subjects Performance IQ exceeded Verbal IQ. Thus, verbal difficulties may contribute to poor outcome overall. Verbal ability has been shown to be an important predictor of both educational (Hughes & Smith, 1990) and vocational success (Faas & D'Alonzo, 1990) among adults with SLD. Hence, even within a sample of individuals with SLD who are very able, verbal ability is likely to play an important role in outcome.

Predictors of outcome beyond academic and cognitive skills

Raskind et al. (1999) reported on a 20-year, longitudinal study of 41 individuals who, as children, attended the Frostig Treatment Center in California for learning disabilities. The mean age at follow-up was 32.1 years. Results indicated that while the participants with SLD made continuous progress in maths and reading skills over time, they were still below expected levels in educational and vocational attainment. Other areas of difficulty were also noted, with 42% of the sample described as having psychological difficulties serious enough to warrant a DSM-IV diagnosis. The study participants were classified as 'successful' or 'unsuccessful' based on a variety of outcome measures (e.g. employment, education, independence, etc.). Attributes such as self-awareness, perseverance and emotional stability were more predictive of success than academic skills. Thus, remediation efforts need to encompass more than just academic skill development.

Findings from longitudinal follow-up studies indicate that females with SLD generally do less well than males (Levine & Nourse, 1998). In a follow-up study reported by Maughan & Hagell (1998), for example, males who were poor readers (many of whom were likely to have RD) showed no marked differences compared to competent readers on measures of social functioning and self-esteem in adulthood. While males who were poor readers were more likely to show avoidant personality problems, anxiety and depression, the clearest systematic differences occurred in the area of independent living. More men who were poor readers were still living with their parents into their late twenties, and more appeared to have done so throughout their early adult lives. However, although this pattern applied to a sizeable minority of the men who were poor readers (about a fifth), it was by no means typical of the group as a whole.

For women, outcomes tend to be less positive in a number of respects. Previous studies (Bruck, 1985) have suggested that young women with histories of reading difficulties are more likely to show adjustment problems in adulthood when compared with women who are competent readers. The poor readers had greater problems in social functioning in their early twenties than the comparison group, and they also appeared to have an increased risk of psychiatric disorders and relationship problems (Maughan & Hagell, 1998). Young women with self-reported literacy problems have also been found to have children at an earlier age than those who report themselves to be competent readers (ALBSU, 1987; Ekynsmith & Brynner, 1994).

It is possible that the greater number of options available to young men once they leave school may play a part in enabling more positive social functioning in adulthood. By being selective about their particular adult activities, they may be able to minimize the functional implications of ongoing literacy difficulties and build on other skills and talents (Maughan & Hagell, 1998).

Self-perceptions and aspirations

While academic self-esteem has consistently been shown to be lower in children and adolescents with SLD, findings on global self-esteem are mixed (Bryan & Bryan, 1990; Huntington & Bender, 1993). In adulthood, early academic difficulties or SLD alone do not necessarily predict lower self-worth. For example, Maughan & Hagell (1998) reported that adults who were poor readers in childhood did not differ from normal reading controls in global self-worth ratings. Similarly, Lewandowski & Arcangelo (1994) reported no differences in self-concept between adults with and without SLD. Why is it that children with LD are consistently shown to have self-concept problems while adults with SLD are not? One possibility is that many of the difficulties encountered in childhood (e.g. stigmatization for academic problems within the school setting) are no longer an issue in adulthood. Conversely, measures of self-concept in adulthood rarely examine academic self-concept, the specific area that is most often found to be lower in children with SLD. More research is needed to determine if adults with SLD are truly less likely to show the self-esteem deficits so often present in childhood.

McCall, Evahn & Krantzer (1992) found that high-school underachievers had lower educational and career aspirations than their peers. Similarly, Maughan et al. (1994), found that poor readers were less likely to have positive work plans and held more modest ambitions in their twenties than peers. Even the minority who acquired formal qualifications, entered relatively unskilled jobs. In a related publication, Maughan (1995; p. 362) concluded that 'some poor readers appear to set self-imposed boundaries on their occupational choices'.

Mental health outcomes

Anxiety and Depression

Surprisingly little has been written about the relationship between SLD and the internalizing disorders of anxiety and depression. Huntington & Bender (1993) reviewed the literature focusing on the emotional well being of adolescents with SLD and concluded that: (1) adolescents with SLD have a less positive academic self-concept than their non-disabled peers; (2) adolescents with SLD attribute both success and failure more internally than comparison groups; (3) adolescents with SLD experience higher levels of trait anxiety and have a significantly higher prevalence of minor somatic complaints than peers without SLD; (4) studies of children in classes for the learning disabled and of adolescents with SLD reported high rates of depression on self-report measures; and (5) while a link between suicide and SLD has been suggested by other authors (e.g. Peck, 1985; Pfeffer, 1986), empirical data to support these suppositions are unavailable. Given the paucity of studies of internalizing disorders involving comparisons of children and adolescents with and without SLD, few firm conclusions can be drawn.

Conduct disorders/delinquency

The association between RD and behaviour problems is weak, with some evidence that behaviour difficulties predate RD and no evidence that RD predate aggressive behaviour (Cornwall & Bawden, 1992). In addition, there is evidence that antisocial behaviours associated with RD are secondary to other variables, such as family dysfunction and low socio-economic status (Fergusson & Lynskey, 1997). However, the possibility that RD may worsen pre-existing externalizing behaviour problems as reported by McGee et al. (1986), needs to be further investigated.

When aggressive behaviour and learning problems have been linked during the early school years it is chiefly through comorbidity with attention deficit hyperactivity disorder (ADHD) (Frick et al., 1991). However, by adolescence, clear links have emerged between frankly antisocial behaviour and verbal deficits and underachievement. A recent study comparing rates of antisocial behaviour in young adult males with and without a childhood history of language impairment found significantly increased rates among males with a childhood history of language impairment (Beitchman et al., 2001). The basis for this association has been the subject of some controversy. Three hypotheses have been proposed: (1) the school failure hypothesis, which states that a lack of educational success produces low self-esteem, frustration and acting out behaviour (Grande, 1988); (2) the differential treatment (or detection) hypothesis, that young people with SLD engage in the same number of antisocial acts as young people without SLD but are treated differently by the justice system (Zimmerman et al., 1979); and (3) the susceptibility hypothesis, which states that SLD is accompanied by personality characteristics that predispose the individual to delinquent behaviour (Larson, 1988).

Support exists for all three hypotheses but the evidence appears strongest for the third. For instance, language-based learning disabilities seem to play an important role in delinquent behaviour, supporting the susceptibility hypothesis. Language deficits have been linked to deficient verbal mediation, which is believed to result in difficulties in social problem-solving (Kazdin, 1987) and a series of related deficiencies, such as problems with delay of gratification, that may heighten the risk for delinquent outcomes. The evidence in support of the remaining two hypotheses is contradictory, though some work by Lynam, Moffitt & Stouthamer-Loeber (1993) and Moffitt & Silva (1988) provides support for the school failure hypothesis and challenges the differential detection hypothesis.

Social competencies

A wide assortment of social skill deficits has been found in individuals with SLD regardless of age (Vaughn et al., 1990; Gerber & Reiff, 1994). While these cause problems in their own right, they can exacerbate academic achievement problems and present a major stumbling block to successful transition into adulthood (e.g. LaGreca & Stone, 1990; Mellard & Hazel, 1992). In a meta-analysis of 152 studies examining social skill deficits and SLD, Kavale & Forness (1996) reported that about 75% of students with SLD manifest social skill deficits that distinguish them from non-SLD controls.

Given the frequency of these difficulties and the potentially debilitating effect they can exert on functioning in adulthood, intervention specific to enhancing social competencies in individuals with SLD throughout childhood and into adulthood, is recommended. Various approaches to intervention have been suggested, depending on the presumed nature of the underlying deficits. Gresham (1986) for example, proposed a model in which four possible sources of difficulty are identified, including deficits in social skills, social performance, self-control skills and self-control performance. After identifying the specific source of the social difficulty, interventions are tailored to fit the deficits. For example, deficits in self-control skills, related to a lack of skill development because of problems with anxiety, anger, etc., are addressed through techniques to manage and reduce the underlying arousal problems (e.g. cognitive techniques) combined with teaching procedures (modelling, coaching, feedback, etc.) to promote the deficient skills.

Regardless of the skill-training approach taken, the setting in which the instruction occurs is also an important consideration. Mellard & Hazel (1992) recommend that instruction is provided regarding the social skill demands of a variety of settings including secondary school, colleges and the workplace, to help improve the chances that the adult with SLD will be successful in these diverse situations. They argue that instruction in interpersonal skills, work tolerance and work skills should be incorporated into the existing secondary and post-secondary curriculum, as well as in work place training programmes.

Interventions

The most comprehensive analysis of interventions for individuals with SLD is the meta-analysis of Swanson, Hoskyn & Lee (1999). This covers over 30 years of intervention research and includes the results of 272 data-based group and single-case studies of intervention outcomes in students with SLD. The authors examined over 300 variables, and generated general findings and recommendations for intervention, as follows:

- A Combined Direct Instruction and Strategy Instruction Model is the most effective procedure for remediating SLD. The important components of this treatment approach include attention to sequencing, drill–repetition–practice, segmenting information into parts or units for later synthesis, controlling task difficulty using prompts and cues, making use of technology (e.g. computers), systematically modelling problem-solving steps, and using small, interactive groups.

- Regardless of the treatment, students with SLD performed most like non-SLD students when the intervention included strategy instructions. The Strategy Instruction and Direct Instruction models were shown to operate independently of each other but to be particularly effective when combined.

- In the area of treatment for RD, both whole word and phonics approaches were shown to make a significant contribution and neither clearly supersedes the other on transfer measures (e.g. reading comprehension, reading novel words).

- Both lower-order (e.g. phonics) and higher-order (e.g. metacognition or strategy) skills were shown to interact in order to influence treatment outcomes. Thus, intervention methods that combine both of these approaches are recommended.

  While youngsters with SLD are clearly at risk for developing psychosocial problems in adulthood, many do not. For males in particular, the level of dysfunction appears to decrease with age. This may reflect the range of opportunities available to seek positive vocational and social environments that do not emphasize literacy skills to the same degree as school. Further, compensation and accommodation may enable the adult to build on other areas of strength that enable a more positive outcome.

  Improvements in reading skills, while likely to be important and helpful for

Table 3.1. Clinical implications of specific learning difficulties (SLD)

- SLD tend to persist throughout development well into adulthood
- Despite this persistence, individuals with SLD vary widely in their adult functioning
- Verbal ability may play a particularly important role in vocational success even when specific learning problems persist
- Attributes such as self-awareness, perseverance, and emotional stability are important contributors to a successful outcome in individuals with SLD, over and above academic skills
- In addition to well-designed academic programmes, most individuals with SLD would benefit from intervention to improve social competencies
- Results from a large scale, meta-analysis indicates that a combination of Direct Instruction and Strategy Instruction approaches is the most effective remediation procedure

vocational functioning, are in themselves not predictive of psychosocial outcomes (Maughan & Hagell, 1998). Thus interventions, especially at the secondary level and beyond, should include both remediation for the academic difficulties and enhancement of personality and motivational characteristics that increase the chances of good outcome (e.g. perseverance, self-awareness) as indicated by Raskind et al. (1999). Enhancement of social skills is an important area of focus across age groups and settings. Finally, given that SLD are lifelong conditions that have an impact on functioning well beyond the academic arena, individuals with SLD need to be taught self-advocacy skills to enhance their chances of success throughout life.

See Table 3.1 for a summary of the clinical implications of SLD.

REFERENCES

Adult Literacy and Basic Skills Unit (ALBSU) (1987). *Literacy, Numeracy and Adults: Evidence from the National Child Development Study*. London: ALBSU.

American Psychiatric Associaion (1994). *Diagnostic and Statistical Manual of Mental Disorders*, Fourth Edition. Washington, DC: American Psychiatric Association.

Beitchman, J.H., Nair, R., Clegg, M., Ferguson, B. & Patel, P.G. (1986a). Prevalence of psychiatric disorders in children with speech and language disorders. *Journal of the American Academy of Child Psychiatry*, **25**: 528–35.

Beitchman, J.H., Nair, R., Clegg, M. & Patel, P. G. (1986b). Prevalence of speech and language disorders in 5-year old kindergarten children in the Ottawa-Carleton region. *Journal of Speech and Hearing Disorders*, **51**: 98–110.

Beitchman, J.H., Wilson, B., Brownlie, E. B., Walters, H. & Lancee, W. (1996). Long-term consistency in speech/language profiles. I. Developmental and academic outcomes. *Journal of the American Academy of Child and Adolescent Psychiatry*, **35**: 804–24.

Beitchman, J.H., Wilson, B., Johnson, C.J., Atkinson, L., Young, A., Escobar, M. & Douglas, L. (2001). Fourteen-year follow-up of speech/language impaired and control children: psychiatric outcomes. *Journal of the American Academy of Child and Adolescent Psychiatry*, **40**: 75–82.

Bell, L. C. & Perfetti, C. A. (1994). Reading skill: some adult comparisons. *Journal of Educational Psychology*, **86**: 244–55.

Bishop, D.V.M. & Adams, C. (1990). A prospective study of the relationship between specific language impairment, phonological disorders and reading retardation. *Journal of Child Psychology and Psychiatry*, **31**: 1027–50.

Blackorby, J. & Wagner, M. (1996). Longitudinal postschool outcomes of youth with disabilities: findings from the National Longitudinal Transition Study. *Exceptional Children*, **62**: 399–413.

Brady, S.A. (1997). Ability to encode phonological representation: an underlying difficulty of poor readers. In *Foundations of Reading Acquisition and Dyslexia*, ed. B.A. Blachman, pp. 21–47. Hillsdale, NJ: Lawrence Erlbaum Associates, Inc.

Brady, S.A. & Shankweiler, D. (1991). *Phonological Processes in Literacy: A Tribute to Isabelle Y. Liberman*. Hillsdale, NJ: Lawrence Erlbaum Associates, Inc.

Bruck, M. (1985). The adult functioning of children with specific learning disabilities: a follow-up study. In *Advances in Applied Developmental Psychology*, ed. I. Sigel, pp. 91–129. Norwood, NJ: Ablex.

Bruck, M. (1992). Persistence of dyslexics' phonological awareness deficits. *Developmental Psychology*, **28**: 874–86.

Bryan, T.H. & Bryan, J.H. (1990). Social factors in learning disabilities: an overview. In *Learning disabilities: Theoretical and Research Issues*, ed. H.L. Swanson & B.K. Keogh, pp. 131–8. Hillsdale, NJ: Lawrence Erlbaum Associates, Inc.

Cardon, L.R., Smith, S.D., Fulker, D.W., Kimberling, W.J., Pennington, B.F. & DeFries, J.C. (1994). Quantative trait locus for reading disability on chromosome 6. *Science*, **266**: 276–9.

Cornwall, A. & Bawden, H.N. (1992). Reading disabilities and aggression: a critical review. *Journal of Learning Disabilities*, **25**: 281–88.

Denckla, M.B. (1993). The child with developmental disabilities grown up: adult residua of childhood disorders. *Behavioral Neurology*, **11**: 105–25.

Ekynsmith, C. & Brynner, J. (1994). The basic skills of young adults: some findings from the 1970 British cohort study. London: ALBSU.

Elbro, C., Nielsen, I. & Petersen, D. K. (1994). Dyslexia in adults: evidence for deficits in non-word reading and in the phonological representation of lexical items. *Annals of Dyslexia*, **44**: 205–26.

Faas L.A. & D'Alonzo, B.J. (1990). WAIS-R scores as predictors of employment success and failure among adults with learning disabilities. *Journal of Learning Disabilities*, **23**: 311–16.

Fairweather, J.S. & Shaver, D.M. (1991). Making the transition to postsecondary education and training. *Exceptional Children*, **57**: 264–69.

Fawcett, A.J. & Nicolson, R.I. (1995). Persistence of phonological awareness deficits in older children with dyslexia. *Reading and Writing: An Interdisciplinary Journal*, **7**: 361–76.

Fergusson D.M. & Lynskey M.T. (1997). Early reading difficulties and later conduct problems. *Journal of Child and Adolescent Psychiatry,* **38**: 899–907.

Fletcher, J.M., Francis, D.J., Rourke, B.P., Shaywitz, S.E. & Shaywitz, B.A. (1993). Classification of learning disabilities. In *Better Understanding of Learning Disabilities,* ed. G.R. Lyon, D.B. Gray, J.F. Kavanagh & N.A. Krasnegor, pp. 27–55. Baltimore: Paul H. Brookes Publishing Co.

Flowers, D.L. (1993). Brain basis for dyslexia: a summary of work in progress. *Journal of Learning Disabilities,* **26**: 575–82.

Foorman, B.R., Francis, D.J., Fletcher, J.M., Schatschneider, C. & Mehta, P. (1998). The role of instruction in learning to read: preventing reading failure in at-risk children. *Journal of Educational Psychology,* **90**: 37–55.

Fourqurean, J.M., Meisgeier, C., Swank, P.R. & Williams, R.E. (1991). Correlates of postsecondary employment outcomes for young adults with learning disabilities. *Journal of Learning Disabilities,* **24**: 400–05.

Frick, P.J., Kamphaus, R.W., Lahey, B.B., et al. (1991). Academic underachievement and the disruptive behavior disorders. *Journal of Consulting and Clinical Psychology,* **59**: 289–94.

Gajar, A.H. (1992). Adults with learning disabilities: current and future research priorities. *Journal of Learning Disabilities,* **25**: 507–19.

Galaburda, A.M., Sherman, G.F., Rosen, G.D., Aboitiz, F. & Geschwind, N. (1985). Developmental dyslexia: four consecutive cases with cortical anomalies. *Annals of Neurology,* **18**: 222–33.

Gerber, P.J. & Reiff, H.B. (1994). *Learning Disabilities in Adulthood: Persisting Problems and Evolving Issues.* Boston: Andover Medical.

Grande, C.G. (1988). Delinquency: the learning disabled student's reaction to academic school failure? *Adolescence,* **23**: 209–19.

Greenbaum, B., Graham, S. & Scales, W. (1996). Adults with learning disabilities: occupational and social status after leaving college. *Journal of Learning Disabilities,* **29**: 167–73.

Gresham, F.M. (1986). Conceptual issues in the assessment of social competence in children. In *Children's Social Behavior: Development, Assessment, and Modification,* ed. P.S. Strain, M.J. Guralnick & H.M. Walker, pp. 143–79. New York: Academic Press.

Grigorenko, E.L., Wood, F.B., Meyer, M.S., Hart, L.A., Speed, W.C. & Shuster, A. (1997). Susceptibility loci for distinct components of developmental dyslexia on chromosomes 6 and 15. *American Journal of Human* Genetics, **60**: 27–39.

Hoffman, F.J., Sheldon, K.L., Minskoff, E.M., Surtter, S.W., Steidel, E.F., Baker, D.P., Bailey, M.B. & Echols, L.D. (1987). Needs of learning disabled adults. *Journal of Learning Disabilities,* **20**: 43–53.

Holliday, G.A., Koller, J.R. & Thomas, C.D. (1999). Post-high school outcomes of high IQ adults with learning disabilities. *Journal for the Education of the Gifted,* **22**: 266–81.

Hughes, C.A. & Smith, J.O. (1990). Cognitive and academic performance of college students with LD: A synthesis of the literature. *Learning Disability Quarterly,* **13**: 66–79.

Huntington, D.D. & Bender, W.N. (1993). Adolescents with learning disabilities at risk? Emotional well-being, depression, suicide. *Journal of Learning Disabilities,* **26**: 159–66.

Hynd, G.W. & Semrud-Clikeman, M. (1989). Dyslexia and brain morphology. *Psychological Bulletin,* **106**: 447–82.

Jernigan, T.L., Hesselink, J.R., Sowell, E. & Tallal, P.A. (1991). Cerebral structure on magnetic resonance imaging in language- and learning-impaired children. *Archives of Neurology*, **46**: 539–45.

Kaufman, W.E. & Galaburda, A.M. (1989). Cerebro-cortical microdysgenesis in neurologically normal subjects: a histopathologic study. *Neurology*, **39**: 238–44.

Kavale, K.A. & Forness, S.R. (1996). Learning disability grows up: rehabilitation issues for individuals with learning disabilities. *Journal of Rehabilitation*, **62**: 34–40.

Kazdin, A.E. (1987). Treatment of antisocial behavior in children: current status and future directions. *Psychological Bulletin*, **102**: 187–203.

LaBuda, M. & DeFries, J.C. (1989). Differential prognosis of reading-disabled children as a function of gender, socioeconomic status, IQ and severity: a longitudinal study. *Reading and Writing: An Interdisciplinary Journal*, **1**: 25–36.

LaGreca, A.M. & Stone, W.L. (1990). Children with learning disabilities: the role of achievement in social, personal, and behavioral functioning. In *Learning disabilities: Theoretical and research issues*, ed. H.L. Swanson & B.K. Keogh, pp. 333–52. Hillsdale, NJ: Erlbaum.

Larson, K.A. (1988). A research review and alternative hypothesis explaining the link between learning disability and delinquency. *Journal of Learning Disabilities*, **21**: 357–63, 369.

Levine, P. & Edgar, E. (1995). An analysis by gender of long-term postschool outcomes for youth with and without disabilities. *Exceptional Children*, **61**: 282–300.

Levine, P. & Nourse, S.W. (1998). What follow-up studies say about postschool life for young men and women with learning disabilities: a critical look at the literature. *Journal of Learning Disabilities*, **31**: 212–33.

Lewandowski, L. & Arcangelo, K. (1994). The social adjustment and self-concept of adults with learning disabilities. *Journal of Learning Disabilities*, **27**: 598–605.

Lovett, M.W. (1992). Developmental dyslexia. In *Handbook of Neuropsychology*, vol. 7, *Child Neuropsychology*, ed. S.J. Segalowitz & I. Rapin, pp. 163–85. Amsterdam: Elsevier.

Lovett, M.W. & Steinbach, K.A. (1997). The effectiveness of remedial programs for reading disabled children of different ages: Is there decreased benefit for older children? *Learning Disability Quarterly*, **20**: 189–210.

Lynam, D., Moffitt, T. & Stouthamer-Loeber, M. (1993). Explaining the relation between IQ and delinquency: class, race, test motivation, school failure, or self-control? *Journal of Abnormal Psychology*, **102**: 187–96.

MacDonald, G.W. & Cornwall, A. (1995). The relationship between phonological awareness and reading and spelling achievement eleven years later. *Journal of Learning Disabilities*, **28**: 523–27.

Maughan, B. (1995). Annotation: long-term outcomes of developmental reading problems. *Journal of Child Psychology and Psychiatry*, **36**: 357–71.

Maughan, B. & Hagell, A. (1998). Poor readers in adulthood: psychosocial functioning. In *Annual Progress in Child Psychiatry and Child Development, 1997*, ed. M.E. Hertzig & E.A. Farber, pp. 171–91. Philadelphia: Brunner/Manzel, Inc.

Maughan, B., Hagell, A., Rutter, M. & Yule, W. (1994). Poor readers in secondary school. *Reading and Writing: An Interdisciplinary Journal*, **6**: 125–50.

McCall, R.B., Evahn, C. & Krantzer, L. (1992). *High School Underachievers: What Do They Achieve as Adults?* Newbury Park: Sage Publications.

McGee, R., Williams, S., Share, D.L., Anderson, J. & Silva, P.A. (1986). The relationship between specific reading retardation, general reading backwardness, and behavioral problems in a large sample of Dunedin boys: A longitudinal study from five to eleven years. *Journal of Child Psychology and Psychiatry*, **27**: 597–610.

Mellard, D.F. & Hazel J.S. (1992). Social competencies as a pathway to successful life transitions. *Learning Disability Quarterly*, **15**: 251–66.

Michelsson, K., Byring, R. & Bjoerkgren, P. (1985). Ten-year follow-up of adolescent dyslexics. *Journal of Adolescent Health Care*, **6**: 31–34.

Moffitt, T.E. & Silva, P.A. (1988). IQ and delinquency: a direct test of the differential detection hypothesis. *Journal of Abnormal Psychology*, **97**: 330–33.

Morais, J. (1987). Segmental analysis of speech and its relation to reading ability. *Annals of Dyslexia*, **37**: 126–41.

Naylor, C.E., Felton, R.H. & Wood, F.B. (1990). Adult outcome in developmental dyslexia. In *Perspectives on Dyslexia*, vol. 2, ed. G.Th. Pavlidis, pp. 215–29. London: John Wiley.

Olson, R.K., Wise, B., Ring, J. & Johnson, M. (1997). Computer-based remedial training in phoneme awareness and phonological decoding: effects on the posttraining development of word recognition. *Scientific Studies of Reading*, **1**: 235–54.

Patton, J.R. & Polloway, E.A. (1992). Learning disabilities: the challenges of adulthood. *Journal of Learning Disabilities*, **25**: 410–15, 447.

Peck, M. (1985). Crisis intervention treatment with chronically and acutely suicidal adolescents. In *Youth suicide*, ed. M. Peck, H.L. Farberow & R.E. Litman, pp. 112–22. New York: Springer.

Pennington, B.F., Van Orden, G.C., Smith, S.D., Green, P.A. & Haity, M.M. (1990). Phonological processing skills and deficits in adult dyslexics. *Child Development*, **61**: 1753–78.

Pfeffer, C.R. (1986). *The Suicidal Child*. New York: Guilford.

Pratt, A.C. & Brady, S. (1988). Relation of phonological awareness to reading disability in children and adults. *Journal of Educational Psychology*, **80**: 319–23.

Raskind, M.H., Goldberg, R.J., Higgins, E.L. & Herman, K.L. (1999). Patterns of change and predictors of success in individuals with learning disabilities: results from a twenty-year longitudinal study. *Learning Disabilities Research & Practice*, **14**: 35–49.

Ryan, A.G. & Price, L. (1992). Adults with learning disabilities in the 1990s. *Intervention in School and Clinic*, **28**: 6–20.

Scanlon, D.M. & Vellutino, F.R. (1997). A comparison of the instructional backgrounds and cognitive profiles of poor, average, and good readers who were initially identified as at risk for reading failure. *Scientific Studies of Reading*, **1**: 191–216.

Shaywitz, S.E., Escobar, M.D., Shaywitz, B.A., Fletcher, J.M. & Makuch, R. (1992). Evidence that dyslexia may represent the lower tail of a normal distribution of reading ability. *New England Journal of Medicine*, **326**: 145–50.

Shepherd, M.J. & Uhry, J.K. (1993). Reading disorder. *Child and Adolescent Psychiatric Clinics of North America*, **2**: 193–208.

Siegel, L.S. (1992), An evaluation of the discrepancy definition of dyslexia. *Journal of Learning Disabilities,* **22**: 469–78, 486.

Sitlington, P.L. & Frank, A.R. (1990). Are adolescents with learning disabilities successfully crossing the bridge into adult life? *Learning Disability Quarterly,* **3**: 97–111.

Snowling, M.J., Goulandris, N. & Defty, N. (1996). A longitudinal study of reading development in dyslexic children. *Journal of Educational Psychology,* **88**: 653–69.

Spreen, O. (1989). Learning disability, neurology, and long-term outcome: some implications for the individual and for society. *Journal of Clinical and Experimental Neuropsychology,* **11**: 389–408.

Stanovich, K.E. (1986). Matthew effects in reading: Some consequences of individual differences in the acquisition of literacy. *Reading Research Quarterly,* **21**(4): 360–406.

Stanovich, K.E. (1991). Changing models of reading and reading acquisition. In *Learning to Read: Basic Research and Its Implications,* ed. L. Rieben & C.A. Perfetti, pp. 19–31. Hillsdale: Erlbaum.

Stanovich, K.E. (1994). Annotation: does dyslexia exist? *Journal of Child Psychology and Psychiatry,* **55**: 579–95.

Swanson, H.L., Hoskyn, M. & Lee, C. (1999). *Interventions for Students with Learning Disabilities: A Meta-Analysis of Treatment Outcomes.* New York: The Guilford Press.

Torgesen, J.K., Wagner, R.K. & Rashotte, C.A. (1994). Longitudinal studies of phonological processing and reading. *Journal of Learning Disabilities,* **27**: 276–86.

Torgesen, J.K., Wagner, R.K. & Rashotte, C.A. (1997). Prevention and remediation of severe reading disabilities: Keeping the end in mind. *Scientific Studies of Reading,* **1**(3): 217–34.

Vaughn, S., Hogan, A., Kouzekanam, D. & Shapiro, S. (1990). Peer acceptance, self-perceptions, and social skills of learning disabled students prior to identification. *Journal of Educational Psychology,* **82**: 101–06.

Vogel, S.A. & Adelman, P.B. (1990). Intervention effectiveness at the postsecondary level for the learning disabled. In *Intervention Research in Learning Disabilities,* ed. T. Scruggs & B. Wong, pp. 329–44. New York: Springer-Verlag.

Vogel, S.A. & Adelman, P.B. (1992). The success of college students with learning disabilities: factors related to educational attainment. *Journal of Learning Disabilities,* **25**: 430–41.

Wagner, R.K., Torgesen, J.K. & Rashotte, C.A. (1994). Development of reading-related phonological processing abilities: new evidence of bidirectional causality from a latent variable longitudinal study. *Developmental Psychology,* **30**: 73–87.

White, W. (1992). The post school adjustment of persons with learning disabilities: Current status and future projections. *Journal of Learning Disabilities,* **25**: 448–55.

Wise, B.W., Ring, J., Sessions, L. & Olson, R.K. (1997). Phonological awareness with and without articulation: a preliminary study. *Learning Disability Quarterly,* **20**(3): 211–25.

Young, A.R., Beitchman, J.H., Johnson, C., Douglas, L., Atkinson, L., Escobar, M. & Wilson, B. (in press). Young adult academic outcomes in a longitudinal sample of early identified language impaired and control children. *Journal of Child Psychology and Psychiatry.*

Zimmerman, J., Rich, W.D., Keilutz, I. & Broder, P.K. (1979). *Some Observations on the Link Between Learning Disabilities and Juvenile Delinquency* (LDJ D–003). Williamsburg, VA: National Center for State Courts.

4

Metabolic disorders

Anupam Chakrapani and John Walter

Most inherited inborn errors of metabolism are perceived as paediatric diseases, presenting early in life and resulting in significant morbidity and mortality in infancy and childhood. Several of these conditions profoundly affect the nervous system, and in the past have resulted in considerable neurological debility in later life. However, advances in early diagnosis and therapy have significantly altered the natural course of many conditions, permitting prolonged survival. It is now well established that a number of disorders such as phenylketonuria and homocystinuria can be compatible with near-normal neurological and intellectual functioning. Nevertheless, as growing numbers of individuals advance into adolescence and adulthood, the full profile of the long-term outcome of such early-treated disorders is only now being unravelled. Older individuals with metabolic disorders frequently have abnormalities of intellectual function on formal testing, and unexpected neurological deterioration has occasionally been reported. Additionally, therapeutic interventions such as severely restricted diets and bone marrow transplantation are themselves commonly associated with psychological problems.

The spectrum of metabolic disorders is enormous. In this chapter we will discuss only the common conditions that are likely to be seen in a general neuropsychological setting.

Phenylketonuria

Phenylketonuria (PKU) is one of the commonest inborn errors of metabolism, occurring with a frequency of 1 : 12 000 in populations of European extraction. The enzyme deficiency results in very high blood phenylalanine levels ($> 1200\,\mu mol/l$; normal levels $< 120\,\mu mol/l$), which are toxic to the developing brain. Screening programmes around the world have virtually eliminated severe mental retardation from PKU, but individuals often have subtle neuropsychological problems even when treated early.

Aetiology

PKU results from an autosomal recessive deficiency of phenylalanine hydroxylase, an enzyme that catalyses the conversion of phenylalanine to tyrosine. The disorder is extremely heterogeneous, with over 400 different causative mutations identified in the gene, which is located at chromosome 12q24.1. The enzyme deficiency results in elevated blood phenylalanine levels (hyperphenylalaninaemia), along with the accumulation and urinary excretion of abnormal metabolites such as the phenylketones and phenylamines.

Hyperphenylalaninaemia is believed to interfere with brain development and function by various mechanisms. Disturbances of myelination have been demonstrated in mouse models and it has been postulated that increased myelin turnover is not compensated for by an increased rate of myelin synthesis, a process referred to as 'dysmyelination' (Dyer et al., 1996). High phenylalanine levels have been shown to decrease neurotransmitter receptor density, thereby interfering with cell connectivity. Hyperphenylalaninaemia may also competitively inhibit the transport of the neurotransmitter precursors tryptophan and tyrosine across the blood–brain barrier by the shared large neutral amino acid (LNAA) transport system (Knudsen et al., 1995). Additionally, direct inhibition of the enzymatic synthesis of serotonin, dopamine and GABA by high levels of phenylalanine and its metabolites may also occur (Pietz et al., 1995). The clinical and pathological findings in PKU can be explained by some or all of these hypotheses, but the complete pathophysiology of the condition is not yet fully understood. In addition to these biological factors, the psychological effects of a highly restrictive diet and the emotional stress experienced by the patients and their families also contribute to the overall neuropsychiatric and social morbidity of the condition.

Clinical features

The most common manifestation of untreated PKU is global learning difficulties, with almost all individuals having eventual IQ scores of less than 50 (Paine, 1957; Smith & Wolff, 1974). Other features include irritability, vomiting, an eczematoid rash, fair skin and hair and a peculiar musty body odour. Additionally, about a third of individuals have spastic cerebral palsy, and another third have mild neurological signs such as positive Babinski responses and brisk tendon reflexes. Hyperactivity, behavioural problems, seizures and microcephaly are common in older individuals. With the advent of newborn screening and early treatment since the late 1960s, these manifestations of PKU are rarely seen today. Children with PKU are now treated with a low-phenylalanine diet from the neonatal period, and grow up to have normal IQ levels in adulthood (Scriver et al., 1995). They can expect to have normal social and career ambitions, and usually, no serious long-term neurological sequelae occur.

Treatment

The principle of treatment for PKU is the provision of a diet sufficiently low in phenylalanine so that plasma levels fall within a range that permits normal brain growth and development. This is usually accomplished using a low protein diet. Phenylalanine levels of $< 360 \ \mu mol/l$ are necessary through early childhood to prevent learning difficulties. The pathological effects of hyper-phenylalaninaemia diminish with age, and for older individuals it is recommended that they maintain plasma phenylalanine levels of $< 700 \ \mu mol/l$ (Smith & Lee, 2000). The deficit in protein intake is made up by providing a phenylalanine-free amino acid supplement along with vitamins and minerals. Close monitoring of blood phenylalanine levels is required, especially in infancy and early childhood. Recently, MRI (magnetic resonance imaging) spectroscopic methods that directly measure brain phenylalanine levels have been developed (Avison et al., 1990; Kreis et al., 1995). This technique is being evaluated as a potentially useful means of monitoring long-term dietary therapy (Moats et al., 2000).

Parents of children diagnosed as having PKU on newborn screening usually experience significant distress on being told the diagnosis. They often find it difficult to assimilate facts, and have feelings of anxiety and disbelief. The understanding and administration of the diet is quite complex. Considerable professional and family support is therefore necessary not only in the initial stages, but even later as strict dietary control is essential to prevent intellectual disability. Parent and child education forms a very important part of management, and helps improve long-term dietary adherence. Compliance with treatment is often a problem in teenagers (Schuett, Brown & Michals, 1985; Gleason et al., 1992; Schulz & Bremer, 1995; Weglage et al., 1996). A number of different factors may contribute to the loss of dietary control in adolescence, including time constraints, social pressures, financial limitations and growing independence from the family. The degree of metabolic control in individuals of this age group has been found to correlate positively with two psychosocial factors: the level of social support and a positive attitude to dietary treatment (Levy & Waisbren, 1994). Strategies that may help improve dietary adherence include rigorous diet and disease-specific education of children and parents (Weglage et al., 1992); practical dietary training closely supervised by dietitians (Weglage et al., 1992); early acceptance of the responsibility of dietary treatment and monitoring by the individuals themselves (Wendel & Langenbeck, 1996); and peer-support programmes (Levy & Waisbren 1994).

A multidisciplinary approach involving close liaison between dietitians, health visitors, clinicians, nurse specialists and biochemists is necessary to maintain an effective PKU treatment programme. Currently, lifelong dietary treatment is recommended (Medical Research Council Working Party, 1993).

Outcome in childhood

The majority of children and adolescents with PKU are of normal intelligence and have no obvious physical disability. The introduction of newborn screening with early diagnosis and treatment has resulted in a marked reduction in intellectual disabilities from over 80% to around 4–8%. This is, however higher than the 2% prevalence of mental retardation in the general population. Studies from around the world have consistently revealed that children and adolescents with PKU have mean IQ levels about 4–8 points lower than their unaffected siblings and the general population. The quality of dietary treatment in the pre-school years (including the age at initiation of diet, the average phenylalanine levels and the duration of low phenylalanine levels) is a major determinant of subsequent IQ levels. Termination of dietary treatment after the age of 12 years does not appear to affect final IQ levels (Pietz et al., 1998).

It has emerged in the last 20 years that deficits in subtle aspects of intellectual function are common in early-treated patients who have terminated dietary treatment (Dobson et al., 1976; Koff, Boyle & Pueschel, 1977; Brunner, Jordan & Berry, 1983). Several studies since the early 1980s have focused on neuro-psychological function in early-treated children and adolescents. Most have reported deficits in various aspects of information processing (Brunner et al., 1983; Pennington et al., 1985; Seashore et al., 1985; Brunner & Berry, 1987; Brunner, Burch & Berry, 1987; Welsh et al., 1990; Lou et al., 1992). Neuro-psychological function in PKU has been assessed using either problem solving tasks or tests of attention and reaction times (Waisbren et al., 1994). Early studies of problem-solving abilities reported that early-treated PKU patients who were off dietary treatment showed deficits when required to integrate information, whether the tasks required visual, motor or mental utilization of information (Brunner et al., 1983; Pennington et al., 1985; Seashore et al., 1985). More recent studies have found abnormalities on tests of higher level problem solving, or 'executive function', which is believed to reflect prefrontal lobe dysfunction (Welsh et al., 1990; Diamond et al., 1997; Arnold et al., 1998). Deficits are also reported in the attention area of information processing (Lou et al., 1992; Schmidt et al., 1994). Although on simple reaction time tests (tests of visual motor speed) individuals with PKU do not show a difference from normal controls, as the complexity of the task increases they do make more errors and slow down significantly. Areas that do not appear to be adversely affected include speech, language, pure motor tasks, memory and basic logic (Waisbren et al., 1994). The neuropsychological abnormalities have been shown to significantly improve with reinstitution of dietary treatment (Krause et al., 1985; Clarke et al., 1987). It has also been found that performance correlates well with blood phenylalanine levels, both concurrent and within the preceding two years (Brunner et al., 1983; Krause et al., 1985; Clarke et al., 1987; Sonneville et al., 1990; Pietz et al., 1993).

Children and adolescents with PKU also appear to be at high risk of developing behavioural problems. Smith et al. (1988) reported the results of behavioural assessment on a large cohort of 8-year-old children with early-treated PKU, using the Rutter behaviour questionnaire (B2 scale) (Rutter, Graham & Yule, 1970). Children on a strict phenylalanine-controlled diet were at least 1.5 times more likely than age and sex-matched controls to show deviant behaviour; the risk was significantly higher in those with a poorly controlled diet. Children with PKU more often had mannerisms (twitching, thumb sucking), hyperactivity, and signs of anxiety ('worried', 'fearful', 'miserable'). They were also less responsive and more solitary than controls. On the other hand, antisocial behaviour (school refusal, disobedience, destructiveness, lying, truancy, aggressiveness) was not more common. Another study on 34 adolescents with PKU focused on psychosocial findings compared with age- and sex-matched controls using standardized questionnaires (Weglage et al., 1992). Individuals with PKU were significantly less motivated, had less desire for autonomy, less frustration tolerance and a more negative self-image than the controls. They displayed less masculinity in their attitudes and were less carefree, less orientated towards success, less extroverted and had more physical complaints. Seventy-seven per cent found adherence to the diet extremely difficult and 94% wished to stop the diet immediately; 80% adhered to the diet more strictly before their phenylalanine levels were checked; and 59% were unable to manage the diet without the help of their mothers, of whom 68% rated themselves as overprotective. It was concluded that the strictness of the dietary restrictions influenced the personality characteristics of affected individuals, and that their restrictive upbringing resulted in feelings of insufficiency, social incompetence and a negative self-image.

The psychosocial outcome of PKU therefore appears to depend on two aetiological factors: the biological effects of elevated phenylalanine on the brain cells; and the psychological effects of a highly restricted diet. The inevitable concomitants of chronic disease, such as regular blood tests and frequent hospital visits may also play a role. Counselling and psychological support are essential from the time of diagnosis.

Outcome in adulthood

Studies on the cognitive outcome in adults with PKU reveal findings very similar to those in children and adolescents. Though mean IQ levels have been consistently 4–8 points below those of controls, the majority of early-treated adults with PKU are of normal intelligence. Adult IQ levels are largely determined by the quality of dietary control during childhood but appear to be independent of biochemical control beyond the age of 12 years (Pietz et al., 1998). However, as in the case of children and adolescents, detailed neuropsychological testing has revealed reversible subtle cognitive deficits in sustained attention, reaction times and planning skills in adults who have elevated phenylalanine levels (Lou et al., 1985; Pietz et al., 1993; Schmidt et al., 1994).

Adults with PKU also appear to be at increased risk of psychiatric morbidity. In a study utilizing a standardized interview on 35 adults with early treated PKU, Pietz et al. (1997) reported 'clearly observable' psychiatric symptoms in 25% of patients, whilst the prevalence in controls was 16%. Though the difference was not statistically significant, further analysis revealed that the individuals with PKU had exclusively internalizing symptoms (25.7% of PKU group vs. 8.3% of controls). The mean score for functional and emotional disturbances (such as depressed mood, phobias, general anxiety and hypochondriac worries) was significantly elevated in the group with PKU, but the antisocial symptoms were significantly reduced (0% vs. 7.8%). There was no correlation between these symptoms and concurrent or past biochemical control. Ris et al. (1997) found that 20% of adult PKU patients demonstrated significant psychiatric morbidity on a self-report inventory of psychiatric symptoms. These adults were particularly troubled by unwanted impulsive thoughts, as well as feelings of alienation and discomfort in interpersonal relationships.

Minor neurological abnormalities such as intention tremor and brisk tendon reflexes are commonly seen in adults who have terminated dietary treatment. Isolated cases of neurological deterioration with prominent pyramidal tract features have also been reported (Villasana et al., 1989; Thompson et al., 1990). Additionally, MRI studies in adults with PKU on unrestricted diets have almost universally found symmetrical patchy areas of enhanced signal intensity in the posterior periventricular white matter which extend to the frontal and subcortical white matter in the more severely affected cases (Bick et al., 1991, 1993;

Leuzzi et al., 1993; Thompson et al., 1993; Pietz et al., 1996). These changes correlate strongly with concurrent blood phenylalanine levels but not with early dietary control in childhood (Cleary et al., 1994). No relationship has been found between MRI changes and performance (Lou et al., 1992). These radiological changes and many of the abnormalities of executive function are reversible with re-institution of dietary treatment and reduction of phenylalanine levels to < 900 µmol/l (Cleary et al., 1995). The long-term implications of these findings are unknown, as the oldest early-treated adults with PKU are, at present, only in their fourth decade of life. The Medical Research Council, therefore, currently recommends dietary treatment of PKU for life (Medical Research Council Working Party, 1993).

Galactosaemia

Classical galactosaemia, the major disorder of galactose metabolism, was first described in detail by Mason & Turner in 1935 (Segal & Berry, 1995). Reversal of the acute toxicity of the syndrome in newborns and infants by elimination of galactose from the diet was recognized early, and led to the belief that it was a benign disorder once stringent dietary treatment was instituted. A number of clinical observations in the 1970s, however, suggested that even well-treated patients went on to develop learning disabilities and speech impairment, and ovarian failure was frequently noted to occur in affected females. Since then, further evidence of late-onset neurological problems has emerged, and it is now well established that dietary treatment has no effect on the long-term neuro-degenerative and ovarian pathology in classical galactosaemia.

Aetiology

Classical galactosaemia occurs due to an autosomal recessive deficiency of the enzyme galactose-1-phosphate uridyl transferase (GALT). GALT catalyses the second step in galactose–glucose interconversion, the normal metabolic pathway for galactose utilization (Figure 4.1). The gene is situated on chromosome 9. Over 150 different mutations have been described worldwide, and some genotype–phenotype correlation has been found. In the United Kingdom (UK), one common mutation (Q188R) accounts for over 80% of mutant alleles (Tyfield et al., 1999; Shield et al., 2000). Homozygosity for the Q188R mutation results in substantial or complete loss of GALT activity and is associated with a relatively poor cognitive outcome. Several variants of transferase deficiency, such as the Duarte variant, the Los Angeles variant, and the 'Negro' variant, described in the past, are now known to represent milder mutations on the

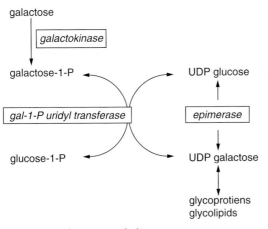

Figure 4.1. Galactose metabolism.

transferase gene (Segal & Cautrecasas, 1968; Segal & Berry, 1995; Berry et al., 1997). These are all associated with some residual enzyme activity and a relatively good long-term outcome.

Direct biochemical consequences of GALT deficiency include accumulation of galactose-1-phosphate, which in turn is metabolized to galactitol and galactonate, both of which accumulate in abnormal quantities in tissues. Galactitol is an osmotically active compound that causes cataracts by increasing the water content of the lens (Segal & Berry, 1995). Galactonate is believed to play a role in the acute hepatic and renal toxicity. The elimination of galactose from the diet to reduce levels of these compounds forms the basis of treatment of the acutely presenting neonate.

The pathogenesis of long-term neurological damage and of ovarian failure in well-treated patients is not clearly understood. Three principal theories have been proposed (Segal, 1995a). The first is that of chronic intoxication with galactose, the sugar being produced endogenously from either UDP galactose formed from UDP glucose via the epimerase reaction (Figure 4.1), or from galactoprotein and galactolipid turnover. The second theory is that of depletion of key metabolites such as UDP galactose, which has an important role in galactosylation of complex galactoproteins and galactolipids. A third possibility is in utero neurological damage due to abnormal prenatal galactose metabolism, supported by the demonstration of abnormalities such as low brain weight, low brain DNA, abnormal brain inositol metabolism and decreased number of oocytes in the offspring of pregnant rats that have been fed a high galactose diet (Segal, 1995b).

Clinical features

Galactosaemia occurs in about 1 in 45 000 newborns in the UK (Walter, Collins & Leonard, 1999). Estimates of prevalence in other populations range from 1:18 000 to 1:180 000 (Segal & Berry, 1995). It commonly manifests as a life-threatening illness in the neonatal period, with poor feeding, failure to thrive, vomiting, jaundice, cataracts, encephalopathy, liver failure, septicaemia particularly due to *Escherichia coli*, and renal tubular dysfunction. Improvement occurs on stopping feeds and commencing intravenous fluids (Badawi et al., 1996). After diagnosis, institution of a galactose-free diet eliminates the risk of acute toxicity, and normal early growth and development can be achieved.

Treatment

A minimal-lactose diet is essential throughout life. Follow-up by a specialist centre for clinical, biochemical and dietary supervision is necessary (Walter et al., 1999). Soya-based infant formulae provide adequate calcium in infancy, but supplementation is necessary later. Many medications, particularly tablets, contain lactose and must be checked before prescribing. Small amounts of galactose, however, are insignificant compared with endogenous production and may be allowed for short periods (Walter et al., 1999). Growth and puberty in girls require close monitoring, preferably by an endocrinologist. Most females require hormone replacement therapy at some stage.

Outcome in childhood

Lactose restriction in classical galactosaemia prevents cataracts, liver failure and death from *E. coli* sepsis, though mild growth retardation is common. However, data collated over the last 30 years has demonstrated that dietary treatment does not affect the development of neuropsychological problems and ovarian failure in later life (Segal, 1995). The first manifestation of neurological dysfunction is usually a delay in speech acquisition (Nelson et al., 1991). Severe learning difficulties are rare in galactosaemia but intellectual deficits are common. There is evidence that although DQ or IQ levels are normal in infancy, there is a progressive decline in performance through childhood and adolescence. Amongst 134 cases with galactosaemia, Schweitzer et al. (1993) found DQ or IQ levels of < 85 in 12% of those below the age of 6 years and in 83% of those aged over 12 years. In another survey, Waggoner, Buist & Donnell (1990) reported the results of IQ tests on 350 individuals with galactosaemia performed at different ages. Children tested at 3–5 years of age ($n = 85$) had a mean IQ of 92 (range 50–138), those tested at 6–9 years of age

($n = 88$) had a mean IQ of 87 (range 39–152), whereas at 10–16 years ($n = 67$) the mean IQ was 80 (range 26–115). Children who had IQ tests at both 3–5 years and 6–9 years ($n = 42$) showed a mean drop of 6.2 IQ points, and those tested at both 6–9 years and 10–16 years ($n = 46$) had a mean decrease of 4.4 points. Speech abnormalities with a characteristic verbal dyspraxia occurred in about 60% of children over the age of 3 years in both surveys. Neither survey found any significant relationship between IQ and the age at which treatment was initiated. In addition children with galactosaemia often have specific learning difficulties involving visual–spatial relationships and mathematics (Segal & Berry, 1995).

Lee (1972) studied the psychological aspects of galactosaemia in 60 children aged between 2 and 17 years, and found emotional disturbances in 50% using the Bristol Social Adjustment Guide (Stott, 1965). On this scale, 23% scored as 'maladjusted' and 27% as 'unsettled', with high scores on scales of 'unforthcomingness', 'depression' and 'hostility to adults'. Another study (Fishler et al., 1966) that used projective tests reported significant personality disturbances in a group of 34 children with galactosaemia aged from 2 months to 17 years. The older children (aged 12–17 years) were generally tense, over-anxious or over-sensitive with poor self-image. They were said to have passive, over-dependent personalities and difficulty in accepting the limits of authority, both in and outside the home. Most of those aged 5–9 years had signs of emotional disturbances, such as bed-wetting, nail-biting and repetitive head-scratching. They were described as shy, restrained and withdrawn in interpersonal contacts, with difficulty in handling hostility, which they were said to repress by trying to please those who had evoked such feelings in the first place. The males had poor masculine identification and displayed feminine interests. Early recognition of the cognitive and psychological problems in children with galactosaemia is essential to enable appropriate interventions such as speech therapy, special educational programmes and counselling.

Outcome in adulthood

The speech and learning difficulties and behavioural problems may persist into adulthood to varying degrees. A further drop in IQ during adulthood may be expected based on the studies in children and adolescents (Waggoner et al., 1990; Schweitzer et al., 1993). Abnormal neurological signs, such as intention tremor and ataxia, are often found in adults, and progressive ataxia and extrapyramidal signs have also been reported (Waggoner et al., 1990). Nelson et al. (1992) have reported brain MRI scan abnormalities in the form of abnormal white matter signal, cerebral atrophy, cerebellar atrophy or scattered small cerebral white matter lesions in a majority of galactosaemic patients. The long-term neurological effects of galactosaemia, therefore appear to be due to a progressive neurodegenerative syndrome that does not respond to dietary treatment. Additionally, almost all women with galactosaemia develop premature ovarian failure irrespective of treatment. Hypergonadotrophic hypogonadism can be found even in early childhood, and most females go on to develop primary or secondary amenorrhea. Diminished or absent ovarian tissue can be demonstrated on ultrasonography, and older women often have streak ovaries. Premature menopause usually occurs by the third decade. Despite the common occurrence of ovarian failure, occasional successful pregnancies have been observed without any maternal or fetal complications. Male gonads are not affected.

Homocystinuria

The amino acid homocysteine is formed during the metabolic conversion of the essential sulphur-containing amino acid methionine to the non-essential amino acid cysteine (Figure 4.2). Depending on metabolic demands, homocysteine is normally either converted back to methionine or catabolized to cysteine. Defects on either of these pathways can result in elevated blood homocysteine levels (hyperhomocystinaemia) and its excretion in the urine (homocystinuria) (Finkelstein, 1998). The commonest cause of homocystinuria is the genetic deficiency of the enzyme cystathionine β-synthase (CBS), also referred to as 'classical homocystinuria'. Homocystinuria can also be caused by other rarer enzyme deficiencies that result in defective metabolism of the cofactors involved in these pathways, folic acid and cobalamin (Table 4.1).

Aetiology

CBS deficiency is autosomal recessively inherited, and the gene has been localized to chromosome 21q22.3. Over 90 different mutations are known (Kraus et al., 1999). Pyridoxine (vitamin B6) is a cofactor for the enzyme. The clinical and biochemical variations, such as pyridoxine responsiveness, are genetically determined and related to specific mutations. The various defects of folate and cobalamin metabolism are also probably autosomal recessive traits, though the gene for only one of them, methylenetetrahydrofolate reductase deficiency, has so far been identified.

The neurological and psychiatric manifestations of homocystinuria are thought to arise from two principal mechanisms. The oxidative by-products of homocysteine, such as homocysteic acid and homocysteine sulphinic acid may cause excitotoxic damage to neurons via stimulation of the NMDA receptors

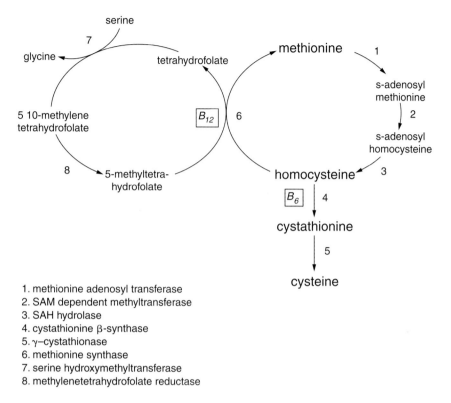

1. methionine adenosyl transferase
2. SAM dependent methyltransferase
3. SAH hydrolase
4. cystathionine β-synthase
5. γ–cystathionase
6. methionine synthase
7. serine hydroxymethyltransferase
8. methylenetetrahydrofolate reductase

Figure 4.2. Homocysteine metabolism.

(Santosh-Kumar et al., 1994). An additional mechanism may be related to impaired methylation. S-Adenosylmethionine (Figure 4.2) is a key metabolite in the transfer of single-carbon metabolites (i.e. methylation) in the synthesis of various vital substances, including some neurotransmitters. In homocystinuria, alterations in the S-adenosylmethionine: S-adenosylhomocysteine ratio result in impairment of this pathway, with consequent effects on the synthesis of dopamine, noradrenalin and serotonin (Bottiglieri et al., 1994, Li & Stewart, 1999). The abnormal S-adenosylmethionine: S-adenosylhomocysteine ratio also possibly affects β-adrenergic, muscarinic and GABAergic receptors in the brain (Li & Stewart, 1999). Hyperhomocysteinaemia is directly responsible for the pathogenesis of most of the other clinical abnormalities (Mudd, Levy & Skovby, 1995).

Clinical features

CBS deficiency occurs in all ethnic groups with varying frequency, from about 1 : 50 000 in Ireland to fewer than 1 : 800 000 in Japan. The overall incidence is estimated to be 1 : 344 000 live births (Mudd et al., 1995).

Table 4.1. Homocystinuria due to defects of folate and vitamin B12 metabolism

Disorder	Metabolic defect	Clinical features	Biochemical findings	Treatment
Methylene tetrahydrofolate reductase (MHTFR) deficiency	Defective recycling of folate	Developmental delay, motor and gait abnormalities, seizures, psychiatric problems	Hyperhomocysteinaemia, homocystinuria, low blood methionine and folate	Folates, betaine, methionine
Cobalamin E and G defects	Defective methylcobalamin synthesis	Developmental delay, seizures, cerebral atrophy, megaloblastic anaemia	Hyperhomocysteinaemia, homocystinuria, low blood methionine, normal folate	Hydroxycobalamin, folinic acid, betaine
Cobalamin C, D and F defects	Defective adenosylcobalamin and methylcobalamin synthesis	Failure to thrive, developmental delay, seizures, retinopathy, megaloblastic anaemia	Hyperhomocysteinaemia, homocystinuria, methylmalonic aciduria	Hydroxycobalamin, folinic acid, betaine

The most common clinical features of untreated classical homocystinuria include myopia due to lens dislocation, osteoporosis, skeletal deformities, a marfanoid appearance (tall stature with long and thin hands and feet), learning difficulties, psychiatric disturbances and vascular complications. Cerebrovascular disease, coronary artery disease and deep vein thrombosis are also commonly seen and have a significant bearing on the long-term outcome (Mudd et al., 1995). CBS deficiency shows considerable phenotypic heterogeneity and the age of presentation can vary from early childhood to adulthood, depending on the genotype and a number of environmental factors. Many cases are now diagnosed on newborn screening. About half of the affected individuals show a response to treatment with pyridoxine, and this group tends to have relatively milder clinical manifestations (Mudd et al., 1995). Psychiatric manifestations are commmon in untreated adults with homocystinuria (see below). Adults and children with defects of folate or cobalamin metabolism tend to have predominantly neurological manifestations. Most of these patients present in infancy with developmental delay, hypotonia, seizures, microcephaly or progressive encephalopathy; those presenting later in childhood and adulthood often have prominent psychiatric manifestations. Megaloblastic anaemia and methylmalonic aciduria may be present in those with defects of cobalamin metabolism.

Treatment

Pyridoxine and folic acid treatment of pyridoxine-responsive patients with CBS deficiency usually prevents further deterioration (Mudd et al., 1985). Daily pyridoxine requirements vary considerably, from as little as 10 mg to over 500 mg. Folate depletion may limit the response to pyridoxine, and folate supplementation is therefore necessary. Pyridoxine-unresponsive patients require a low-methionine diet. This is achieved by restricting dietary protein and supplying other essential amino acids as a synthetic methionine-free supplement. Dietary adherence is often a problem in adolescence and young adulthood (Walter et al., 1998). Close monitoring of plasma homocysteine levels is essential in order to prevent long-term complications. Betaine, a methyl donor, is a useful adjunctive treatment in doses of 150–250 mg/kg/day, especially if dietary compliance is unsatisfactory. Anticoagulant therapy may be required for patients who develop vascular complications. Homocystinuria due to defects of folate and cobalamin metabolism is treated with a combination of folic acid and vitamin B12.

Outcome in childhood

The natural history of untreated homocystinuria was defined in a large international survey published in 1985 (Mudd et al., 1985). The major determinant of outcome appeared to be responsiveness to pyridoxine, with responders having significantly lower rates of lens dislocation (55% of pyridoxine responsive cases at 10 years of age versus 82% of non-responders), thromboembolic events (12% incidence in pyridoxine-responders at age 15 years versus 23% in non-responders), spinal osteoporosis (36% in responders, 64% in non-responders at age 15 years) and mortality by age 30 years (4% in responders, 23% in non-responders). Important advances have since been made in early diagnosis by newborn screening and in homocysteine-lowering treatment, and more recent reports have shown a significantly lower morbidity and mortality in early-treated cases with good compliance.

In a retrospective study from Northern Ireland (Yap & Naughten, 1998), where newborn screening for homocystinuria is routinely performed, 25 cases were diagnosed over a 25-year period of which only one case was pyridoxine-responsive. All patients who were diagnosed and treated early and who had good compliance were of normal intelligence at ages ranging from 2.5 to 23.4 years. No thromboembolic events were recorded in 365.7 patient-years of treatment, which in the majority of cases was commenced within 6 weeks of birth. Other complications such as lens dislocation, learning disabilities and osteoporosis occurred only in the seven cases who were either poorly compliant or who were missed on screening. Studies from Australia (Wilcken & Wilcken, 1997) and the Netherlands (Kluijtmans et al., 1999) have reported similarly low rates of thromboembolism and other complications amongst patients on effective homocysteine-lowering treatment. Psychosocial difficulties relating to dietary restriction may arise in children and adolescents who do not respond to pyridoxine therapy, as they need a lifelong methionine-restricted diet. Though most reports of psychiatric disturbances in homocystinuria relate to adults, a few cases of children with psychiatric symptoms have also been recorded (Turner, 1967; Grobe, 1980).

Outcome in adulthood

The adult outcome of homocystinuria largely depends on the time of initiation of treatment and the responsiveness to pyridoxine. The adult IQ levels in the survey by Mudd et al. (1985) varied widely, ranging from 10 to 138, though median IQ levels were found to be lower in the non-responsive group than the responders (64 and 78, respectively). Individuals who are late-diagnosed are at risk of developing any of the complications, and cerebrovascular events may result in a wide range of neurological findings. Psychiatric disturbances are particularly common in untreated cases. Omenn (1978) estimated that about 50% of adults with untreated homocystinuria suffered from psychiatric disorders. Abbott et al. (1987) reported a similar incidence of 51%, with four diagnostic categories predominating: episodic depression (10%); chronic disorders of behaviour (17%); chronic obsessive–compulsive disorders (5%); and chronic personality disorders (19%). Though there are only a few reports of homocystinuric patients diagnosed as having schizophrenia, psychotic symptoms have been frequently described. These have included violent behaviour, autism, thought disorder, loss of contact with surroundings, hallucinations, delusions, catatonic posturing and sociopathic behaviour (Schimke et al., 1965; Rahman, 1971; Freeman, Finkelstein & Hudd, 1975). These symptoms respond favourably to appropriate homocysteine-lowering treatment. Homocystinuria should therefore be considered in the differential diagnosis of unexplained neuropsychiatric disorders, particularly in patients with a family history of homocystinuria, learning difficulties, a past history of thromboembolic episodes, vascular diseases, or clinical and laboratory features of vitamin B12 or folate deficiency.

X-linked adrenoleukodystrophy

The term adrenoleukodystrophy (ALD) describes a group of disorders that cause adrenal dysfunction and associated white matter degeneration in the nervous system. ALD may result from two distinct groups of genetic disorders that affect the peroxisomes, which are small intracellular structures with a variety of biochemical functions, including the oxidation of very long chain fatty acids (VLCFA). One, neonatal ALD, is a rare autosomal recessive disorder affecting the assembly of peroxisomes, with clinical and biochemical manifestations resembling Zellweger syndrome. This disorder will not be discussed further. The genetic abnormality in the other form is X-linked (X-linked ALD, XALD), associated with disordered VLCFA oxidation in intact peroxisomes. Though XALD was first described nearly 80 years ago, the gene has only recently been identified and cloned. The pathogenesis and phenotypic variability of the condition remain poorly understood and treatment options are limited. Genetic counselling of family members is essential, and prenatal diagnosis is possible and must be offered.

Aetiology

The XALD gene (ALDP) has been localized to Xq28. It encodes a transport protein located on the peroxisomal membrane (Mosser et al., 1993). Biochemically, there is a defect in the activity of VLCFA coenzyme A synthase (VLCAS), an enzyme that catalyses the attachment of coenzyme A to VLCFA, the initial step in the degradation of VLCFA (Hashmi, Stanley & Singh, 1986). The exact function of the ALD protein remains to be ascertained, but it is believed to have a role in transporting across the peroxisomal membrane either the VLCAS enzyme itself or a cofactor required for its activity (Mosser et al., 1993; Smith et al., 1999).

The primary defect in ALD is the inability to degrade VLCFA within peroxisomes, with resultant accumulation of these compounds in all body fluids and tissues. CT (computed tomography) or MRI scan studies of the brain in cerebral forms of ALD show symmetric high signals in the parietal and occipital periventricular white matter (Melhem et al., 1999). Histologically, demyelination and sclerotic lesions are seen in affected areas along with significant inflammation (Schaumburg et al., 1975). This inflammatory reaction is characteristic of ALD and may play a role in pathogenesis; the rapidity of progression of the cerebral forms relates to the degree of inflammation (Moser, Smith & Moser, 1995). VLCFA excess is believed to directly or indirectly induce this inflammatory response (van Geel et al., 1997).

Over 200 mutations on the ALD gene are known to cause XALD (Smith et al., 1999). There is, however, no genotype–phenotype correlation, and a given mutation may result in many different clinical phenotypes, as evidenced by the remarkable variability of the condition within families. The reason for this is not entirely clear. As the severity of the brain inflammatory lesions seems to correlate with outcome, it has been proposed that an as yet unidentified modifier gene that regulates the inflammatory response may have a significant bearing on the phenotypic expression of ALD mutations (Maestri & Beaty, 1992).

Clinical features

XALD has been reported to occur in all races and geographic locations. Estimates of minimum incidence have varied from 0.5 to 1.6 per 100 000 births in different populations (Moser et al., 1995).

The clinical spectrum of XALD is very broad, ranging from a severe neurodegenerative disorder of childhood to an asymptomatic adult. Six phenotypes have been described (Bezman & Moser, 1998) based on the site of neurological involvement, the age at onset and the rate of progression of the disorder (Table 4.2; Moser et al, 1991b; van Geel et al., 1997; Bezman & Moser, 1998).

In the most common form, childhood cerebral ALD (CCALD), behavioural

Table 4.2. Adrenoleukodystrophy (ALD) – spectrum of clinical phenotypes

	CCALD	Adolescent CALD	ACALD	AMN	Addison only	Asymptomatic
Relative frequency (%)	30–50	4–7	1–5	25–40	12–17	5–13
Age at onset of neurological symptoms (years)	< 10	10–21	> 21	20–40	–	–
Main CNS involvement	Cerebral	Cerebral	Cerebral	Spinal cord	None	None
Rate of neurological progression	Rapid	Rapid	Rapid	Slow	–	–
Behavioural disturbances	Common	Common	Common	Infrequent	–	–
Cognitive dysfunction	Common	Common	Common	Common	–	–
Pyramidal involvement	Late	Late	Common	Present by definition	–	–
Endocrine dysfunction	AD in most	AD in most	AD in most	AD in most	Present by definition	Subnormal response to ACTH 60%

CCALD, childhood cerebral ALD; ACALD, adult cerebral ALD; AMN, adrenomyeloneuropathy; AD, arenal insufficiency; CNS, central nervous system; ACTH, adrenocorticotrophin.

disturbances, school difficulties, impaired hearing, visual problems or inco-ordination are common manifestations in boys aged 4–8 years. Attention deficit disorder is diagnosed initially in many patients. Rapid neurological deterioration occurs, with seizures, dementia and spasticity becoming apparent within months. Most patients die 2–5 years after the onset of neurological symptoms.

The adolescent and adult forms of cerebral ALD (CALD) are rare. The clinical features and progression resemble CCALD, but onset is much later. Adult CALD may be mistaken for a psychiatric disorder such as schizophrenia with dementia. Adrenomyeloneuropathy (AMN) is comparatively common, usually presenting in the third or fourth decade, with symptoms and signs of spinal cord involvement. Characteristic features are stiffness, clumsiness and weakness of the legs, voiding dysfunction, impotence, symptoms of adrenal insufficiency and paraperesis. About 10% of adults with ALD have isolated adrenocortical dysfunction (Moser, 1995). It is estimated that in developed countries, up to 40% of males with Addison's disease may have ALD (Moser et al., 1991a). Most of these go on to develop neurological symptoms after several years, usually manifesting the AMN phenotype. Some individuals have no neurological or endocrine manifestations of ALD, but are diagnosed biochemi-cally and/or genetically as having ALD during family screening. These individ-uals run a high risk of neurological disease later in life, with the phenotype determined by age and the site of principal nervous system pathology.

Unusual forms of ALD have been described, such as isolated gonadal insufficiency (Powers & Schaumburg, 1980), predominant cerebellar involve-ment (Marsden, Obeso & Lang, 1982) and symptoms resembling olivo-ponto-cerebellar degeneration (Ohno et al., 1983).

A majority of female heterozygotes develop manifestations because of the process of random X-chromosome inactivation (Moser et al., 1995). Neurologi-cal abnormalities resemble AMN, but generally occur later, are milder and progress is slower. Cerebral involvement and adrenal dysfunction are rare.

There is a striking intrafamilial variation in phenotypic manifestations (Moser et al., 1995), with the different forms of ALD occurring even within the same nuclear family (Martin et al., 1980, Erlington et al., 1989).

Treatment

Corticosteroid replacement treatment is essential for adrenal insufficiency, but it does not change the neurological course. Currently, the most effective treatment for the cerebral forms of ALD is bone marrow transplantation (BMT). If transplantation is performed early, there is a high probability of prolonged remission of the disease process, as opposed to death within a few years without transplant (Krivit et al., 1995). BMT is not successful if performed later in the neurological course, and in many such cases has led to rapid deterioration and death. As it is impossible to predict the disease course in asymptomatic cases, BMT is usually performed as soon as the first signs of neurological involvement appear. Frequent neurological surveillance with clinical examination and MRI scanning is therefore necessary in asymptomatic individuals. A five-year follow-up of 12 patients with early CCALD (defined as IQ < 80) treated with BMT has revealed not only stabilization of neurological disease and MRI changes, but also continued recovery of verbal and perform-ance abilities (Krivit et al., 1999). Over 120 children worldwide have undergone BMT for cerebral ALD with about 60% five-year survival. It has been suggested that normalization of plasma VLCFA levels using Lorenzo's oil (see below) prior to transplantation may reduce the complications and improve survival (Krivit et al., 1999).

The discovery of elevated VLCFA levels in the blood, brain and other body tissues in ALD has led to the development of several forms of dietary therapy. Treatment with Lorenzo's oil, a 4 : 1 mixture of glyceryl trioleate and glyceryl trierucate, is very effective in lowering plasma VLCFA levels, and most patients started on this product have normalization of plasma VLCFA levels within a month (Moser et al., 1995). The neurological progression of CCALD and AMN, however, is not altered by this treatment (Auborg et al., 1993; Rizzo, 1993; Asano et al., 1994; Korenke et al., 1995). There is no evidence to support the use of dietary therapy in asymptomatic males to delay or prevent the onset of neurological disease. Newer approaches to treatment that are being evaluated in the treatment of XALD include lovastatin (Singh et al., 1998), 4-phenyl-butyrate (Kemp et al., 1998), beta-interferon (Korenke et al., 1996), and gene therapy (Doeflinger et al., 1998).

Outcome in childhood

The problems faced by families of individuals with ALD are typical of meta-bolic disorders in which there is a period of normal development followed by rapid deterioration and death within a few years. The presenting features of ALD often comprise alterations of behaviour, affect, attention and sleeping patterns. Psychiatric disorders may be suspected, and children placed in special schools for learning and emotional difficulties. Because of these initial problems and subsequent impairment of cognitive abilities, co-ordination of school services is essential with the aim of improving the quality of life and providing as much normalization as is possible. Once symptomatic, children with

CCALD tend to deteriorate rapidly with loss of cognitive skills and neurological disability, and death usually occurs within a few years. When it is no longer appropriate for the child to attend school, the parents require considerable support with handling, positioning, feeding and transporting the child. With further deterioration, children may lose auditory and visual perception, and support has to be provided to help them interpret environmental stimuli. Progressive bulbar dysfunction often necessitates nasogastric or gastrostomy feeding and regular oropharyngeal suctioning in the later stages.

From the psychosocial point of view, parents and families often experience grief, anger and frustration about the lack of effective treatment. They have to deal with a child with a rapidly deteriorating condition, and the terminal stages may be particularly difficult. Factors that may add to the psychological stress include the maternal inheritance of ALD and the fact that there may be other affected members in the family. Should there be other affected but asymptomatic individuals in the family, a programme for monitoring disease progression through regular neuroimaging and neuropsychometric testing is required. BMT is the treatment of choice in the early stages, and if feasible, places further stress on the family. The psychosocial aspects of BMT are discussed in the section on lysosomal disorders.

Parent and family organizations are particularly useful in providing an opportunity for families to exchange information regarding personal experiences, and in helping them with coping strategies.

A co-ordinated multidisciplinary approach involving health professionals, social workers and support organizations is therefore essential in the effective management of a patient with ALD.

Outcome in adulthood

Patients with the childhood onset forms of ALD do not survive to adulthood. However, as mentioned previously, the disorder is very heterogenous and may present much later in life, with primary involvement of the brain, the spinal cord or the adrenals. The common adult form of ALD is adrenomyeloneuropathy, which presents with spinal symptoms, with slow progression leading to death in 10–15 years. The adult cerebral forms are rare, but these often present with a variety of psychiatric symptoms such as schizophrenia and dementia, with rapid progression and death as in CCALD.

Lysosomal storage disorders

The lysosomes are specialized intracellular structures containing about 70 different enzymes (including glycosidases, nucleases, proteases and lipases), their principal function being the degradation of a variety of macromolecules. Genetic deficiencies of any of the lysosomal enzymes can result in abnormal storage of these complex molecules. About 40 different lysosomal storage disorders are known, and they are classified according to the type of material stored (lipidoses, mucolipidoses, glycoproteinoses, mucopolysaccharidoses; see Tables 4.3, 4.4 and 4.5).

Clinical features

The clinical spectrum of the storage disorders is very wide, ranging from prenatal manifestation as severe fetal oedema and ascites (hydrops fetalis) to very mild symptomatology in adulthood (Rapola, 1994). Characteristically, there is an asymptomatic phase, which may last weeks to decades, followed by the development of progressive symptoms and signs. Conditions in which storage occurs in the central nervous system show regression of acquired skills over a variable period, resulting in eventual inanition and death, though milder variants of most such disorders are well recognized. The diagnosis is usually suspected clinically. Suggestive signs include coarsening of facial features, neurological deterioration and hepatosplenomegaly. Radiologically, patients with storage disorders often have a characteristic skeletal dysplasia (dysostosis multiplex) with a large skull, spinal deformities and short, thick tubular bones. Depending on the individual disorder, specific enzyme analysis requires analysis of serum, leukocytes or cultured skin fibroblasts. Prenatal diagnosis by mutation analysis and enzyme studies on amniocytes or chorion villus cells is usually possible.

Treatment

Fully effective treatment is not yet available for these disorders. Extensive genetic counselling and family support are necessary. Symptomatic treatment and palliative care are required for disorders with neurological involvement and those with orthopaedic problems.

Enzyme replacement therapy has proven to be very effective in non-neuronopathic forms of Gaucher disease (Grabowski, Leslie & Wenstrup, 1998). Therapeutic trials are ongoing for other conditions that may be amenable to this form of treatment, such as Fabry disease and Pompe disease. A major limitation of enzyme replacement is the difficulty in delivering large

Table 4.3. Lipidoses

Disorder	Enzyme defect	Genetics	Clinical features	Outcome
GM1 Gangliosidosis	β-galactosidase	AR	Neurodegeneration, dysostosis multiplex, coarse features hepatosplenomegaly, cherry red spot. Infantile, juvenile and adult forms recognized	Infantile – death by 2 years Juvenile – death 3–10 years Adult – onset 2nd–4th decade, slow neurodegeneration
GM2 Gangliosidosis Sandhoff	Total hexosaminidase	AR	Mental and motor retardation at 6–9 months, myoclonic seizures, no hepatosplenomegaly, cherry red spot. Juvenile and adult forms also seen	Infantile – death in infancy Juvenile – death in 2nd decade Adult – variable onset & course
Tay-Sachs	Hexosaminidase A	AR	Same as Sandhoff	Same as Sandhoff
Fabry	α-galactosidase	XLR	Painful crises, angiokeratoma, renal impairment, later cerebrovascular disease	Onset in late childhood Males die of renal failure in 4th–5th decade
Krabbe	Galactocerebrosidase	AR	Irritability, hypertonia, fits, optic atrophy, neuropathy	Onset 3–6 months Death by 1–2 years
Metachromatic leukodystrophy	Arylsulphatase A	AR	Ataxia, learning disability, quadriparesis. Psychiatric presentation in adult form	Infantile – Onset 1–3 years, death in late childhood Juvenile – onset by 6 years, death by 20 years Adult – prolonged course
Gaucher	β-glucosidase	AR	Hepatosplenomegaly, bone and lung infiltration. Neurological(type II), Non neurological (type I) and intermediate (type III) forms	Type I (common) – prolonged survival, death due to pulmonary or haematological complications Type II – death in infancy Type III – variable survival into childhood

Disease	Enzyme/defect	Inheritance	Clinical features	Outcome
Niemann-Pick types A and B	Sphingomyelinase	AR	Hepatosplenomegaly, lung infiltration, neurological (A) and non-neurological (B) types	Type A – death in infancy; Type B – relatively normal life span
Niemann-Pick C	Cholesterol esterification defect	AR	Neonatal hepatitis, hepatosplenomegaly, vertical ophthalmpolegia, ataxia, later neurodegeneration	Death 1–3 decades after onset of neurodeneration
Wolman, Cholesterol ester storage disease	Acid esterase	AR	Hepatosplenomegaly, steatorrhea, failure to thrive, adrenal calcification, neurodegeneration. Cholesterol ester storage disease a mild variant, causing hepatic fibrosis in adults	Wolman's – death in infancy; Cholesterol ester storage disease – death from liver failure in adulthood
Farber	Ceramidase	AR	Psychomotor deterioration, subcutaneous nodules, painful and deformed joints	Death in infancy; late onset variants known

Table 4.4. Mucolipidoses and glycoprotein storage diseases

Disorder	Genetics	Enzyme defect	Clinical features	Outcome
Mucolipidosis I (Sialidosis)	AR	α-neuraminidase	Myotonic seizures, cherry red spot, psychomotor retardation, hepatosplenomegaly and dysostosis multiplex	Severe cases – death in early childhood Milder cases – survival into adulthood, severely retarded
Mucolipidosis II (I-cell disease)	AR	N-acetylglucosamine-1-phosphatase	Coarse facies, kyphoscoliosis, joint contractures, gingival hyperplasia, cardiomyopathy, dysostosis. Onset in infancy.	Death by 4–6 years from cardiopulmonary disease
Mucolipidosis III	AR	N-acetylglucosamine-1-phosphatase	Stiff joints, kyphoscoliosis, short stature, low-normal intelligence. Presentation by 3–4 years	Usually survive into adulthood with severe orthopaedic problems and mild cardiac involvement
Mucolipidosis IV	AR	unknown	Psychomotor retardation, corneal opacities, retinal degeneration	Survival into adulthood usual with severe retardation. Rare disorder
Galactosialidosis	AR	Neuraminidase and β-galactosidase	Similar to Mucolipidosis I, onset usually in late childhood	Survival into adulthood usual with variable degree of mental retardation
Fucosidosis	AR	α-fucosidase	Psychomotor retardation, mild dysostosis multiplex, angiokeratoma, visceromegaly. Onset in early childhood	Severe form (type I) – death by late childhood Mild form (type II) – survival into adulthood, variable degree of mental retardation

α-Mannosidosis	AR	α-mannosidase	Deafness, mild Hurler phenotype, mental retardation. Onset in infancy or early childhood	Slow intellectual deterioration, eventual developmental level at 5–7 year. Survival into adulthood usual.
β-Mannosidosis	AR	β-mannosidase	Mental retardation, seizures, quadriplegia, angiokeratoma in late onset cases	Severe cases – death in infancy Mild cases – longer survival
Aspartyl-glycosaminuria	AR	Aspartyl-glycosaminidase	Mental retardation, coarse features, presentation at 1–5 years	Slow neurological deterioration, death by 30–40 years from pulmonary disease
Schindler	AR	α-N-acetylgalactosaminidase	Mental retardation, no visceromegaly or dysostosis. Angiokeratoma in mild variant	Severe form – rapid deterioration, profound retardation by 3–4 year Mild form – slow progression of neurological disease

Table 4.5. Mucopolysaccharidoses (MPS)

Disorder	Genetics	Enzyme defect	Clinical features	Outcome
MPS I (Hurler or Scheie)	AR	α-iduronidase	Hurler: psychomotor retardation, coarse facial features, growth retardation, dysostosis multiplex, corneal clouding, visceromegaly. Milder features in Scheie syndrome	Hurler: death by 8–10 year Scheie: normal lifespan; orthopaedic problems common
MPS II (Hunter)	XLR	Iduronate sulphatase	Symptoms similar to Hurler syndrome, no corneal clouding. Rare milder variant with no mental retardation	Death by mid-teens Milder variant: normal life span
MPS III (San Fillipo)	All AR			
Type A		Heparan-N-sulphatase	Commonest MPS disorder in UK, identical phenotype in all types. Marked mental retardation, severe behavioural and sleep disturbance. Mild somatic involvement, mild coarse features, no corneal clouding.	Survival into late teens or adulthood with severe mental retardation
Type B		α-acetyl-glucosaminidase		
Type C		AcetylCoA: α-glucosaminide-N-acetyltransferase		
Type D		N-acetylglucosamine 6-sulphatase		

MPS Type	Inheritance	Enzyme deficiency	Clinical features	Prognosis
MPS IV (Morquio) Type A	Both types AR	N-acetylglucosamine 6-sulphatase	Both types phenotypically similar. No mental retardation, severe skeletal deformities and growth	Survival into adulthood common if death does not occur earlier due to cervical myelopathy.
Type B		β-galactosidase	retardation, cervical myelopathy a potentially fatal hazard, mild corneal clouding	Cardiopulmonary compromise later due to thoracic deformity
MPS VI (Maroteaux–Lamy)	AR	Arylsulphatase B	Skeletal deformities similar to Hurler syndrome, but no mental retardation. Variable cardiac involvement, mild corneal clouding	Severe forms – survive into late teens Mild form – normal life span
MPS VII (Sly)	AR	β-glucuronidase	Variable phenotype ranging from hydrops fetalis to mild adult type similar to MPS I	Variable depending on severity

quantities of enzyme across the blood–brain barrier and it is not very useful in disorders with neurological involvement. BMT has been successful in preventing the onset of central nervous system disease in a number of lysosomal disorders, including Hurler syndrome, metachromatic leukodystrophy and Krabbe's disease (Krivit et al., 1999). Studies on the outcome of BMT in storage disorders have demonstrated that though the overall results are mixed, stabilization of the disease process can be achieved if the procedure is successful. However, the mortality and morbidity from BMT remain high. Gene therapy may offer the best chance of successful treatment, but is still several years away from clinical use.

Outcome

The cognitive outcome of lysosomal storage disorders is highly variable, and largely dependent on the extent of central nervous system involvement. Some disorders, such as Morquios syndrome and Maroteaux–Lamy syndrome are associated with normal intelligence, whereas others like Hurler syndrome result in progressive neuroregression after a period of normal early development. Conductive deafness is common in storage disorders, and may result in delayed acquisition of verbal skills.

The psychosocial morbidity of these disorders may be related to the physical, behavioural and/or the therapeutic aspects of the particular condition involved. Some disorders, such as Morquio syndrome and the mild form of Hunter syndrome, mainly affect physical appearance and patients may suffer from associated stigmatization (Young & Harper, 1981). Adaptation to adult life after special schooling is particularly difficult, and long-term support for the individuals and their families is necessary.

Children with San Filippo syndrome, on the other hand, usually are of normal appearance but characteristically develop disruptive behaviour and neuroregression after a period of normal early development. Three phases have been described in the progression of the neuropsychiatric disturbances (Cleary & Wraith, 1993). The first phase, between the ages of 1 and 4 years, is mainly characterized by mild developmental and speech delay. Behavioural disturbances become prominent in the second phase, which begins around 3–4 years of age. Children have increasingly frequent temper tantrums and hyperactivity, reversal of the sleep–wake cycle, aggression, destructive behaviour and panic attacks. The final phase of the illness, which begins when children are about 10 years old, is characterized by feeding difficulties, imbalance, worsening spasticity and seizures. Individuals are wheelchair-bound by the mid-teens and death usually occurs due to respiratory infection by the end of the second decade. Symptomatic treatment is helpful, and usually includes medications for the sleep disturbance (melatonin, chloral hydrate, trimeprazine), for daytime hyperactivity and aggression (thioridazine, haloperidol) and for reducing oral secretions (hyoscine patches, glycopyrrolate). In addition, the family require considerable support, and the provision of respite care is essential to enable parents to have adequate periods of rest.

BMT has been used to treat a number of lysosomal disorders. Though psychosocial factors do not influence the outcome of BMT, they significantly contribute to the overall morbidity. Important factors that must be considered before transplantation include the child's emotional responses to previous hospitalization and procedures, the guilt and misgivings of the parents, stresses within the family and the potential social disruption caused by prolonged hospitalization (Harris, 2000). During the procedure, the child and one parent face a stressful period of isolation, and the child may experience significant emotional and behavioural disturbances. The child's and the family's responses to other patients are also important; the death of another child on the transplant unit can have a negative influence. Following successful transplantation, the discharge has to be carefully planned as parents often have anxieties regarding possible complications, the safety of the home environment, the return to school and participation in group activities. After discharge, the family continues to need close support. The issue of neuropsychiatric sequelae due to the neurotoxic effects of chemotherapy and total body irradiation remains unresolved. Kramer et al. (1997) found significant reductions in IQ levels one year after BMT in a cohort of 67 children with a mean age of 45 months; there was no further reduction when the children were tested 3 years post-transplant. However, other studies have found either no change in cognitive functioning post-transplant (Simms et al., 1998) or cognitive sequelae only in children transplanted before the age of 3 years (Phipps et al., 2000). Additionally, individuals often have problems with social competence, self-esteem and emotional well being and find re-adjustment to normal life particularly difficult in the first year after BMT (Phipps et al., 1995). There may also be adverse psychological effects on the siblings resulting in symptoms of post-traumatic stress, and these must also be taken into consideration (Packman et al., 1997). In summary, considerable work with the family is needed to optimize the neuropsychological outcome after BMT.

Conclusion

Individuals with many childhood onset metabolic disorders now routinely survive into adolescence and adulthood because of vastly improved diagnosis and treatment. Such individuals are prone to developing neuropsychological problems as a result of the underlying condition as well as various therapeutic interventions. We have described some of the more common disorders that are compatible with prolonged survival in this chapter. The scope is constantly expanding, with descriptions of new disorders and variants of classical entities appearing regularly in medical literature. A comprehensive account of inherited metabolic disorders can be found in the standard reference textbook *The Metabolic and Molecular Basis of Inherited Disease*, edited by Scriver et al. (2001) (see 'Further Reading').

Acknowledgement

The authors wish to thank Dr. Emma Worwood for her very helpful suggestions about the content and layout of this chapter.

REFERENCES

Abbott, M.H., Folstein, S.E., Abbey, H. & Pyeritz, R.E. (1987). Psychiatric manifestations of homocystinuria due to cystathionine β-synthase deficiency: prevalence, natural history and relationship to neurologic impairment and vitamin B6-responsiveness. *American Journal of Medical Genetics*, **26**: 959–69.

Arnold, G.L., Kramer, B.M., Kirby, R.S., Plueau, P.B., Blakely, E.M., Sanger Cregan, L.S. & Davidson, P.W. (1998). Factors affecting cognitive, motor, behavioural and executive functioning in children with phenylketonuria. *Acta Paediatrica*, **87**: 565–70.

Asano, J., Suzuki, Y., Yajima, S. et al. (1994). Effects of erucic acid therapy on Japanese patients with X- linked adrenoleukodystrophy. *Brain Development*, **16**: 454–8.

Auborg, P., Adamsbaum, C., Lavallard-Rousseau, M.-C. et al. (1993). A two-year trial of oleic and erucic acids ("Lorenzo's oil") as a treatment for adrenomyeloneuropathy. *New England Journal of Medicine*, **329**: 745–52.

Avison, M.J., Novotny, E.J., Petroff, C. et al. (1990). Proton NMR observation of phenylalanine and an aromatic brain metabolite in the rabbit brain in vivo. *Pediatric Research*, **27**: 566–70.

Badawi, N., Calahane, S.F., McDonald, M., Mulhair, P., Begi, B., O'Donohue, A. & Naughten, E. (1996). Galactosaemia – a controversial disorder. Screening and outcome. Ireland 1972–1992. *Irish Medical Journal*, **89**: 16–17.

Berry, G.T., Nissin, I., Gibson, J.B. et al. (1997). Quantitative assessment of whole body galactose metabolism in galactosemic patients. *European Journal of Pediatrics*, **156** (Suppl 1): S43–S49.

Bezman, L. & Moser, H.W. (1998). Incidence of X-linked adrenoleukodystrophy and the relative frequency of its phenotypes. *American Journal of Medical Genetics*, **76**: 415–19.

Bick, U., Fahrendorf, G., Ludolph, A.C., Vassallo, P., Weglage, J. & Ullrich, K. (1991). Disturbed myelination in patients with treated hyperphenylalaninaemia: evaluation with magnetic resonance imaging. *European Journal of Pediatrics*, **150**: 185–9.

Bick, U., Ullrich, K., Stober, U. et al. (1993). White matter abnormalities in patients with treated hyperphenylalaninaemia: magnetic resonance relaxometry and proton spectroscopy findings. *European Journal of Pediatrics*, **152**: 1012–20.

Bottiglieri, T., Hyland, K. & Reynolds, E.H. (1994). The clinical potential of ademethionine (S-adenosylmethioine) in neurological disorders. *Drugs*, **48**: 137–52.

Brunner, R.L. & Berry, H.K. (1987). Phenylketonuria and sustained attention: the continuous performance test. *International Journal of Clinical Neuropsychology*, **9**: 68–70.

Brunner, R.L., Burch, D.B. & Berry, H. (1987). Phenylketonuria and complex spatial visualization: an analysis of information processing. *Developmental Medicine and Child Neurology*, **29**: 460–8.

Brunner, R.L., Jordan, M.K. & Berry, H.K. (1983). Early-treated phenylketonuria: neuro-psychologic consequences. *Journal of Pediatrics*, **102**: 831–5.

Clarke, J.T., Gates, R.D., Hogan, S.E., Barrett, M. & MacDonald, G.W. (1987). Neuropsychological studies on adolescents with phenylketonuria returned to phenylalanine restricted diets. *American Journal of Mental Retardation*, **92**: 255–62.

Cleary, M.A., Walter, J.H., Wraith, J.E., Jenkins, J.P., Alani, S.M., Tyler, K. & Whittle, D. (1994). Magnetic resonance imaging of the brain in phenylketonuria. *Lancet*, **344**: 87–90.

Cleary, M.A., Walter, J.H., Wraith, J.E., White, F., Tyler, K. & Jenkins, J.P. (1995). Magnetic resonance imaging in phenylketonuria: reversal of cerebral white matter change. *Journal of Pediatrics*, **127**: 251–5.

Cleary, M.A. & Wraith, J.E. (1993). Management of mucopolysaccharidosis type III. *Archives of Diseases in Childhood*, **69**: 403–6.

Diamond, A., Prevor, M.B., Callender, G. & Druim, D.P. (1997). Prefrontal cortex cognitive deficits in children treated early and continuously for phenylketonuria. *Monographs of the Society for Research in Child Development*, **62**: 1–208.

Dobson, J.C., Khushida, E., Williamson, M. & Friedman, E.G. (1976). Intellectual performance of 36 PKU patients and their non affected siblings. *Pediatrics*, **58**: 53–8.

Doeflinger, N., Miclea, J.M., Lopez, J. et al. (1998). Retroviral transfer and long-term expression of the adrenoleukodystrophy gene in human CD34 + cells. *Human Gene Therapy*, **9**: 1025–36.

Dyer, C.A., Kendler, A., Philibotte, T., Gardiner, P., Cruz J. & Levy, H.L. (1996). Evidence for central nervous system glial cell plasticity in phenylketonuria. *Journal of Neuropathology and Experimental Neurology*, **55**: 795–814.

Erlington, G.M., Bateman, D.E., Jeffrey, M. & Lawton, N.F. (1989). Adrenoleukodystrophy: heterogeneity in two brothers. *Journal of Neurology, Neurosurgery and Psychiatry*, **52**: 310–13.

Finkelstein, J.D. (1998). The metabolism of homocysteine: pathways and regulation. *European Journal of Pediatrics*, **157** (Suppl 2): S40–S44.

Fishler, K., Koch, R., Donnell, G. & Graliker, B.V. (1966). Psychological correlates in galactosemia. *American Journal of Mental Deficiency*, **71**: 117–25.

Freeman, J.M., Finkelstein, J.D. & Mudd, S.H. (1975). Folate-responsive homocystinuria and 'schizophrenia'. *New England Journal of Medicine*, **292**: 491–6.

Gleason, L.A., Michals, K., Matalon, R., Langenberg, P. & Kamath, S. (1992). A treatment program for adolescents with phenylketonuria. *Journal of the American Dietetic Association*, **86**: 1203–7.

Grabowski, G.A., Leslie, N. & Wenstrup, R. (1998). Enzyme therapy for Gaucher disease: the first 5 years. *Blood Reviews*, **12**: 115–33.

Grobe, H. (1980). Homocystinuria (cystathionine beta synthase deficiency): results of treatment I late-diagnosed patients. *European Journal of Pediatrics*, **135**: 199–203.

Harris, J.C. (2000). Psychosocial care of the child and family. In *Inborn Metabolic Diseases: Diagnosis and Treatment*, 2nd edn, ed. J. Fernandes, J.M. Saudubray & G. van den Berghe, pp. 63–74. Berlin: Springer-Verlag.

Hashmi, M., Stanley, W. & Singh, I. (1986). Lignoceryl CoASH ligase: enzyme defect in fatty acid beta-oxidation system in X-linked childhood adrenoleukodystrophy. *FEBS letters*, **196**: 247.

Kemp, S., Wei, H.-M., Lu, J.-F. et al. (1998). Gene redundancy and pharmacological gene therapy: potential for X-linked adrenoleukodystrophy. *Nature Medicine*, **4**: 1261–8.

Kluijtmans, L.A., Boers, G.H., Kraus, J.P., van der Heuvel, L.D., Cruysberg, J.R., Trijbels, F.J. & Blom, H.J. (1999). The molecular basis of cystathionine beta synthase deficiency in Dutch patients with homocystinuria: effect of CBS genotype on biochemical control and on response to treatment. *American Journal of Human Genetics*, **65**: 59–67.

Knudsen, G.M., Hasselbach, S., Toft, P.B., Christensen, E., Paulson, O.B. & Lou, H. (1995). Blood-brain barrier transport of amino acids in healthy controls and in patients with phenylketonuria. *Journal of Inherited Metabolic Disease*, **18**: 653–64.

Koff, E., Boyle, P. & Pueschel, S. (1977). Perceptual-motor functioning in children with phenylketonuria. *American Journal of Diseases in Children*, **131**: 1084–7.

Korenke, G.C., Christen, H., Hunneman, D.H. & Hanefield, F. (1996). Failure of beta interferon therapy in X- linked adrenoleukodystrophy. *European Journal of Pediatrics*, **155**: 833.

Korenke, G.C., Hunneman, D.H., Kohler, J., Stockler, S., Landmark, K. & Hanefield, F. (1995). Glyceroltrioleate/glyceroltrierucate therapy in 16 patients with X-chromosomal adrenoleukodystrophy/adrenomyeloneuropathy: effect on clinical, biochemical and neuropsychological parameters. *European Journal of Pediatrics* **154**: 64–70.

Kramer, J.H., Crittenden, M.R., DeSantes, K. & Cowan, M.J. (1997). Cognitive and adaptive behavior 1 and 3 years following bone marrow transplant. *Bone Marrow Transplant*, **19**: 606–13.

Kraus, J.P., Janosic, M., Kosich, V. et al. (1999). Cystathionine beta-synthase mutations in homocytinuria. *Human Mutation*, **13**: 362–75.

Krause, W., Halminski, M., McDonald, L. et al. (1985). Biochemical and neuropsychological effects of elevated plasma phenylalanine in patients with treated phenylketonuria: a model for the study of phenylalnine and brain function in man. *Journal of Clinical Investigation*, **75**: 40–8.

Kreis, R., Pietz, J., Penzien, J., Herschkowitz, N. & Boesch, C. (1995). Identification and quantitation of phenylalanine in the brain of patients with phenylketonuria by means of localised in vivo ¹H magnetic resonance spectroscopy. *Journal of Magnetic Resonance Imaging B*, **107**: 242–51.

Krivit, W., Auborg, P., Shapiro, E. & Peters, C. (1999). Bone marrow transplantation for globoid cell leukodystrophy, adrenoleukodystrophy, metachromatic leukodystrophy, and Hurler syndrome. *Current Opinion in Hematology*, **6**: 377–82.

Krivit, W., Lockman, L.A., Watkins, P.A. et al. (1995). The future for treatment by bone marrow transplantation for adrenoleukodystrophy, globoid cell leukodystrophy and Hurler syndrome. *Journal of Inherited Metabolic Disease*, **18**: 398–412.

Lee, D.H. (1972). Psychological aspects of galactosaemia. *Journal of Mental Deficiency Research* **16**: 173–91.

Leuzzi, V., Gualdi, G.F., Fabbrizi, F., Trasimeni, G., Di Biasi, C. & Antonozzi, I. (1993). Neuroradiological (MRI) abnormalities in phenylketonuric subjects: clinical and biochemical correlations. *Neuropediatrics*, **24**: 302–6.

Levy, H.L. & Waisbren, S.E. (1994). PKU in adolescents: rationale and psychosocial factors in diet continuation. *Acta Paediatrica Supplement*, **407**: 92–7.

Li, S.C.H. & Stewart, P.M. (1999). Homocystinuria and psychiatric disorder: a case report. *Pathology*, **31**: 221–4.

Lou, H.C., Guttler, F., Lykkelund, C., Bruhn, P. & Niederweiser, A. (1985). Decreased vigilance and neurotransmitter synthesis after discontinuation of dietary treatment for phenylketonuria in adolescents. *Journal of Pediatrics*, **144**: 17–20.

Lou, H.C., Toft, P.B., Andersen, J. et al. (1992). An occipito-temporal syndrome in adolescents with optimally controlled hyperphenylalaninaemia. *Journal of Inherited Metabolic Disease*, **15**: 687–95.

Maestri, N.E. & Beaty, T.H. (1992). Predictions of a 2-locus model for disease heterogeneity: applications to adrenoleukodystrophy. *American Journal of Medical Genetics*, **44**: 576–82.

Marsden, C.D., Obeso, J.A. & Lang, A.E. (1982). Adrenomyeloneuropathy presenting as spinocerebellar degeneration. *Neurology*, **32**: 1031–2.

Martin, J.J., Dompas, B., Ceuterick, C. & Jakobs, K. (1980). Adrenomyeloneuropathy and adrenoleukodystrophy in two brothers. *European Neurology*, **19**: 281–7.

Medical Research Council Working Party on Phenylketonuria (1993). Medical Research Council Working Party on Phenylketonuria due to phenylalanine hydroxylase deficiency: an unfolding story. *British Medical Journal*, **306**: 115–19.

Melhem, E.R., Barker, P.B., Raymond, G.V. & Moser, H.W. (1999). X-linked adrenoleukodystrophy in children: review of genetic, clinical, and MR imaging characteristics. *American Journal of Radiology*, **173**: 1575–81.

Moats, R.A., Koch, R., Moseley, K., Guldberg, P., Guttler, F., Boles, R.G. & Nelson, Jr. M.D. (2000). Brain phenylalanine concentration in the management of adults with phenylketonuria. *Journal of Inherited Metabolic Disease*, **23**: 7–14.

Moser, H.W. (1995). Clinical aspects of adrenoleukodystrophy and adrenomyeloneuropathy. *Journal of Neuropathology and Experimental Neurology*, **54**: 740–5.

Moser, H.W., Bergin, A., Naidu, S. & Landenson, P.W. (1991a). Adrenoleukodystrophy: new aspects of adrenal cortical disease. *Endocrinology and Metabolism Clinics of North America*, **20**: 297–318.

Moser, H.W., Moser, A.B., Naidu, S. & Bergin, A. (1991b). Clinical aspects of adrenoleukodystrophy and adrenomyeloneuropathy. *Developmental Neurosciences*, **13**: 254–61.

Moser, H.W., Smith, K.D. & Moser, A.B. (1995). X-Linked adrenoleukodystrophy. In *The Molecular and Metabolic Basis of Inherited Disease*, 7th edn, ed. C.R. Scriver, A.L. Beaudet. D. Valle & W.S. Sly, pp. 2325–49. New York: McGraw Hill.

Mosser, J., Douar, A.M., Sarde, C.O. et al. (1993). Putative X-linked aadrenoleukodystrophy gene shares unexpected homology with ABC transporters. *Nature*, **361**: 726–30.

Mudd, S.H., Levy, H.L. & Skovby, F. (1995). Disorders of transsulfuration. In *The Metabolic Basis of Inherited Disease*, ed. C.R. Scriver, A.L. Beaudet, D. Valle & W.S. Slys, pp. 1279–328. New York: McGraw-Hill.

Mudd, S.H., Skovby, F., Levy, H.L. et al. (1985). The natural history of homocystinuria due to cystathionine-beta synthase deficiency. *American Journal of Human Genetics*, **37**: 1–37.

Nelson, C.D., Waggoner, D.D., Donnell, G.N., Tuerck, J.M. & Buist, N.R.M. (1991). Verbal dyspraxia in treated galactosemia. *Pediatrics*, **88**: 346.

Nelson, M.D., Wolff, J.A., Cross, C.A., Donnell, G.N. & Kaufman, F.R. (1992). Galactosemia: evaluation with MR imaging. *Radiology*, **184**: 255–61.

Ohno, T., Tsuchia, H., Fukuhara, N., Yuasa, T., Tsuji, T. & Miyatake, T. (1983). Adrenoleukodystrophy: new clinical variant presenting as olivopontocerebellar atrophy. *Annals of Neurology*, **14**: 147–48.

Omenn, G.S. (1978). Inborn errors of metabolism: clues to understanding human behavioural disorders. *Behavioural Genetics*, **6**: 263–84.

Packman, W.L., Crittenden, M.R., Schaeffer, E. et al. (1997). Psychosocial consequences of bone marrow transplantation in donor and nondonor siblings. *Journal of Developmental and Behavioral Pediatrics*, **18**: 244–53.

Paine, R.S. (1957). The variability of manifestations of untreated patients with phenylketonuria (phenylpyruvic aciduria). *Pediatrics*, **20**: 290–302.

Pennington, B.F., van Doorninck, W.J., McCabe, L. & McCabe, E.R.B. (1985). Neuropsychological deficits in early treated phenylketonuric children. *American Journal of Mental Deficit*, **89**: 467–74.

Phipps, S., Brenner, M., Heslop, H., Krance, R., Jayawardene, D. & Mulhern, R. (1995). Psychological effects of bone marrow transplantation on children and adolescents: preliminary report of a longitudinal study. *Bone Marrow Transplant*, **15**: 829–35.

Phipps, S., Dunavant, M., Srivastava, D.K., Bowman, M. & Mulhern, R.K. (2000). Cognitive and academic functioning in survivors of bone marrow transplantation. *Journal of Clinical Oncology*, **18**: 1004–11.

Pietz, J., Dunckelman, R., Rupp, A. et al. (1998). Neurological outcome in adult patients with early-treated phenylketonuria. *European Journal of Pediatrics*, **157**: 824–30.

Pietz, J., Fatkenheuer, B., Burgard, P., Armbuster, M., Esser, G. & Schmidt, H. (1997). Psychiatric disorders in adult patients with early-treated phenylketonuria. *Pediatrics*, **99**: 345–55.

Pietz, J., Landwehr, R., Kutscha, A., Scmidt, H., de Sonneville, L. & Trefz, F.K. (1995). Effect of tyrosine supplementation on brain function in adults with phenylketonuria. *Journal of Pediatrics*, **127**: 936–43.

Pietz, J., Schmidt, E., Kutscha, A. & Meyding-Lamade, U. (1996). Sustained attention deficits and white matter changes (MRI) in phenylketonuria (PKU) *Radiology*, **201**: 413–20.

Pietz, J., Schmidt, E., Matthis, P., Kobialka, B., Kutsch, A. & de Sonneville, L.M.J. (1993). EEGs in phenylketonuria, 1: Follow-up to adulthood; 2: Short-term diet-related changes in EEG and cognitive function. *Developmental Medicine and Child Neurology*, **35**: 54–64.

Powers, J.M. & Schaumburg, H.H. (1980). A fatal cause of sexual inadequacy in men: adrenoleukodystrophy. *Journal of Urology*, **124**: 583–5.

Rahman, M. (1971). Homocystinuria: a review of four cases. *British Journal of Ophthalmology*, **55**: 338–42.

Rapola, J. (1994). Lysosomal storage diseases in adults. *Pathology Research Practice*, **190**: 759–66.

Ris, M.D., Weber, A.M., Hunt, M.M., Berry, H.K., Williams, S.E. & Leslie, N. (1997). Adult psychosocial outcome in early treated phenylketonuria. *Journal of Inherited Metabolic Disease*, **20**: 499–508.

Rizzo, W.B. (1993). Lorenzo's oil: hope and disappointment. *New England Journal of Medicine*, **329**: 801–2.

Rutter, M., Graham, P.J. & Yule, W. (1970). *A Neuropsychiatric Study in Childhood*. London: Heinemann.

Santosh-Kumar, C.R., Hassell, K.L., Deutch, J.C. & Kolhouse, J.F. (1994). Are neuropsychiatric manifestations of folate, cobalamin and pyridoxine deficiency mediated through imbalances in excitatory sulphur amino acids? *Medical Hypotheses*, **43**: 244–9.

Schaumburg, H.H., Powers, J.M., Raine, C.S., Suzuki, K. & Richardson, E.P. (1975). Adrenoleukodystrophy: a clinical and pathological study of 17 cases. *Archives of Neurology*, **32**: 577–91.

Schimke, R.N., McKusick, V.A., Huang, T. & Pollack, A.D. (1965). Homocystinuria: studies of 20 families with 38 affected members. *JAMA*, **193**: 711–19.

Schmidt, E., Rupp, A., Burgard, P., Pietz, J., Weglage J. & de Sonneville, L. (1994). Sustained attention in adult phenylketonuria: the influence of concurrent phenylalanine level. *Journal of Clinical and Experimental Neuropsychology*, **16**: 681–8.

Schuett, V.E., Brown, E. & Michals, K. (1985). Reinstitution of diet therapy in PKU patients from twenty-two US clinics. *American Journal of Public Health*, **75**: 39–42.

Schulz, B. & Bremer, H.J. (1995). Nutrient intake and food consumption of adolescents and young adults with phenylketonuria. *Acta Paediatrica*, **84**: 743–8.

Schweitzer, S., Shin, Y., Jakobs, C. & Brodehl, J. (1993). Long-term outcome in 134 patients with galactosaemia. *European Journal of Pediatrics*, **152**: 36–43.

Scriver, C.R., Kaufman, S., Eisensmith, R.C. & Woo, S.L.C. (1995). The Hyperphenylalaninaemias. In *The Metabolic and Molecular Basis of Inherited Disease*, 7th edn, ed. C.R. Scriver, A.L. Beaudet, D. Valle & W.S. Sly, pp. 1015–76. New York: McGraw-Hill.

Seashore, M.R., Friedman, E., Novelly, R.A. & Bapat, V. (1985). Loss of intellectual function in children with phenylketonuria after relaxation of dietary phenylalanine restriction. *Pediatrics*, **75**: 226–32.

Segal, S. (1995a). Galactosemia unsolved. *European Journal of Pediatrics*, **154**(Suppl 2): S97-S102.

Segal, S. (1995b). In utero galactose intoxication in animals. *European Journal of Pediatrics*, **154** (Suppl 2): 582–86.

Segal, S. & Berry, G.T. (1995). Disorders of galactose metabolism. In *The Metabolic and Molecular Basis of Inherited Disease*, 7th edn, ed. C.R. Sriver, A.L. Beaudet, D. Valle & W.S. Sly, pp. 967–99. New York: McGraw-Hill.

Segal, S. & Cautrecasas, P. (1968). The oxidation of c14 galactose by patients with congenital galactosemia: Evidence for a direct oxidative pathway. *American Journal of Medicine*, **44**: 340–4.

Shield, J.P., Wadsworth, E.J., Macdonald, A. et al. (2000). The relationship of genotype to cognitive outcome in galactosaemia. *Archives of Diseases in Childhood*, **83**: 248–50.

Simms, S., Kazak. A.E., Gannon, T., Goldwein, J. & Bunnin, N. (1998). Neuropsychological outcome of children undergoing bone marrow transplantation. *Bone Marrow Transplant*, **22**: 181–4.

Singh, I., Khan, M., Key, L. et al. (1998). Lovastatin for X-linked adrenoleukodystrophy. *New England Journal of Medicine*, **339**: 702–3.

Smith, I., Beasley, M.G., Wolff, O.H. & Ades, A.E. (1988). Behaviour disturbance in 8-year old children with early treated phenylketonuria. *Journal of Pediatrics*, **112**: 403–8.

Smith, I. & Lee, P. (2000). The hyperphenylalaninaemias. In *Inborn Metabolic Diseases: Diagnosis and Treatment*, 2nd edn. ed. J. Fernandes, J.M. Saudubray & G. Van den Berghe, pp. 171–84. Berlin: Springer-Verlag.

Smith, I. & Wolff, O.H. (1974). Natural History of phenylketonuria and influence of early treatment. *Lancet*, **2**: 540–4.

Smith, K.D., Kemp, S., Braiterman, L.T. et al. (1999). X-linked adrenoleukodystrophy: genes, mutations, and phenotypes. *Neurochemistry Research*, **24**: 521–35.

Sonneville, L.M.J. de, Schmidt, E., Michel, U. & Batzler, U. (1990). Preliminary neuropsychological test results of the German phenylketonuria collaborative study. *European Journal of Pediatrics*, **149**(Suppl 1): S39–S44.

Stott, D.H. (1965). *The Social Adjustment of Children*, 3rd edn. London: University of London Press.

Thompson, A.J., Smith, I., Branton, D. et al. (1990). Neurological deterioration in young adults with phenylketonuria. *Lancet*, **336**: 602–5.

Thompson, A.J., Tillotson, S., Smith, I., Kendall, B., Moore, S.G. & Brenton, D.P. (1993). Brain MRI changes in phenylketonuria. Associations with dietary status. *Brain*, **116**: 811–21.

Turner, B. (1967). Pyridoxine treatment in homocystinuria. *Lancet*, **2**: 1151.

Tyfield, L., Reichardt, J. & Fridovich-Keil, J. (1999). Classical galactosaemia and mutations at the galactose–1-phosphate uridyl transferase gene (GALT) *Human Mutation*, **13**: 417–30.

van Geel, B.M., Assies, J., Wanders, R.A.J. & Barth, P.G. (1997). X linked adrenoleukodystrophy: clinical presentation, diagnosis, and therapy. *Journal of Neurology, Neurosurgery and Psychiatry*, **63**: 4–14.

Villasana, D., Butler, I.J., Williams, J.C. & Roongta, S.M. (1989). Neurological deterioration in adult phenylketonuria. *Journal of Inherited Metabolic Disease*, **12**: 451–7.

Waggoner, D.D., Buist, N.R.M. & Donnell, G.N. (1990). Long-term prognosis in galactosaemia: Results of a survey of 350 cases. *Journal of Inherited Metabolic Disease*, **13**: 802–18.

Waisbren, S.E., Brown, M.J., de Sonneville, L.M.J. & Levy, H.L. (1994). Review of neuro-psychological functioning in treated phenylketonuria: an information processing approach. *Acta Paediatrica Supplement*, **407**: 98–103.

Walter, J.H., Collins, J.E. & Leonard, J.V. (1999). Recommendations for the management of galactosaemia. *Archives of Disease in Childhood*, **80**: 93–6.

Walter, J.H., Wraith, J.E., White, F.J., Bridge, C. & Till, J. (1998). Strategies for the treatment of cystathionine β synthase deficiency: the experience of the Willink Biochemical Genetics Unit over the past 30 years. *European Journal of Pediatrics*, **157** (Suppl 2): S71–S76.

Weglage, J., Funders, B., Ullrich, K., Rupp, A. & Schmidt, E. (1996). Psychosocial aspects in phenylketonuria. *European Journal of Pediatrics*, **155** (Suppl 1): S101–S104.

Weglage, J., Funders, B., Wilken, B., Scubert, D., Schmidt, E., Burgard, P. & Ullrich, K. (1992). Psychological and social findings in adolescents with phenylketonuria. *European Journal of Pediatrics*, **151**: 522–5.

Welsh, M.C., Pennington, B.F., Ozonoff, S., Rouse, B. & McCabe, E.R.B. (1990). Neuropsychology of early-treated phenylketonuria: Specific executive function deficits. *Child Development*, **61**: 1697–713.

Wendel, U. & Langenbeck, U. (1996). Towards self-monitoring and self-treatment in phenyl-ketonuria – a way to better diet compliance. *European Journal of Pediatrics*, **155** (Suppl 1): S105–S107.

Wilcken, D.E. & Wilcken, B. (1997). The natural history of vascular disease in homocystinuria and the effects of treatment. *Journal of Inherited Metabolic Disease*, **20**: 295–300.

Yap, S. & Naughten, E. (1998). Homocystinuria due to cystathionine beta-synthase deficiency: 25 years' experience of a newborn screened and treated population with reference to clinical outcome and biochemical control. *Journal of Inherited Metabolic Disease*, **21**: 738–47.

Young, I.D. & Harper, P.S. (1981). Psychosocial problems in Hunter's syndrome. *Child Care Health Development*, **7**: 201–9.

Further reading

Applegarth, D.A., Dimmick, J.E. & Hall, J. (Eds) (1997). *Organelle Diseases: Clinical Features, Diagnosis, Pathogenesis and Management*, 1st edn. London: Chapman & Hall Medical.

Fernandes, J., Saudubray, J.M. & van den Berghe, G. (Eds). (2000). *Inborn Metabolic Diseases: Diagnosis and Treatment*, 2nd edn. Berlin: Springer-Verlag.

Scriver, C.R., Beaudet, A.L., Valle, D. & Sly, W.S. (Eds) (2001). *The Metabolic and Molecular Basis of Inherited Disease*, 8th edn. New York: McGraw-Hill.

5

Hemiplegic cerebral palsy

Robert Goodman

Introduction

Cerebral palsy (CP) is the single largest cause of severe physical disability in childhood. CP is not a single condition but an 'umbrella term' for a heterogeneous group of congenital and early-acquired brain disorders that meet three criteria. Firstly, the disorders are long-lasting rather than short-lived. While most types of CP are life-long, some children with mild CP in early childhood do eventually outgrow their symptoms. Secondly, the underlying brain lesions are static, though the clinical manifestations may change as the child grows up. This criterion rules out progressive neurodegenerative conditions or brain tumours. Thirdly, the clinical manifestations include impairments of motor function, including weakness, stiffness, poor co-ordination or involuntary movements. These motor problems are often accompanied by other clinical manifestations of brain disorders, including epilepsy, learning problems and sensory impairments. The American term 'static encephalopathy' is roughly equivalent to CP, except that motor involvement is not obligatory.

The subclassification of CP is based on the type and distribution of motor problems. Spasticity – involving stiffness and weakness of affected muscles – is usually the dominant motor problem. This spasticity affects: just one side of the body in hemiplegic CP; both legs to a severe extent and both arms to a mild extent in diplegic CP; and all four limbs severely in quadriplegic CP (which is also known as tetraplegia or double hemiplegia). Less commonly, the motor problems are dominated by ataxia (incoordination) or by dyskinesia (involuntary jerking or writhing movements). The aetiology of CP is largely unknown, though there are some recognized associations, e.g. between severe jaundice in the newborn period and dyskinetic CP, and between a variety of severe generalized brain insults and quadriplegic CP. Heredity seems particularly relevant to ataxic CP. Prematurity is an important risk factor for diplegic CP (and also, to a lesser extent, for others varieties of CP). Further background information about CP is available from textbooks of paediatric neurology (e.g. Menkes, 1995; Brett, 1997; Aicardi et al., 1998).

What is hemiplegia?

Hemiplegia refers to weakness and stiffness affecting just one side of the body – either the left or the right side. Children with hemiplegic CP can be divided into two main groups: those with *congenital hemiplegia*, whose brain disorder dates back to pregnancy, birth or the first few weeks after birth; and those with *acquired hemiplegia*, who acquire brain disorders later in development, typically between one and 60 months of age. Congenital hemiplegia accounts for about 80% of all hemiplegic CP. The nature of the underlying brain disorder varies – including malformations dating back to the first third of pregnancy, strokes occurring late in pregnancy (usually without an obvious cause), and damage to the white matter of the brain following very premature birth. Acquired hemiplegias also have many possible origins, ranging from brain infections (meningitis or encephalitis) to child abuse, and from traffic accidents to strokes.

Up to one child in a thousand has hemiplegic CP, making it the commonest variety of CP. Slightly more children have hemiplegias affecting the right side of the body than the left side, and males are slightly more likely to be affected than females. The reasons for these laterality and gender imbalances are unknown. Epilepsy, learning difficulties and perceptual problems each affect a substantial minority of children with hemiplegic CP. Physical and psychological aspects of hemiplegic CP are reviewed in Neville & Goodman (2000).

Why focus on hemiplegic CP?

The rest of this chapter focuses on the psychological consequences of hemiplegic CP not only because it is the commonest subtype of CP, but also because its psychological consequences have been studied in greater depth than those of other forms of CP. Hemiplegic CP has been relatively intensively studied because several factors make it a particularly suitable 'model' for investigating brain-behaviour links in childhood in general. Firstly, it is considerably more common than many other neurodevelopmental disorders. Secondly, since the majority of affected children is of normal intelligence and attends mainstream school, it is possible to examine psychological problems that are not secondary to intellectual impairment or segregated schooling. Thirdly, the relatively mild motor disability does not preclude the use of ordinary psychological and psychiatric assessment techniques. When assessing hyperactivity, for example, it is just as appropriate to ask about overactivity and fidgetiness in a child with hemiplegic CP as it would be for any other child. By contrast, it would make little sense to ask the same questions about a child with severe dyskinetic CP who was not independently mobile and who was constantly writhing as a result of the involuntary movements. Finally, a focus on hemiplegic CP provides an opportunity to examine whether psychological consequences vary with the side of the brain that is affected, or with the age at onset of the brain disorder (which ranges from the early prenatal period to later childhood).

Early studies of psychological difficulties associated with hemiplegic CP in childhood

Evidence that hemiplegic CP is associated with an increased rate of emotional and behavioural difficulties in childhood goes back some 50 years. Some of the earliest reports are about children with hemiplegic CP who had a hemispherectomy operation for the control of seizures (Neville, 2000). The operation can be dramatically successful, with complete cure of seizures in many cases and no deterioration in motor control. Many descriptions of the outcome of hemispherectomy also make it clear that the seizure problems had often been accompanied by behavioural problems and that the operation frequently improved behaviour as well as relieving seizures. For example, in the pioneering description by Krynauw (1950) of hemispherectomy for children with hemiplegic CP and intractable epilepsy, he emphasized the severity of the behavioural and social problems, stating that it was often 'the mental state, rather than the hemiplegia and epilepsy, which has led the parents to seek advice' (p. 243). In many children, both in Krynauw's study and in subsequent studies, the hemispherectomy operation not only abolished seizures but also led to a marked improvement in behaviour.

Children requiring hemispherectomy were clearly not typical of children with congenital hemiplegia in general, but other early studies showed that behavioural problems were not simply confined to those children with intractable seizures. The two classical descriptions of the hyperkinetic syndrome – involving severe and pervasive hyperactivity and inattention – both demonstrated a link with hemiplegic CP. Ounsted (1955) reported a high rate of hyperkinesis among children with epilepsy, associated with hemiplegia: 31% of children with epilepsy and hemiplegia also showed the hyperkinetic syndrome, as compared with 7% of those with epilepsy alone. In Ingram's (1955) study of a representative sample of children with CP, he also noticed a high rate of hyperkinesis, affecting 12% of the children with hemiplegic CP as compared with 5% of children with other types of CP. In a subsequent paper, Ingram (1956) provided more details on eight children with hemiplegic CP and hyper-kinesis; it was particularly noteworthy that five of the eight children did not have seizures. The link between hemiplegic CP and hyperactivity clearly could not be attributed solely to the consequences of epilepsy or anti-epileptic medication.

Early studies also made it clear that chronic neurodevelopmental problems were associated with a broad range of psychological problems and not just with hyperactivity. Ingram (1955) reported that the majority of his representative sample of children with CP showed behavioural disorders at some time or another.

The conclusion that many children with CP have associated psychiatric problems was confirmed by the subsequent neuropsychiatric study by Rutter, Graham & Yule (1970) on the Isle of Wight (UK): psychiatric disorders were present in 44% of children with CP who had an IQ of at least 50, as compared with 12% of children with chronic physical disorders not involving the cerebral hemispheres, and 7% of children with no physical disorders. This Isle of Wight study was a landmark in demonstrating that children with chronic neur-odevelopmental disorders were at a substantially higher risk of developing psychiatric problems than were other children, even when these other children had chronic physical disorders. Subsequent studies have provided further evidence for direct brain-behaviour links over and above the psychological distress related to any form of chronic disability or illness (Seidel, Chadwick & Rutter, 1975; Breslau, 1985; Howe et al., 1993; Austin et al., 1996). The Isle of Wight study further demonstrated that chronic neurodevelopmental disorders were associated with an increased rate of many different sorts of psychiatric problems, including emotional, hyperactivity and conduct disorders. There was no one 'brain damage syndrome'.

More recent studies of the psychological difficulties in hemiplegic CP

Studies of the frequency of psychological problems in hemiplegic CP need to be done on representative rather than clinic samples. This is to avoid selection bias, which typically leads to children with complex and severe problems being over-represented. There have been two large and representative samples of children with hemiplegic CP that have been studied from a behavioural perspective – one in Sweden (Uvebrant, 1988) and one in the UK (Goodman & Graham, 1996). Uvebrant (1988) recorded severe hyperkinetic behaviour and attention deficit in 6 of 111 (5.4%) children with hemiplegic CP in the absence of intellectual disability. Though no control group was included, this is probably three to five times more common than would be expected in a comparable sample of children without any physical disability.

The London Hemiplegia Register (LHR) (Goodman & Graham, 1996) looked at the rate, type and persistence of psychological problems in a large and representative sample of children with hemiplegic CP. Most of the rest of this chapter is based on findings of the LHR study, supplemented by clinical experience from the Maudsley Hospital's Brain and Behaviour Clinic (London, UK) for the psychological complications of hemiplegic CP.

In the LHR study, the children were ascertained from multiple sources including hospital and community paediatricians, orthopaedic surgeons, neurosurgeons, hospital and community physiotherapists, special schools and voluntary organizations. A total of 461 individuals under the age of 17 years was recruited from the Greater London area, and all were assessed using parent and teacher questionnaires. Subsequently, 149 of these individuals, all aged between 6 and 10 years, were individually assessed from neurological, psychological and psychiatric perspectives. Judging from demographic, medical, cognitive and behavioural variables, the characteristics of the sample as a whole closely resembled those of previous epidemiological samples of children with hemiplegic CP (Goodman & Yude, 1996). Standardized behavioural screening questionnaires had been completed by the parents and teachers of 428 children who were between 2 years 6 months and 16 years old at the time of assessment. The proportion of children scoring above the 'caseness' cut-off on these questionnaires was used to estimate the proportion with psychiatric disorders. Across the entire age band, the proportion with psychiatric disorders was 54% as judged from parental reports and 42% as judged by the reports of teachers or other professionals. There were no consistent age trends, with rates of disorder being high throughout the pre-school period, middle childhood years and teenage years (Goodman & Graham, 1996). A questionnaire follow-up, carried out an average of 4 years later, found that around 70% of children thought to have psychiatric disorders initially were still scoring within the disorder range at follow-up (Goodman, 1998).

Although the questionnaire findings from the LHR study suggest a high rate of psychiatric disorder throughout childhood, questionnaires are best seen as 'quick and dirty' assessment tools whose findings need to be confirmed by detailed individual assessments. When such assessments were carried out on 6- to 10-year-olds from the LHR sample, 61% were judged to have at least one diagnosable psychiatric disorder (Goodman & Graham, 1996). Common types of disorders included anxiety or depressive disorders in 25% of children;

conduct disorders involving disruptive and irritable behaviour in 24%; severe hyperactivity and inattention in 10%; and autistic disorders in 3%. Some children had more than one type of disorder, with hyperactivity and conduct disorders often occurring together. The common and rare types of disorders are described in more detail in the subsequent sections. Although the LHR study did not involve a control group of children without any physical disability, the overall rate of psychiatric disorder in children with hemiplegic CP was probably at least three times higher than in children without a physical disability; hyperactivity and autistic disorders were particularly over-represented.

Childhood fears and worries

Many children with hemiplegic CP meet the diagnostic criteria for at least one anxiety disorder. The commonest disorders are specific phobias and separation anxiety, though some children are affected by social phobia, panic attacks, generalized anxiety and mixed anxiety disorders.

The intense separation anxiety of some children with hemiplegic CP is a major problem for them, causing them great distress and restricting their lives. In addition, it can be a major burden for the key attachment figure, commonly the mother, who can come to feel like a prisoner under constant surveillance.

Childhood misery

Many children with hemiplegic CP feel miserable at times, which is understandable given the difficulties they have to surmount, e.g. their physical disability, any associated learning difficulties, or teasing. In some cases this misery amounts to a depressive disorder in which marked and persistent low mood is accompanied by disrupted sleep and appetite, loss of interest and energy, feelings of worthlessness and hopelessness, and suicidal thoughts or behaviours.

Difficult behaviour in childhood

The diagnostic terms *Oppositional–Defiant Disorder* and *Conduct Disorder* cover three main types of difficult behaviour in childhood: defiant and negativistic behaviour; aggressive behaviour; and antisocial behaviour such as stealing, robbing and fire-setting. Children with hemiplegic CP do commonly show markedly defiant and negativistic behaviour, often beginning with severe and frequent temper tantrums in infancy, and continuing with marked irritability throughout childhood accompanied by a great reluctance to do as they are told.

On some occasions, these traits can lead to marked aggression, e.g. hitting people and throwing things in the course of a temper outburst. This sort of aggression is not the sort of deliberate aggression shown by bullies; it is sometimes described as *irritable aggression* as opposed to *instrumental aggression*. In ordinary child mental health clinics, professionals are used to seeing irritability and defiance going along with antisocial behaviour. Fortunately, this is rarely the case in children with hemiplegic CP, who are very unlikely to enter upon the 'delinquent way of life'.

Childhood inattention and overactivity

Many children with hemiplegic CP have their lives, and particularly their education, curtailed by a mixture of fidgetiness, restlessness, poor concentration and easy distractibility. Typically, they will only spend a few minutes on any one task – even if it is one that they enjoy and are good at – before breaking off to do something else. Even when they are engaged in a task, this is often accompanied by a lot of wriggling, fidgeting, standing up and sitting down. They typically have difficulty staying seated for an entire meal, and often wander off on outings. True hyperactivity and inattention are evident both at home and at school.

Autism and autistic features in childhood

Autistic disorders such as infantile autism and Asperger syndrome only affect around 3% of children with hemiplegic CP, though this is some 10 times higher than the rate of similar disorders in the non-disabled population. By comparison to the relative rarity of full-blown autism, a considerably larger number of children with hemiplegic CP have some autistic features. Of the children referred to the Maudsley Hospital's Brain and Behaviour Clinic for the psychological complications of hemiplegic CP, roughly a fifth have prominent autistic features (Frampton & Goodman, unpub. data). These commonly involve intense preoccupations, some of which are an exaggeration of ordinary childhood interests, e.g. a focus on specific cartoon characters to the exclusion of everything else. In other cases, the preoccupation is with an unusual topic, e.g. washing machines, lawn mowers or yoghurt pots. These preoccupations are often associated with impoverished pretend play. Some of these children do not engage in any pretend play at all, but the majority will tend to enact the same simple scenarios over and over again with little variation. Difficulty in social understanding is often shown by a lack of interest in other children or by clumsy attempts to join in with other children, frequently involving telling their peers what to do and not being willing to follow their lead. However, delay and deviance in language development, which are characteristics of typical autism, are relatively uncommon in children with hemiplegic CP.

Other child psychiatric disorders

A few children with hemiplegic CP develop obsessions and compulsions, often involving checking things such as electric switches or doing things to avoid contamination, e.g. repeated hand washing. These obsessions and compulsions are often part of a broader anxiety or depressive disorder.

Anorexia nervosa does affect a small number of individuals with hemiplegic CP – mostly teenage girls. The rate is sufficiently low that it may simply be a coincidence that the same individual has both hemiplegic CP and an eating disorder. Anecdotally, though, it is possible that the disturbance in body image is partly related to the visuospatial problems that are so common in hemiplegic CP. Anorexic individuals typically see themselves as fat even when other people think they are far too thin. Perhaps this is more likely to happen to individuals whose visuospatial problems make it very hard for them to judge the volume of anything, whether it is glass or a box or their own body.

Psychotic illnesses, involving hallucinations or delusions, appear to be extremely rare. This is both fortunate and theoretically interesting, given that some other childhood neurological disorders are associated with an increased risk of psychotic problems (Ounsted, Lindsay & Richards, 1987).

Mind-reading skills

Over recent years, developmental psychologists have become increasingly interested in the way children acquire the ability to understand another person's point of view and predict what another person will be feeling or thinking (Theory of Mind). There is increasingly good evidence that children with autism have particular difficulties with mind-reading skills (Happé, 1994). Preliminary data suggest that children with hemiplegic CP commonly have subtle difficulties with mind-reading skills (Balleny, 1996). Somewhat surprising, many of these children do not have autistic traits, though they are commonly seen as emotionally and socially immature by their families and others. Typically, these immature children tend to play with younger children or seek out the company of adults, finding it far harder to relate to children of their own age. Their parents often describe them as naïve in interpersonal relationships and unable to 'read between the lines' in stories and television dramas; they are able to follow the outline of the plot but find it harder than younger siblings to make sense of irony, deceit or other situations where people mean something rather different from what they say or do. Clearly, difficulty deciphering these sorts of situations will make it much harder for children to participate on equal terms in the fast-moving social world of the playground.

Social relationships in childhood

The LHR study examined the peer relationships of a representative sample of 9- to 10-year olds with hemiplegic CP attending mainstream school. By comparison with their classmates, the children with hemiplegic CP were twice as likely to be rejected, twice as likely to have no friends, and five times as likely to be severely victimized (Yude, Goodman & McConachie, 1998). It was very striking that this excess of peer problems occurred in a group whose age and circumstances might have been expected to favour social integration – they were generally in stable peer groups where they had been with the same classmates for 5 years or more. Not all the excess of peer relationship problems could be attributed to learning and behavioural difficulties. The constitutional difficulties in social understanding described in the previous section probably also played a part. Children's prejudices against disabled classmates may also be relevant, and in this respect, children with relatively mild physical disabilities may be worse off than children with severe physical disabilities – the latter are more likely to have appropriate allowances made for them, while children with milder disabilities are often unfairly expected to compete on entirely equal terms.

Why do children with hemiplegic CP have more psychiatric problems?

The fact that children with neurological disorders have a higher rate of emotional, behavioural and social difficulties reflects the operation both of organic factors and of psychosocial factors (Goodman, 2002). Since the brain is the organ of thought and feeling as well as the organ of movement and perception, it is not surprising that disorders of the brain can directly affect thoughts and feelings as well as movements and perceptions. Equally, it is important not to lose sight of how stressful it can be in our society to be physically disabled and experience teasing or school failure due to unrecognized specific learning difficulties. In many cases, psychiatric problems result from the combination and interaction of both organic and psychosocial factors.

In the LHR study, a higher rate of psychiatric disorder was associated with more involvement of the affected side of the body, with some degree of involvement of the 'good' side of the body, with the presence of seizures and with lower IQ. All of these variables were highly correlated with one another, but IQ was the most powerful predictor in multivariate analyses, with the other variables adding nothing extra once IQ had been allowed for. The most likely explanation for this is that IQ is a particularly sensitive index of the amount of underlying cerebral damage (Goodman & Graham, 1996).

The psychiatric problems of children with hemiplegic CP are associated with a higher rate of parental anxiety and depression and with more parental criticism of the child (Goodman & Graham, 1996). Longitudinal studies suggest that this association primarily occurs because the child's problems impose a stress on parents, rather than because family stresses cause the child's problems (Goodman, 1998). This is not to argue that the child's environment is unimportant, but stresses in the classroom or playground often seem more relevant than stresses in the home.

One of the potential interests in studying children with hemiplegic CP is the possibility of comparing children with left and right-sided hemiplegias, thereby providing a window on the differential specialization of the two hemispheres. Although various studies of small and unrepresentative groups of children with hemiplegic CP have claimed side-specific differences in the rate or type of psychiatric problems, this has not been confirmed by studies of large and representative samples (Goodman & Yude, 1997). For clinicians and parents, the main implication is that the side of hemiplegia is irrelevant as far as psychological complications are concerned. For the theoretician, the main implication is that the neuroplasticity unleashed by early brain lesions is sufficiently powerful to override any pre-existing difference between the two hemispheres. Indeed, it is possible that some of the adverse psychological consequences of early brain damage stem from neuroplasticity, reflecting the adverse effects of new but maladaptive neuronal connections formed in response to the early injury (Goodman, 1989).

Treatment of childhood psychological and psychiatric problems

This section is based primarily on experience acquired at the Maudsley Hospital's Brain and Behaviour Clinic in the course of treating around 150 children with the psychological complications of hemiplegic CP. Since the LHR study was an epidemiological rather than an intervention study, it did not provide much information about treatment besides establishing that the great majority of children with hemiplegic CP and associated psychiatric disorders receive no treatment at all. In part, this may simply mirror the fact that most children with psychiatric problems get no help, whether or not they have additional disabilities. In addition, both paediatricians and child psychiatrists sometimes feel out of their depth dealing with problems that cross the brain–behaviour divide. In most respects, treating the psychological complications of children with hemiplegic CP is similar to ordinary child mental health work. One positive difference is that the families of children with hemiplegic CP are often easier to engage and help than the average family referred to child mental health services. Hemiplegic CP affects a random cross-section of families – it is not particularly associated with the sorts of social disadvantage and family disruption that are so familiar to child mental health professionals. In addition, the families of children with hemiplegic CP have long been in contact with paediatric services and are generally willing to accept the advice of well-informed professionals.

When planning psychological treatment, the fact that the child also has hemiplegic CP is relevant in four main respects. Firstly, it is often a great relief to parents to learn that the main cause of their child's behavioural problems is the hemiplegic CP itself (or rather the same underlying brain disorder that has caused the hemiplegic CP). Parents have often supposed that their children's emotional or behavioural problems stem from the way they have been brought up, so it can be very heartening for them to hear that many other children with hemiplegic CP have almost identical problems, despite having grown up in very different families. Further relief comes from sharing experiences directly with other families through newsletters and meetings organized by parents of other children with hemiplegic CP (Yude, 2000). Knowing that emotional and behavioural difficulties have biological origins is obviously not an excuse for doing nothing about them. Parents and professionals sometimes fall into the trap of assuming that because the underlying brain disorder is irreversible, nothing can be done about the psychological consequences. But just as physiotherapy or anti-epileptic medication can reduce or eliminate some of the physical consequences of the brain disorder, so appropriate treatment can reduce or eliminate the psychological complications. Reducing unnecessary guilt by emphasizing the role of brain–behaviour links need not be at the cost of abandoning other forms of treatment.

Secondly, the presence of hemiplegic CP may influence the treatment of psychological complications, in that it is sometimes essential to focus not on the behaviour but on the child's epilepsy. When the child has behavioural problems and poorly controlled epilepsy, improving seizure control through changes in medication or even neurosurgery is often accompanied by a dramatic improvement in behaviour. The child's behaviour sometimes may be worsened by a particular anti-epileptic medication, with parents usually having noticed that the behavioural difficulties have waxed and waned as the dose of a particular anti-epileptic medication has altered. Barbiturates used to be the common culprits, but nowadays it is more likely that behavioural-worsening is associated with benzodiazapines, valproate or vigabatrin, though any anti-epileptic medication can be responsible. On occasions, frequent ultra-brief epileptic discharges (transient cognitive impairments) can mimic the attention difficulties seen in hyperactivity. EEGs are not normally needed when assessing the psychological complications of hemiplegic CP, but they are sometimes indicated if the history or direct observation suggest that the child's attention is frequently interrupted by what could be frequent brief seizures.

Hemiplegic CP can also be relevant to the treatment of psychological complications in a third way if the affected individual, commonly in the teenage years, is tacitly or explicitly denying the physical disability. Particularly if the physical disability is mild, the teenager may refuse to acknowledge it or to accept the sort of help needed to circumvent it. For example, writing may be extremely difficult for someone with hemiplegic CP plus some degree of involvement of the 'good' side of the body, in which case regular access to a laptop computer in school can make an enormous difference. However, some teenagers refuse to accept this because it would make them look different from their classmates and they prefer to be 'ordinary failures' who write a few illegible lines with difficulty rather than being successes who openly acknowledge and attempt to cope with a potential disability. It is not easy to get round teenagers' understandable desire to 'be one of the crowd', but their failure to acknowledge their disability often buys temporary relief at the cost of greater long-term stress.

The fourth point is the inverse of the previous point. If failure to accept appropriate help for circumventing physical problems can sometimes lead to worsened stress and adverse psychological consequences, so too can the imposition of inappropriate or excessive help. For example, inappropriately intense physiotherapy programmes may consume much of the child's time without any corresponding benefit (Scrutton, 2000). Apart from wasting time the child could otherwise be spending with friends or getting on with age-appropriate activities, it is also likely to build up resentment towards parents and professionals.

After allowing for these factors that are relatively specific to hemiplegic CP or related conditions, the treatment of psychological and psychiatric difficulties makes use of the same specific techniques that are employed in child mental health practice in general (Goodman & Scott, 1997). Goodman & Yude (2000) provide more details of the ways these approaches can be harnessed to helping the emotional, attentional or behavioural problems of children with hemiplegic CP.

Adults with hemiplegic CP

Since the survival of mildly and moderately disabled children with CP is not much lower than that of unaffected children (Hutton, Cooke & Pharoah, 1994), it is surprising how little is known about the adult outcome of CP. One reason that research in this area has been so neglected is that it is not easy to find representative samples of adults with CP. The main difficulty is that it is precisely those individuals with prominent problems who are the most likely to be known to adult services – many others will have 'disappeared' into the general population because they are successfully circumventing their disability. Consequently, a study that locates adults with CP via adult services is bound to provide a gloomy picture of outcome since it will focus primarily on the most severely affected individuals. By contrast, it is relatively easy to find a representative sample of individuals with CP in childhood since, regardless of severity, nearly all affected individuals are known to school health services and most are in regular contact with paediatricians or physiotherapists. Consequently, one of the most straightforward approaches to locating a representative sample of adults with CP is to find them in childhood and then follow them up as adults. The disadvantage, of course, is that this strategy will initially only provide information on young adults – it will take a great deal of patience and funding to trace adequate numbers of adults with CP into mid-life or old age.

The LHR study used the follow-up approach to investigate a representative sample of individuals who had first been recruited into an epidemiological study of hemiplegic CP several years earlier when they were still of school age. This study will be presented in detail since it is the only one of its kind (Goodman, O'Neill & Beecham, 1998). The original LHR study had located a sample of 461 individuals with hemiplegic CP who were initially aged between 0 and 16 years. By the time of the adult follow-up, 114 of these individuals were 18 to 25 years old. Of these 81 (71%) were traced and recruited into the study – a relatively good participation rate given that 18- to 25-year-olds are notoriously difficult to trace and recruit. Of those who were not recruited into the study, eight were seen and declined to participate, nine did not respond to letters and were never at home when the interviewer called, and 16 could not be traced. The 81 participants were compared with the 33 non-participants using information from parent and teacher questionnaires collected about 6 years prior to the follow-up study. Participants and non-participants were very similar in gender, age and estimated IQ, but non-participants were more likely to have grown up in deprived neighbourhoods (higher Townsend score, $t = 2.7$, 112 df, $P < 0.01$), and to have had higher teacher ratings of psychopathology (higher Rutter score, $t = 2.2$, 101 df, $P < 0.05$). Consequently, if sample attrition had any effect on the findings, it would be in the direction of making what was originally a representative sample 'super normal' by differential loss of disruptive and disadvantaged individuals. One result is that the reported rate of problems in the following sections may be a slight underestimate.

Psychiatric disorder in young adult life

The LHR study of young adults with hemiplegic CP (Goodman et al., 1998) used the 12-item version of the General Health Questionnaire (GHQ–12; Goldberg & Williams, 1988) to gauge the rate of current anxiety and depression. Fifty young adults with hemiplegic CP completed a GHQ–12 about themselves; the non-completers were mainly individuals with additional learning difficulties. Using the standard GHQ scoring system, 14% scored 4 or more on the GHQ–12. The corresponding rate in the large community sample of 16- to 24-year-olds surveyed in the 1997 Health Survey for England was 16.5% (McMunn et al., 1998). In other words, those young adults with hemiplegic CP who were able to complete a GHQ–12 did not seem to be at an increased risk of new-onset anxiety or depression. This is encouraging but does not rule out the possibility that young adults with hemiplegic CP suffer from an increased rate of chronic psychiatric or psychosocial problems.

A standardized investigator-based interview, the Maudsley version of the Schedule for Schizophrenia and Affective Disorder – Lifetime (Maudsley SADS-L; Spitzer & Endicott, 1975; Harrington et al., 1988), was used in this same follow-up study to assess which individuals had experienced any psychiatric disorder since their 16th birthday. Fifty-one young adults with hemiplegic CP were interviewed; once again, the non-respondents were mainly individuals with additional learning difficulties. Ten interviewed individuals (20%) had had depressive disorders at some time during their adult life; most of these were brief, self-limiting and had not recurred. The 10 individuals with depression included one individual who had also had anorexia nervosa, and two individuals who had prominent anxiety symptoms at the same time as their depression. In two individuals, the depressive episode was linked to voluntarily discontinuing the use of non-prescribed stimulants taken for recreational purposes. The 20% rate of depressive (plus anxiety) disorders *at some stage* in early adulthood compares favourably with the 25% rate for *current* emotional disorders among 6- to 10-year-olds with hemiplegic CP (Goodman & Graham,

1996). This suggests that a childhood tendency to emotional disorders may become less prominent in adulthood, though it remains possible that continuing anxiety-proneness or sensitivity sometimes interfere with psychosocial functioning even when they do not lead to frank psychiatric disorders.

Information provided by parents was used to diagnose pervasive developmental disorders such as autism or Asperger syndrome in young adult life. Three of the 81 (4%) individuals had pervasive developmental disorders in adult life; these were chronic and severely impairing in all cases. The 4% rate of autistic disorders in adult life is comparable to the 3% rate reported for 6- to 10-year-old children with hemiplegic CP (Goodman & Graham, 1996) – an equivalence that is not surprising since pervasive developmental disorders are generally life-long.

Psychosocial adjustment in young adult life

The same LHR follow-up study of 18- to 25-year-olds with hemiplegic CP also assessed the psychosocial adjustment of the 81 individuals. When they were capable of understanding the questions, the young adults were interviewed in detail about how well they had been functioning in a broad range of activities and roles since the age of 16. The same topics were also covered in detailed interviews with key informants (usually parents). Self-report or informant-based details on adjustment were available on all 81 individuals. Combining information from all available sources, summary 5-point ratings were made for adjustment in five key domains: friendships; love relationships; education/ work; activities of daily living (ADLs); and leisure. The inter-rater reliabilities of these ratings were good, with kappa coefficients for chance-corrected agreement ranging from 0.66 to 0.90. All of the adjustment ratings used the same 5-point scale: seriously impaired (scored 0); impaired (scored 1); fair (scored 2); good (scored 3); and excellent (scored 4); and there are explicit criteria for each rating. Although norms are not available – since comparable ratings were not made on young adults without disabilities – a useful guide to interpretation is that 'impaired' or 'seriously impaired' functioning would be judged a significant problem by most adults.

Tables 5.1 to 5.5 and Figure 5.1 show the distribution of adjustment scores in each domain, both for the sample as a whole, and after splitting the sample into those with and without generalized learning difficulties (as defined by an estimated IQ of under 70). The five separate adjustment scores were summed to generate an overall adjustment rating; inter-rater agreement on this score

Table 5.1. Adjustment ratings for friendships

Rating (and illustrative criteria)	Whole sample (n = 81) %	Individuals with IQ ≥ 70 (n = 57) %	Individuals with IQ < 70 (n = 24) %
Seriously impaired. No friends. Rejected or neglected. Avoidance. Continual discord or arguments	14	7	29
Impaired. Superficial friendships. No support or confiding. Discord/arguments weekly or more. Only meet in school, college or workplace	21	14	38
Fair. Some friendships – significant problems but some successes. Sometimes meet outside, school, college or work. Discord less than weekly	27	28	25
Good. Confiding supportive friendships of limited duration. Discord less than monthly	12	16	4
Excellent. Close enduring friendships. Mutual support and confiding. Discord rare	26	35	4

Table 5.2. Adjustment ratings for close interpersonal (love) relationships

Rating (and illustrative criteria)	Whole sample (n = 81) %	Individuals with IQ ≥ 70 (n = 57) %	Individuals with IQ < 70 (n = 24) %
Seriously impaired. No relationships or extreme violence within relationships	41	32	63
Impaired. Occasional dates but mostly goes out in groups. No regular relationships or commitments. Discord weekly or more	25	24	25
Fair. Short-term relationships, regular dating outside of group. Minimal confiding and support. Discord less than weekly	13	16	8
Good. Long-term relationship. Identified as a couple. Confiding, supportive, some commitment. Discord less than monthly	17	23	4
Excellent. Confiding, supportive, committed. Discord rare	4	5	0

Table 5.3. Adjustment ratings for education or work

Rating (and illustrative criteria)	Whole sample (n = 81) %	Individuals with IQ ≥ 70 (n = 57) %	Individuals with IQ < 70 (n = 24) %
Seriously impaired. Dropped out of education at 16 or earlier. Never worked and not seeking work. Remains at home, not otherwise occupied	4	5	0
Impaired. In education but failing. Dropped out of post-16 education with no clear pathway. Continually changing course or job with no overall plan. Dismissed from job. Attends day centre but unhappy or not participating	3	4	0
Fair. Broad life plan and attempts to adhere to it. Post-16 education or training scheme. If job fails, seeks re-employment or further training. Attends day centre and sometimes participates	37	37	37
Good. Full-time education or has recognised qualifications within ability level. Has definite life plan and adheres to it. Employed or fills breaks between jobs profitably, e.g. with voluntary work. Attends day centre and participates fully	40	31	63
Excellent. Following education to highest level within own ability. Continuous employment. Could be high flyer or someone of lesser ability following stable path in sheltered employment	16	23	0

was excellent, with an intra-class correlation of 0.97. Figure 5.1 shows the distribution of this overall adjustment score, again dichotomizing the sample by IQ – scores of 0–5 can be thought of as poor, 6–10 as fair, 11–15 as good, and 16–20 as excellent. Since individuals with lower IQs were more likely to be rated as poorly adjusted, it is important to emphasize that the adjustment ratings were designed so as not to penalize individuals simply because they had learning difficulties. For example, when rating adjustment in the education/work domain, individuals with learning difficulties could be judged as excellently adjusted to their special colleges or sheltered workplaces.

Table 5.4. Adjustment ratings for activities of daily living (ADLs)

Rating (and illustrative criteria)	Whole sample (n = 81) %	Individuals with IQ ≥ 70 (n = 57) %	Individuals with IQ < 70 (n = 24) %
Seriously impaired. Totally dependent on others for all care needs. Cannot go out alone	5	0	17
Impaired. Highly dependent for help with bathing, washing hair, cutting nails, cutting up food. Requires escort or carer when outside the home	15	3	42
Fair. Moderately dependent for help with personal and domestic tasks. Can make oneself snacks and hot drinks. Able to undertake pre-planned well practised journeys alone	31	30	33
Good. Minimal dependence on others, e.g. some physical tasks, cutting nails. Can plan and organize own transport but sometimes relies on parents or others	22	30	4
Excellent. Independent in all personal and domestic ADLs. Independent with own or public transport	27	37	4

The findings presented in Tables 5.1 to 5.5 support both optimistic and pessimistic conclusions. One optimistic conclusion is that in every domain the psychosocial adjustment of some young adults with hemiplegic CP is good or excellent. Another is that the presence of learning difficulties does not necessarily rule out good or excellent adjustment. These findings provide grounds for optimism when providing a prognosis for the parents of young children with hemiplegic CP, or when answering the questions that teenagers with hemiplegic CP often have about their future. The key message is that hemiplegic CP (with or without learning difficulties) does not necessarily preclude good psychosocial adjustment.

At the same time, the findings also support the pessimistic conclusion that the adjustment of many young adults with hemiplegic CP is poor, particularly if they also have learning difficulties. In the domain of close interpersonal (love) relationships, for example, 56% of individuals of normal intelligence were impaired or seriously impaired, as were 88% of individuals with generalized learning difficulties. At best, this may represent a developmental delay; perhaps

Table 5.5. Adjustment ratings for leisure activities

Rating (and illustrative criteria)	Whole sample (n = 81) %	Individuals with IQ ≥ 70 (n = 57) %	Individuals with IQ < 70 (n = 24) %
Seriously impaired. Mostly alone watching TV, listening to music or playing on computer. Or dependent on others to occupy him/her and structure activity	15	5	37
Impaired. Mostly alone, but occasional group or family activities	37	32	50
Fair. Going out with others most of the time. Sometimes alone not through choice. Participation in family activities not always through choice	22	26	13
Good. Part of a group, sometimes as a pivotal member. Spends leisure time alone or with family through choice	12	18	0
Excellent. Engages in a wide variety of leisure activities alone, with friends and with family	14	19	0

a follow-up into their thirties would find that after a slow start, most adults with hemiplegic CP had adjusted well in this and other domains. At worst, this poor adjustment at the beginning of adulthood may represent the shape of things to come; there are certainly no grounds for complacency.

In summary, although it is encouraging that young adults with hemiplegic CP do not seem to be at particularly high risk of anxiety disorders, depression or schizophrenia, this is only part of the story. The high rate of child psychiatric disorders may contribute to the high rate of maladaptive and restricting personality traits that subsequently interfere with the quality of the individual's life in adulthood. While many young adults with hemiplegic CP lead full and fulfilling lives, others lead unnecessarily restricted lives. Sometimes, this is due to the individual's tendency to withdraw from social situations, perhaps in continuity with earlier separation anxiety. In other instances, earlier irritability and negativism lead on to an abrasive personality style that makes it hard to form and keep friendships. Far too many individuals leave school to live out a very constrained life in the family home, with few opportunities for fulfilment through work, friendships or leisure activities. This is not a necessary conse-

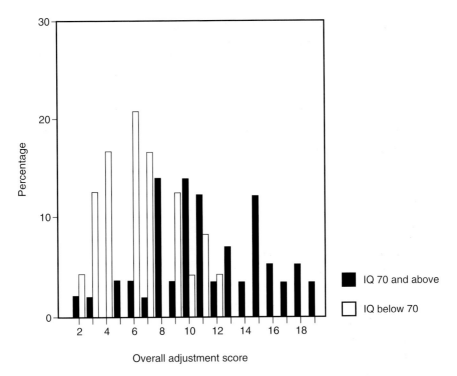

Figure 5.1. Psychosocial adjustment in adulthood by IQ level.

quence of hemiplegic CP even when there are associated problems such as epilepsy or learning difficulties. With appropriate help, some individuals with severe hemiplegia and additional problems are living fulfilling adult lives. Nevertheless, the fact that this is far from universal emphasizes the need for early help when this is called for, and for an education that progressively builds up social and self-help skills in order to prepare each individual for an adult life that is as independent and fulfilling as possible.

The impact on parents

The LHR follow-up study of 18- to 25-year-olds with hemiplegic CP assessed possible impact on parents by asking them to complete the Zarit Burden Inventory (ZBI; Zarit & Zarit, 1990), which is a 22-item scale covering different ways in which caring for a relative might have a negative impact on the carer's life, e.g. resulting in carers being stressed or embarrassed, having too little time for themselves, or having a restricted social life. Each item is scored on a 5-point scale ranging from 'never' (scored 0) to 'nearly always' (scored 4). The total score can therefore range from 0 to 88. Previous studies using the ZBI have mostly looked at the carers of dementing adults.

In the current study, 64 parents completed the ZBI; the mean score was 27 (standard deviation 18). Norms for the ZBI are not available, and would clearly be fairly meaningless since the level of carers' perceived burden is likely to vary markedly with the nature and severity of the relatives' disorder or disability. As a rough guideline to interpretation, however, the results can be compared with a large study of over 300 people caring for dementing relatives. In this study, carers reported a mean score of 44 on the ZBI, with a standard deviation of 16 (Coyne, Reichman & Berbig, 1993). In other words, being the parent of a young adult with hemiplegic CP is generally substantially less burdensome than being the carer for a dementing relative. Nevertheless, it is striking that 22% of the parents in this sample had a burden score of 45 or more, i.e. a fifth of young adults with hemiplegic CP were experienced as more burdensome than an average adult with dementia. Focusing on the ZBI item on possible impact on the carer's health, it is also noteworthy that 14% of the parents in this sample felt that their health had suffered 'quite frequently' or 'nearly always' as a result of their involvement with their son or daughter.

Service-related costs in adult life

The LHR follow-up study of 18- to 25-year-olds with hemiplegic CP was used to calculate the impairment-associated costs in adult life, i.e. the costs related to additional impairment-related use of services provided by health, education, social services and the voluntary sector (Beecham, O'Neill & Goodman, 2001). The average impairment-related cost was estimated to be around £5400 ($8700) each per year at 1996–97 prices. The range of impairment-related costs was wide: zero for a third of the sample, and between £11 ($18) and £43 725 ($70 000) for the remainder – the distribution was very skewed, with nine individuals (11% of the sample) accounting for 71% of the sample's impairment-related costs. The nine high-cost individuals included seven with learning difficulties. Of the two high-cost individuals with an IQ in the normal range, one had an autistic disorder and the other had severe and poorly controlled epilepsy. It is worth emphasizing that all these cost estimates were based on services actually received, i.e. unmet needs cost nothing. Had the estimate been based on the likely expense of providing optimal care packages to each individual, the average cost might well have been substantially higher.

Treatment for psychiatric disorders and poor psychosocial adjustment

In the LHR follow-up, the young adults with hemiplegic CP and their parents were asked whether they thought that additional services were needed. The views of the young adults and their parents were combined to generate a best estimate of client-assessed need. Judging from this 'consumer' perspective, there were unmet needs for psychological services (counsellors, psychologists or psychiatrists) for 23% of individuals. Unfortunately, this consumer perspective cannot be compared with an evidence-based estimate of the need for psychological treatments. The problem is a lack of relevant evidence – there are no treatment-evaluation studies on adults with hemiplegic CP, and neither are there any distillations of clinical experience on the topic (mirroring the virtual absence of specialized services for adults with any form of CP). As described above, in the case of children with hemiplegic CP, clinical experience suggests that although some CP-specific factors do need to be allowed for, psychiatric disorders are often best treated in the same way that they would have been had the child not had CP. It seems plausible that much the same applies to the psychiatric treatment of adults with hemiplegic CP, but for the present this is simply a conjecture rather than an established finding. Setting up specialist clinics for the assessment and treatment of the psychological complications of adults with CP and related life-long neurodisabilities may offer the best chance for acquiring the relevant clinical experience and trial evidence.

REFERENCES

Aicardi, J., Gillberg, C., Ogier, H. & Bax, M. (1998). *Diseases of the Nervous System in Children*, 2nd edn, *Clinics in Developmental Medicine*. London: MacKeith Press.

Austin, J.K., Huster, G.A., Dunn, D.W. & Risinger, M.W. (1996). Adolescents with active or inactive epilepsy or asthma: a comparison of quality of life. *Epilepsia*, **37**: 1228–38.

Balleny, H. (1996). *Are the concepts of 'Theory of Mind' and 'executive function' useful in understanding social impairment in children with hemiplegic cerebral palsy*, Clin Psy D thesis, University of East Anglia, Norwich.

Beecham, J., O'Neill, T. & Goodman, R. (2001). Supporting young adults with hemiplegia: services and costs. *Health and Social Care in the Community*, **9**: 51–9.

Breslau, N. (1985). Psychiatric disorder in children with physical disabilities. *Journal of the American Academy of Child Psychiatry*, **24**: 87–94.

Brett, E.M. (Ed.) (1997). *Paediatric Neurology*, 3rd edn. Edinburgh: Churchill Livingstone.

Coyne, A.C., Reichman, W.E. & Berbig, L.J. (1993). The relationship between dementia and elder abuse. *American Journal of Psychiatry*, **150**: 643–6.

Goldberg, D. & Williams, P. (1988). *A Users Guide to the General Health Questionnaire*. Windsor: NFER-Nelson.

Goodman, R. (1989). Neuronal misconnections and psychiatric disorder: is there a link? *British Journal of Psychiatry*, **154**: 292–9.

Goodman, R. (2002). Brain disorders. In *Child and Adolescent Psychiatry*, 4th edn, ed. M. Rutter, E. Taylor, L. Hersov, pp. 241–60. Oxford: Blackwell Science.

Goodman, R. (1998). The longitudinal stability of psychiatric problems in children with hemiplegia. *Journal of Child Psychology and Psychiatry*, **39**: 347–54.

Goodman, R. & Graham, P. (1996). Psychiatric problems in children with hemiplegia: cross sectional epidemiological survey, *British Medical Journal*, **312**: 1065–9.

Goodman, R., O'Neill, T. & Beecham, J. (1998). Provision for individuals with hemiplegic cerebral palsy: what happens when they outgrow children's services. A final report for the NHS Executive.

Goodman, R. & Scott, S. (1997). *Child Psychiatry*. Oxford: Blackwell Science.

Goodman, R. & Yude, C. (1996). Do incomplete ascertainment and recruitment matter? *Developmental Medicine & Child Neurology*, **38**: 156–65.

Goodman, R. & Yude, C. (1997). Do unilateral lesions of the developing brain have side-specific psychiatric consequences in childhood? *Laterality*, **2**: 103–15.

Goodman, R. & Yude, C. (2000). Emotional, behavioural and social consequences. In *Congenital Hemiplegia: Clinics in Developmental Medicine*, No 150, ed. B.G.R. Neville & R. Goodman, pp. 166–78. London: MacKeith Press.

Happé, F.G.E. (1994). Current psychological theories of autism: the 'Theory of Mind' account and rival theories. *Journal of Child Psychology and Psychiatry*, **35**: 215–29.

Harrington, R., Hill, H., Rutter, M., John, K., Fudge, H., Zoccolillo, M. & Weissman, M. (1988). The assessment of lifetime psychopathology: a comparison of two interviewing styles. *Psychological Medicine*, **18**: 487–93.

Howe, G.W., Feinstein, C., Reiss, D., Molock, S. & Berger, K. (1993). Adolescent adjustment to chronic physical disorders. I. Comparing neurological and non-neurological conditions. *Journal of Child Psychology and Psychiatry*, **34**: 1153–71.

Hutton, J.L., Cooke, T. & Pharoah, P.O.D. (1994). Life expectancy in children with cerebral palsy. *British Medical Journal*, **309**: 431–5.

Ingram, T.T.S. (1955). A study of cerebral palsy in the childhood population of Edinburgh. *Archives of Disease in Childhood*, **30**: 85–98.

Ingram, T.T.S. (1956). A characteristic form of overactive behaviour in brain damaged children. *Journal of Mental Science*, **102**: 550–8.

Krynauw, R.A. (1950). Infantile hemiplegia treated by removing one cerebral hemisphere. *Journal of Neurology, Neurosurgery and Psychiatry*, **13**: 243–67.

McMunn, A., Nazroo J., Primatesta, P. & Bost, L. (1998). *The Health Survey for England 1997*, Chapter 2, Report to the Department of Health. London: Stationery Office.

Menkes, J.H. (1995). *Textbook of Child Neurology*, 5th edn. Philadelphia: Lippincott, Williams & Wilkins.

Neville, B. (2000). Hemispherectomy. In *Congenital Hemiplegia: Clinics in Developmental Medicine*, No. 150, ed. B.G.R. Neville & R. Goodman, pp. 162–5. London: MacKeith Press.

Neville, B.G.R. & Goodman, R. (Eds) (2000). *Congenital Hemiplegia: Clinics in Developmental Medicine*, No 150. London: MacKeith Press.

Ounsted, C. (1955). The hyperkinetic syndrome in epileptic children. *Lancet*, **2**, 303–11.

Ounsted, C., Lindsay, J. & Richards, P. (1987). *Temporal Lobe Epilepsy 1948–1986: A Biographical Study. Clinics in Developmental Medicine*, No. 103. Oxford: Blackwell Scientific Publications.

Rutter, M., Graham, P. & Yule, W. (1970). *A Neuropsychiatric Study in Childhood. Clinics in Developmental Medicine*, Nos 35/36. London: S.I.M.P. with Heinemann.

Scrutton, D. (2000). Physical assessment and aims of treatment. In *Congenital Hemiplegia: Clinics in Developmental Medicine*, No. 150, ed. B.G.R. Neville & R. Goodman, pp. 65–80. London: MacKeith Press.

Seidel, U.P., Chadwick, O.F.D. & Rutter, M. (1975). Psychological disorders in crippled children. A comparative study of children with and without brain damage. *Developmental Medicine & Child Neurology*, **17**: 563–73.

Spitzer, R.L. & Endicott, J. (1975). *Schedule for Affective Disorders and Schizophrenia – Lifetime Version*. New York: Biometrics Research.

Uvebrant, P. (1988). Hemiplegic cerebral palsy aetiology and outcome. *Acta Paediatrica Scandinavica*, Supplement **345**: 1–100.

Yude, C. (2000). Supporting parents of children with hemiplegia. In *Congenital Hemiplegia: Clinics in Developmental Medicine*, No 150, ed. B.G.R. Neville & R. Goodman, London: MacKeith Press.

Yude, C., Goodman R. & McConachie, H. (1998). Peer problems of children with hemiplegia in mainstream primary schools. *Journal of Child Psychology and Psychiatry*, **39**: 533–41.

Zarit, S.H. & Zarit, J.M. (1990). *The Memory and Behavior Problems Checklist and The Burden Interview*. Pennsylvania State University: Gerontology Center.

6

Autistic disorders

Patricia Howlin

Introduction

Autism is a pervasive developmental disorder that is usually apparent from early childhood (Volkmar, Stier & Cohen, 1985). It is characterized by deficits in three domains: communication; social understanding, and rigid and repetitive patterns of behaviour; and it is this *combination* of difficulties that constitutes the basic diagnostic criteria for the disorder (American Psychiatric Association, 1994 – DSM-IV; World Health Organization, 1992 – ICD–10, see Table 6.1).

The condition was first systematically described by Leo Kanner in the United States (US) in 1943, but a remarkably similar account, written by Hans Asperger in Austria, appeared at much the same time (Asperger, 1944; Frith, 1991). Debate continues as to whether autism and Asperger syndrome are quantitatively or qualitatively different (Schopler, Mesibov & Kunce, 1998) and in particular whether Asperger syndrome should be distinguished from high functioning autism (i.e. IQ > 70; Volkmar, Klin & Cohen, 1997). Szatmari, Bartolucci & Bremner (1989a) in a comparative outcome study of 28 individuals with Asperger syndrome and 25 with high functioning autism, concluded that 'there were no substantive, qualitative differences' between them. In contrast, Klin & Volkmar (1997) suggested that there may be certain neuropsychological differences between the two conditions. However, on the basis of present knowledge, it appears that there are few major differences, either in early history or outcome, between these two groups, when IQ is controlled for.

Prevalence and associated features

Once considered to be a very rare condition, affecting only three to four individuals in every 10 000 (Lotter, 1974a,b; Wing & Gould, 1979), recent studies have indicated increasingly higher prevalence rates for autism. Fombonne (1999), in an overview of epidemiological research from 1966 to 1998,

Table 6.1. ICD-10[a] criteria for autism

A. Abnormal or impaired development is evident before the age of 3 years in at least one of the following areas:

   (1) Receptive or expressive language as used in social communication;

   (2) The development of selective social attachments or of reciprocal social interaction;

   (3) Functional or symbolic play.

B. A total of at least six symptoms from (1), (2), and (3) must be present, with at least two from (1) and at least one from each of (2) and (3):

(1) Qualitative abnormalities in reciprocal social interaction are manifest in at least two of the following areas:

   (a) Failure adequately to use eye-to-eye gaze, facial expression, body posture, and gesture to regulate social interaction;

   (b) Failure to develop (in a manner appropriate to mental age, and despite ample opportunities) peer relationships that involve a mutual of interests, activities, and emotions;

   (c) Lack of socio-emotional reciprocity as shown by an impaired or deviant response to other people's emotions; or lack of modulation of behaviour according to social context; or a weak integration of social, emotional, and communicative behaviours;

   (d) Lack of spontaneous seeking to share enjoyment, interests, or achievements with other people (e.g. lack of showing, bringing, or pointing out to other people objects of interest to the individual).

(2) Qualitative abnormalities in communication are manifest in at least one of the following areas:

   (a) Delay in, or total lack of, development of spoken language that is *not* accompanied by an attempt to compensate through the use of gesture or mime as an alternative mode of communication (often preceded by a lack of communicative babbling);

   (b) Relative failure to initiate or sustain conversational interchange (at whatever level of language skills is present), in which there is reciprocal responsiveness to the communications of the other person;

   (c) Stereotyped and repetitive use of language or idiosyncratic use of words or phrases;

   (d) Lack of varied spontaneous make-believe or (when young) social imitative play.

(3) Restricted, repetitive, and stereotyped patterns of behaviour, interests, and activities are manifest in at least one of the following areas:

   (a) An encompassing preoccupation with one or more stereotyped, restricted patterns of interest that are abnormal in content or focus; or one or more interests that are abnormal in their intensity and circumscribed nature though not in their content or focus;

   (b) Apparently compulsive adherence to specific, non-functional routines or rituals;

   (c) Stereotyped and repetitive motor mannerisms that involve either hand or finger flapping or twisting, or complex whole body movements.

   (d) Preoccupations with part-objects or non-functional elements of play materials (such as their odour,the feel of their surface, or the noise or vibration that they generate).

The clinical picture is not attributable to the other varieties of pervasive developmental disorders; specific developmental disorder of receptive language with secondary socio-emotional problems; reactive attachment disorder or disinhibited attachment disorder; mental retardation with some associated emotional or behavioural disorder; schizophrenia of unusually early onset; and Rett syndrome.

[a] WHO (1992).

concluded that prevalence for pervasive developmental disorders is around 18.7 per 10 000. This figure does *not* include cases with Asperger syndrome, and statistics published by the National Autistic Society (1997) suggest that if these are included the rate rises to around 91 per 10 000 – i.e. almost 1% of the population. Whilst the research studies on which some of these data are based are open to criticism (mainly because they involve small samples, which tend to yield higher prevalence rates; Fombonne, 1999), it is clear that autism-related disorders are far more common than once thought. The clinical implications of this, for both child and adult services are evident.

As with almost any condition affecting language-related skills, autism is far more common in males than females. The overall ratio is around 4 : 1 (Fombonne, 1999), but amongst those who are more able or have a diagnosis of Asperger syndrome the gender imbalance is even more marked (possibly in excess of 9 : 1; Howlin & Ashgarian, 1999).

Autism is also significantly associated with intellectual disability. Although the syndrome can occur in individuals of all levels of ability, the majority (about 80%; Fombonne, 1999) has some associated learning disabilities and around 50% have an IQ below 50. Non-verbal IQ scores are typically higher than verbal IQ scores, but this pattern may change with age, and in older, more able individuals verbal IQ scores may be similar to performance IQ (Mawhood, Howlin & Rutter, 2000). The level of intellectual impairment is also closely correlated with the development of language. In those with severe to profound cognitive impairments useful speech is unlikely to develop, but the expressive skills of individuals with an IQ in the normal range usually develop relatively well, even though initially there may have been significant delays.

Causes

Although associated with a range of possible causes, genetic factors are now considered to be implicated in the majority of cases (Bailey, Phillips & Rutter, 1996; International Molecular Genetic Study of Autism Consortium, 1998, 2001; Szatmari et al., 1998). The exact mechanisms involved are far from being understood but it is evident that autism is not a single gene disorder. Probably three or more genes are likely to be involved (Pickles et al., 1995) and many possible chromosome sites have been suggested (Gillberg, 1998). Chromosomes 7q and 15q have been implicated in a number of research investigations, and there may also be associations with 10q, 16q and 17p (Lauritsen et al., 1999). However, far more extensive family research studies are required in order to confirm these findings (Folstein et al., 1998; Maestrini et al., 1998). There is no evidence that medical conditions play a major aetiological role

(Rutter et al., 1994) and these are probably significant only in around 6% of cases (Fombonne, 1999). Although prenatal and obstetric complications are relatively common, these are now thought to be linked to genetic factors influencing fetal development (Bailey et al., 1996). The postulated links with conditions such as phenylketonuria, neurofibromatosis and congenital rubella are also considered to be tenuous (Lord & Rutter, 1994) and although these may sometimes co-occur with autism the picture is generally atypical. The fragile X anomaly has been identified in a small minority of cases, but again the association is weaker than originally suggested (Rutter et al., 1994). The most significant relationship is with tuberous sclerosis and it is estimated that 40–50% of cases with this disorder meet criteria for autism (Smalley, 1998). The association is particularly marked among individuals with tubers in the temporal lobes (de Vries & Bolton, Chapter 11). There are no data to support claims that the MMRI vaccine can cause autism (Taylor et al., 1999). Neither, despite early suggestions by Kanner (1943) that inadequate parenting might be responsible, is there evidence that environmental factors play a significant causal role. The one possible exception is children who are raised in conditions of extreme physical and emotional deprivation, as was the case of the Romanian orphans, legally adopted into British families and followed up by Rutter and colleagues (1999). At the age of 4 years, 6% of these children exhibited 'quasi' autistic features. However, by 6 years most of the cases who were not also severely cognitively delayed no longer met criteria for autism on the Autism Diagnostic Interview (ADI; Lord, Rutter & Le Couteur, 1994).

Early indicators

In the majority of cases the first signs of autism are apparent in infancy (Howlin & Moore, 1997) and many parents have serious concerns about their child's development in the first year of life (Gillberg et al., 1990; Frith, Soares & Wing, 1993; Smith, Chung & Vostanis, 1994). These early anxieties tend to focus around abnormalities in communication, play, social responsiveness, or more general behavioural difficulties; marked ritualistic and repetitive behaviours are less likely to be apparent in the early years (Frith et al., 1993; Smith et al., 1994; De Giacomo & Fombonne, 1998; Howlin & Ashgarian, 1999).

Autism-specific problems

Although autism is associated with a range of behavioural difficulties, including aggression, temper-tantrums, destructiveness, toileting, and eating and sleeping difficulties, these also occur in many other developmental disorders. The primary causes of many common or 'challenging' behaviours in autism can often be traced back to the more fundamental, syndrome-specific problems that characterize the disorder, and it is these that are the focus of the following section (see Howlin, 1998, for further details).

Communication difficulties

It is estimated that around half of all children with autism fail to develop functional speech (Lord & Rutter, 1994). Many of these will have little or no understanding of spoken language, and will fail to develop any compensatory use of gesture. There is also a significant minority of children (probably around 20%, Lord & Bailey, 2001) who seem to develop single word speech normally but then, sometime between 15 and 30 months, cease to make further progress and lose the vocabulary previously acquired. Although a minority of these cases later regains language, their communication skills tend to remain relatively impaired (Howlin, 1998).

Amongst children with autism who do develop language, the acquisition of first words or phrases is usually delayed, although some more able children may acquire speech around the normal age. There are also many unusual features, including repetitive and stereotyped language; semantic errors, such as neologisms and pronoun reversal; abnormalities in voice tone and modulation, and often a formal and pedantic style of speaking. The most characteristic deficit, however, whatever the individual's level of ability, is the lack of reciprocal conversation and the failure to use communication for purely *social* purposes. Receptive language is often much poorer than expressive ability; interpretation of speech may be very literal, and abstract concepts present particular difficulties. Imaginative play, also, is usually extremely limited.

Social abnormalities

Although the nature and extent of social difficulties may vary between individuals, and may also change with age (Wing & Gould, 1979), certain core features tend to prevail whatever the child's developmental level. These include impairments in non-verbal communication (gesture, eye-gaze, greeting behaviours, etc.), lack of reciprocity, impaired empathy, failure to share enjoyment or activities with others and, in particular, an inability to understand other people's feelings, beliefs or emotions, or to respond to these in an appropriate way. This 'mindblindness' (Baron-Cohen, 1995) permeates all social interactions, affecting very able children as well as those who are most handicapped. Because of their lack of appreciation of social rules, the behaviour of both children and adults with autism may often be unacceptable or even offensive to others, and very few are ever able to develop close reciprocal relationships, especially with their peers.

Ritualistic and stereotyped interests or behaviours

Problems in this area also span a wide range, and again vary according to the child's intellectual level. Stereotyped motor behaviours, such as rocking, hand flapping, spinning, flicking, or lining up objects are characteristic of children who are more severely cognitively handicapped. There is also a greater risk of this group developing self injurious behaviours, such as head banging, eye-poking, skin picking and biting (Hall, 1997).

Some children insist on acquiring extensive collections of particular objects (e.g. leaves of a particular shape, Thomas the Tank Engine trains, Mr. Bean videos, woodlice, coke cans, and many, many others). Although the type of object collected is not necessarily unusual, it is the number of items collected, or the child's overwhelming interest in these that gives rise to problems. Many young children with autism also develop intense attachments to certain objects, often of an unusual nature. If these are lost, broken, or otherwise unobtainable severe distress may result. Insistence on routines and marked resistance to change can also lead to severe disruption to normal family life. Some children become distraught by even minor changes to their environment (such as an ornament being moved or a door left open at a different angle). Occasionally, too, compulsive behaviours involving handwashing or constant checking can emerge in later childhood, as may obsessional and intrusive thoughts.

More able children often try to involve other people in their rituals and verbal routines and questioning can be especially difficult to deal with. This group is also more likely to develop intense preoccupations with certain topics, often collecting *facts* rather than objects, and they may acquire a vast amount of knowledge in their particular area. Even when these interests appear to be age appropriate, as for example in sport or computers, their intensity is such that they may still become extremely disruptive.

Autism in adulthood

Initial follow-up studies of adults with autism were largely anecdotal and unsystematic but towards the end of the 1960s Rutter and his colleagues conducted a detailed assessment of 38 young adults first diagnosed as autistic during the 1950s and 1960s. At follow-up (age 16 + years) only three had paid jobs; over half were in long stay hospitals; seven were still living with their parents, with no outside occupation; three were living in special communities; and four attended day centres. However, most had shown improvements in their behaviour as they grew older, and Rutter noted 'it was rare to see marked remissions and relapses as in adult psychotic illnesses'. (See Rutter, Greenfield & Lockyer, 1967; Rutter & Lockyer, 1967; Lockyer & Rutter, 1969, 1970).

Although several other follow-up studies have been conducted since then, many include both children and adults, which makes it difficult to reach clear conclusions about long-term prognosis. Of those that have focused on individuals aged at least 16 years or over (Lotter, 1974a,b; Gillberg & Steffenberg, 1987; Kobayashi, Murata & Yashinaga, 1992) there has been an indication in recent years of some improvements in outcome (Howlin & Goode, 1998), but the majority of individuals remains very dependent on their families for support; rates of employment are low (typically under 25%), and overall ratings of level of functioning are generally in the 'poor' to 'very poor' range. As in Rutter's earlier study, many families note considerable improvements when children are aged between 10 and 15 years, although some (up to 23% in the Japanese survey of Kobayashi et al., 1992) report deterioration in behaviour (such as destructiveness, aggression, self-injury, obsessionality, overactivity, etc) around early adolescence.

In the most detailed of these recent studies, S. Goode, P. Howlin and M. Rutter (unpub. data) followed up 75 individuals (64 males and 11 females), all aged 21 years or over, who had originally been diagnosed in childhood. Eight individuals were living independently or semi-independently, but 25 were still with their parents and 19 lived in sheltered communities, mostly specifically for people with autism; another 10 were in long-stay hospital care. Only eight people were in regular, paid employment; one was self-employed, four others worked in a voluntary capacity, and 10 were in some form of sheltered or supported employment. Two-thirds (50) attended day or residential centres. Few individuals had close friends and although two men had married, one had later divorced. A composite rating of outcome, based on social interactions, level of independence and occupational status, indicated that around 15% (11) could be described as having a 'good' or 'very good' outcome and 21% (16) were rated as functioning moderately well. The remainder of the group was highly dependent, living either in special residential units or long-term hospital care.

There have also been a number of accounts focusing specifically on individuals with Asperger syndrome or high functioning autism (Rumsey, Rapoport & Sceery, 1985; Szatmari et al., 1989b; Lord & Venter, 1992; Howlin, Mawhood &

Rutter, 2000; Mawhood et al., 2000). Sample sizes are generally small (between 14 and 22) but most of the people involved remained socially isolated and continued to show some communication problems. Few had married or entered into a sexual relationship and close, intimate friendships were rare. With access to some form of day centre or to sheltered or supported employment, few individuals were without any daytime occupation, but only a minority was in regular employment and those jobs that did exist were generally low level and poorly paid. In all the studies, most people were still living with their parents and, with the exception of some individuals in the Szatmari group, almost none lived entirely independently. Despite the relatively high IQ levels of the individuals involved, attainments generally were poor. Rumsey et al. (1985) noted that scores on the Vineland Social Maturity Scale were 'strikingly' low and that socially inappropriate behaviours were common. Mawhood et al. (2000) also found that obsessional and ritualistic tendencies continued to give rise to problems. Amongst their group of 19 men in their mid-twenties, composite rating of outcome, based on communication skills, friendships, levels of independence and behavioural difficulties indicated that, overall, only three individuals were considered to have a good outcome; two remained moderately impaired and 14 continued to show substantial impairments. Lord & Venter (1992) comment on the very variable outcome between individuals, and although generally prognosis in autism is determined by innate cognitive and linguistic abilities, they conclude that for adults of this level outcome may be influenced more by the availability of adequate support networks than by individual skills.

Factors related to outcome

In almost all follow-up studies two variables have been consistently associated with later prognosis. The first is the level of language attained by 5–6 years of age – very few of those who remain without speech after this age are reported to have a positive outcome. The second crucial prognostic indicator is IQ. Individuals who are either untestable as children, or who have non-verbal IQ scores within or below the moderately retarded range, almost invariably remain highly dependent. However, relatively good cognitive and communication skills do not necessarily guarantee a successful outcome (Howlin et al. 2000). The presence of *additional* skills or interests, such as specialized knowledge or competence in particular areas (e.g. mathematics, music or computing), which allow individuals to find their own 'niche' in life and which may enable them to be more easily integrated into society, also seems to be of prognostic importance (Kanner, 1973).

Educational placement is another major factor, with the best outcomes generally reported for children who receive mainstream education. However, since this is directly affected by individuals' linguistic and cognitive levels, the influence of schooling, per se, on long-term functioning remains unclear.

The possible impact of many other variables remains uncertain. Although in almost every follow-up study outcome has been poorer for females than males, the number of women involved is generally very small and differences rarely reach significance (Goode et al., unpub. data); the lower IQ of females further complicates the issue (Lord & Schopler, 1985).

The relationship between the severity of autistic symptomatology in early childhood and later outcome is also unclear. Rutter and colleagues (Rutter & Lockyer, 1967; Lockyer & Rutter, 1969, 1970) found no significant correlation between individual symptoms in childhood (other than lack of speech) and adult outcome, although there was a significant relationship with the total number of major symptoms rated. DeMeyer et al. (1973) also reported a relationship between overall severity of autistic symptoms and later progress. However, Lord & Venter (1992) did not find an association between prognosis and total number of early symptoms as rated on the ADI. Of greater predictive value were the degree of language *abnormality* and the level of disruption caused by stereotyped and repetitive behaviours.

In some studies, the development of epilepsy in people with autism seemed to predict a poorer outcome, but again epilepsy is associated to some extent with low IQ in this group. Socio-economic factors and ratings of family adequacy have also been correlated with prognosis in some studies (DeMeyer et al., 1973; Lotter, 1974a). There is little evidence of a direct causal relationship between an impoverished or disruptive family background and later outcome, although, as with any other condition, disruption at home is unlikely to be beneficial.

Do follow-up studies indicate improvements in prognosis over time?

Noting that 11–12% of his original sample had done well in the absence of any specialist intervention or support, Kanner speculated that the outcome for people with autism might well improve in future years as recognition of the disorder, and knowledge about causation, and appropriate educational and therapeutic facilities progressed. A comparison of outcome studies conducted between the 1960s and 1990s suggested that prognosis may have improved with time (Howlin, 1998). However, because of the different ways in which data have been collected, the findings are very variable.

One area in which real improvements appear to have taken place is in the proportion of individuals placed in long-stay hospitals or institutions for people with mental retardation. Over half of all cases in outcome studies pre–1980 were in long-stay hospitals, whereas in the period after 1980 the figure falls to around 8%. There has been a substantial increase, too, in the numbers living independently or with only minimal support. Among the pre–1980 studies, only Kanner's anecdotal report describes any individuals living in their own homes. In the post–1980 studies an average of around 12% had their own homes. This may not be a particularly high figure but it is certainly a great improvement over earlier years.

Work prospects too, seem to have improved, with the average proportion in work rising from around 5% before 1980 to over 20% in the later studies. This figure is even higher if sheltered workshop placements are included, and now few individuals have no access to daytime programmes.

Problems related to adulthood

Behavioural deterioration and/or loss of skills

Generally, the risk of deterioration in adulthood seems to be greater in individuals who are of low IQ and/or who develop epilepsy (Nordin & Gillberg, 1998). Many more able people with autism show significant improvements with age (cf Kanner, 1973). Piven et al. (1995), in a study of 38 high functioning individuals, compared functioning at age 5 years (as reported retrospectively on the ADI) with current functioning when aged between 13 and 28 years. Composite ADI scores for communication and social functioning had improved in 82% of cases and 55% showed improvement in ritualistic/stereotyped behaviours. There was no significant difference in the pattern or extent of change shown by males and females.

Epilepsy

It is estimated that around one-third of individuals with autism develop epilepsy, with onset often occurring in adolescence or early adulthood. Gillberg (1992) suggests that the most common form of seizure disorder is complex-partial (psychomotor) epilepsy. The incidence tends to be greater in individuals of lower IQ, with the rates being highest in those with severe to profound learning difficulties. If these groups are excluded, the overall rate is around 17–20% (Tantam, 1991; Goode, Rutter & Howlin, 1994; Fombonne, 1999), with there being little difference between individuals of normal IQ and those with moderate learning disabilities.

Some adolescents or young adults may have one or two isolated fits but no more, and because of the disadvantages of giving unnecessary medication, drugs are often not prescribed unless there is evidence of more frequent attacks. There is no evidence to suggest that successful control of epilepsy is particularly difficult to achieve for people with autism. However, because individuals are unlikely to report unwanted side effects themselves, careful monitoring of their response to treatment is particularly important.

Mortality

Although Gillberg (1991) has suggested that mortality rates in people with autism below the age of 30 years may be substantially increased (from 0.6% in the general population to almost 2% in autism), Isager, Mouridsen & Rich (1999) concluded that mortality rates from childhood to early/middle adult-hood in autism were not significantly higher than in the general population. Nevertheless, in a 25-year study of 324 patients with autism and related disorders (mean age 31 years) the same authors reported a crude mortality rate of 3.4%, considerably higher than the figure for non-autistic males of the same age. Death rates were higher in those of low IQ, and were often associated with epilepsy. Death in the three 'normal IQ' individuals in the study was in one case due to suicide; in another, accidental drug overdose; and in the third pneumonia (associated with Hodgkin's disease). Deaths reported in other studies have resulted from a range of different causes including head injury as a result of severe self-injury, encephalopathy, nephritic syndrome and asthma (Kobayashi et al., 1992). A number of accidental deaths (e.g. from traffic accidents) has been reported amongst more able individuals (Kanner, 1973; Larsen & Mouridsen, 1997).

Psychiatric disorders
Schizophrenia

Kanner's early views on the relationship between autism and schizophrenia were unequivocal: 'I do not believe that there is any likelihood that early infantile autism will at any future time have to be separated from the schizophrenias' (Kanner, 1949). Nevertheless, Rutter (1972) and Wing (1986) have documented many crucial differences between the two conditions. And although some researchers (e.g. Wolff & McGuire, 1995) have suggested an association between Asperger syndrome and schizoid disorders, this view is largely unsupported (Wing, 1986).

That is not to say, of course, that autism and schizophrenia never co-exist. Wolff & McGuire (1995) noted that 2 out of 17 girls and 2 out of 32 males with a *possible* diagnosis of Asperger syndrome (they were initially diagnosed as 'schizoid') later developed schizophrenia. Clarke and colleagues (Clarke et al., 1989, 1999) identified two cases of schizophrenia amongst 11 men with autism, and Wing (1981) noted one case with an unconfirmed diagnosis of schizophrenia among eight individuals with Asperger syndrome. Petty et al. (1984) also described three cases in whom early onset schizophrenia seems to have been preceded by autism. There is also a number of single case reports on the comorbidity of the two conditions (Szatmari et al., 1986; Sverd, Montero & Gurevich, 1993; and see review by Clarke et al., 1999).

However, larger scale studies of children and adults with autism have failed to find any evidence of increased rates of schizophrenia (Chung, Luk & Lee, 1990; Ghaziuddin, Tsai & Ghaziuddin, 1992). None of the cases followed up by Kanner, over a period of 40 years, was reported as showing positive psychiatric symptoms (delusions or hallucinations). Rumsey et al. (1985), in a detailed psychiatric study of 14 young adults found no evidence of schizophrenia and Volkmar & Cohen (1991) found only one individual with an unequivocal diagnosis of schizophrenia in a sample of 163 cases. In Goode's study of 75 adults with autism, all over 21 years of age, none had developed a schizophrenic illness (Howlin & Goode, 1998).

Schizophrenia also appears to be relatively uncommon amongst more able individuals or those with Asperger syndrome. Asperger noted that only one out of his 200 cases developed schizophrenia (Frith, 1991). Tantam (1991) diagnosed three cases of schizophrenia in 83 individuals with Asperger syndrome but these were all psychiatric referrals. None of the 19 relatively able subjects in the study by Mawhood et al. (2000) had developed a schizophrenic disorder and only one individual in a similar group studied by Szatmari et al. (1989b) was being treated for chronic schizophrenia.

Other psychotic conditions

Although the presence of first rank schizophrenic symptoms is relatively unusual, there are reports of individuals who show isolated psychotic symptoms, including paranoid and delusional thoughts. One young man described by Wing (1981) could not be deterred from his conviction that some day Batman was going to come and take him away as his assistant. Clarke et al. (1989) reported on another case of delusional disorder and one with an unspecified psychosis. Szatmari et al. (1989b) noted several cases of paranoid thinking or possible hallucinations, whilst Tantam described four patients with hallucinations, one with epileptic psychosis and two with obsessive compulsive disorders. Szatmari et al. (1989b) and Rumsey et al. (1985) also identified a number of cases of obsessional or compulsive disorder although Szatmari cautioned: 'We found it very difficult ... to distinguish between obsessive ideation and the bizarre preoccupations so commonly seen in autistic individuals'.

Affective disorders

As early as 1970, Rutter noted the risk of depressive episodes occurring in adolescents or older individuals with autism. Other authors have also reported a high frequency of affective disorders (see Tantam, 1991; Lainhart & Folstein, 1994; Clarke et al., 1999). Tantam (1991) comments that in several cases the illness incorporated a delusional content, often linked with the individual's autistic preoccupations. One man, for example, had thrown himself into the river Thames because the UK government refused to abolish British Summer Time and he believed that watches were damaged by the necessity of being altered twice a year.

Wing (1981) also found that just under a quarter of her group of 18 individuals with Asperger syndrome showed signs of an affective disorder. Three had attempted suicide or talked about doing so. One young man, who had become very distressed by minor changes in his work routine, tried to drown himself but failed because he was a good swimmer. When he tried to strangle himself the attempt also failed because, as he said, 'I am not a very practical person'. Wolff & McGuire (1995) noted that death from suicide was greater in their sample of 'schizoid' individuals (several of whom probably had Asperger syndrome) than in the general population and 10 out of 17 women and 17 out of 32 men had attempted suicide. In the follow-up study by Rumsey et al. (1985) of 14 relatively high functioning individuals, generalized anxiety problems were found in half the sample. Six individuals also showed occasional outbursts of temper, aggression or destructiveness.

Although few hard data are available it is often suggested that the incidence of depressive and anxiety related disorders is especially high amongst individuals with Asperger syndrome. Although sometimes (wrongly) described as a 'mild' variant of autism, the symptoms of Asperger syndrome are, in many cases, just as pervasive and as devastating as those of less able individuals. However, because of their relatively high cognitive ability and *apparently* competent use of language, this group is often least well served or understood. In fact, many individuals have extensive linguistic and comprehension difficulties (especially involving abstract or complex concepts); their understanding of the more subtle aspects of social interaction is often profoundly limited, and their obsessional interests and behaviours may also prove a barrier to social integration. Others' expectations of their social and academic potential tend to be unrealistically high, and when these expectations are not met individuals

Table 6.2. Patterns of diagnosis in cases of autism referred for psychiatric disorder

Total cases[a]	112	%
Psychiatric Diagnoses:		
Psychotic depression	31	28
Bipolar	17	15
Mania/manic episodes	6	5
Other affective disorders (n.o.s.)	18	16
Total affective	72	64
Schizophrenia	13	12
Possible/unconfirmed schizophrenia	4	3.5
Other psychosis (n.o.s.)	4	3.5
Hallucinations/delusions/paranoid thoughts	7	6
Severe withdrawal/catatonia	7	6
Obsessive–compulsive disorder	5	4

[a] Figures based on reviews by Lainhart & Folstein, 1994; Clarke et al., 1999; plus cases reported by Sverd et al., 1993; Rumsey et al., 1985; Szatmari et al., 1989b; Tantam, 1991; Larsen & Mouridsen 1997; Howlin et al., 2000; S. Goode, P. Howlin & H. Rutter (unpub. data).

may be viewed as lazy, lacking in motivation, rude and insensitive. Seemingly so close to 'normality', there is constant pressure for them to 'fit in', in ways that would never be demanded of those who are less able. This can lead to enormous pressure and sometimes intolerable levels of anxiety and stress.

Rates of psychiatric illness

No epidemiological studies of psychiatric morbidity in individuals with autism exist, and hence any estimates must be treated with caution because of problems of sampling and referral bias. However, in an attempt to obtain a clearer picture of the comparative rates of different disorders, the author reviewed 112 clinical case reports (see Table 6.2 for details). This indicated that by far the most common psychiatric diagnosis reported was psychotic depression. This accounted for over a quarter of diagnoses in the studies reviewed and a further 16% were non-specific affective disorders, mostly related to anxiety and depression. Bipolar disorders and mania were the next most common types of disorder, occurring in about 20% of the cases. In the autistic population as a whole, Abramson et al. (1992) suggested that the overall risk of affective disorders is around 33%, a figure similar to Tantam's (1991) combined estimate of the rates for mania (9%), depression (15%) and clinically significant anxiety disorders (7%).

Schizophrenic type diagnoses in the cases reviewed were much less frequent, representing around 12% of all psychiatric diagnoses. Volkmar & Cohen (1991) suggested that the frequency of schizophrenia in individuals with autism is around 0.6%, which is roughly comparable to that in the general population. They concluded that, 'it does not appear that the two conditions are more commonly observed together than would be expected on a chance basis' and there is certainly little evidence to support claims of 'an excess of schizophrenia in later life' (cf Wolff & McGuire, 1995).

In summary, despite a lack of epidemiological data, it is evident that individuals with autistic disorders are at considerable risk of developing depressive and anxiety related illnesses in later life. The difficulties inherent in making a valid diagnosis of psychosis in people with autism also need to be recognized. Impoverished language, literal interpretation of questions, concrete thinking and obsessionality can all give rise to misunderstandings, and possible misdiagnosis, especially in the case of individuals who appear relatively able. For those with more severe intellectual disabilities and little or no speech, the danger is that psychiatric illness will go undiagnosed, even when serious problems arise.

More research into psychiatric conditions in adulthood is badly needed, not only to identify the true level of risk, but also to improve knowledge amongst clinicians about how psychiatric disorders in this group are manifest. It is particularly important for clinicians working in adult services to be aware that autism and psychiatric illnesses can co-exist. However, differential diagnosis cannot be made on the basis of a single face-to-face interview, and a detailed developmental history from parents (or someone who has known the individual well since childhood) will be required in order to distinguish between behaviours caused by the autism and those caused by the additional psychiatric disorder. Better understanding of appropriate intervention strategies, both pharmacological and psychological, is also required. Clinical experience suggests that delays in diagnosing and treating psychiatric disorders in this group are particularly undesirable as behaviour patterns that are established during the course of the illness (e.g. disturbed waking and sleeping patterns) can then be very difficult to alter, even when the patient's condition generally has improved.

Forensic problems

There is little evidence of any excess of crimes amongst more able people with autism, despite occasional and sometimes lurid media publicity suggesting otherwise. However, isolated incidents of offending, often related to obsessional tendencies or impaired social understanding, have been reported. These include injuries to others resulting from an obsession with conducting experiments (Wing, 1981; Tantam, 1991), and attacks on infants and young women apparently associated with a 44-year-old man's preoccupation with finding a girl friend, his dislike of certain styles of dress and the noise of crying (Mawson, Grounds & Tantam, 1985). 'Sexual offending' in the young man with Asperger syndrome described by Chesterman & Rutter (1994) related mainly to his obsession with washing machines and women's night-dresses. A number of cases of arson has also been reported (Everall & Le Couteur, 1990; Tantam, 1991). Tantam (1991) noted that in the group whom he studied, violence, in a fight, in an explosion of rage or in sexual excitement was rare, and property offences were uncommon except as the 'side-effects of the pursuit of a special interest'. Sexual offending, too, was unusual, although some individuals got into trouble for indecent exposure.

Because offending by individuals with autism often seems to be associated with lack of social understanding, rigidity of behaviour or obsessional interests, the crimes committed may be of an unusual or bizarre nature. For example, there is Baron-Cohen's (1988) account of a 21-year-old man who had, over a period of several years violently assaulted his 71-year-old 'girl-friend'. Wing (1986) described one individual who attempted to drive away an unattended railway engine because of an obsession with trains and another who caused explosions and fires because of a preoccupation with chemical reactions. Occasionally, too, crimes are unwittingly, or unwillingly, committed at the instigation of others, such as the young man who was forced by a local gang to lay concrete blocks across a railway line, and another who was coerced into handing over the keys of the jewellery shop where he worked as a janitor (Howlin, 1997).

The only relatively large-scale study of offending by individuals with autism or Asperger syndrome was conducted by Scragg & Shah (1994), who assessed the entire male population of Broadmoor Special Hospital, in the UK. Using a variety of measures they identified nine cases with autism or Asperger syndrome out of a total of 392 patients – a prevalence rate of just over 2%. The offences committed included violence or threats of violence, unlawful killing (including one case of matricide) and fire setting. Six individuals had a fascination with poisons, weapons, murder books or combat. Because the number of patients with an autistic disorder was higher than predicted on the basis of population data, the authors suggest that there is an association with criminality and violence. A similar conclusion was reached by Mawson et al. (1985). However, it is clearly invalid to base estimates of pathology on either single cases or studies of highly selected individuals. Ghaziuddin, Tsai & Ghaziuddin (1991) concluded that the incidence of violence or other offences by people with autism or Asperger syndrome is actually very small. In a review of 132 reports of people with Asperger syndrome, they found that only the three described by Wing (1981), Baron-Cohen (1988) and Mawson et al. (1985) had a clear history of violent behaviour. There may well be more people with autism in prisons or secure accommodation than is realized (Scragg & Shah, 1994) and it is clearly important that such individuals are correctly identified and treated. Nevertheless, in the absence of epidemiological research, there is no reason to suppose that people with autistic disorders are more prone to offending than anyone else. Indeed, because of the very rigid way in which many tend to keep to rules and regulations, they may well be more law-abiding than the population generally.

Similarly, although there are no data on alcohol or drug abuse in autism, many high functioning individuals with autism seem to make strenuous attempts to avoid drugs of any kind (sometimes including those prescribed for a medical condition). Instead, they may get themselves into trouble for remonstrating with people who are smoking or drinking. However, given the rigidity of behaviour patterns in autism, it also seems that if drug or alcohol habits become established, these can then be extremely difficult to modify.

Interventions for autism

Over the past 50 years various treatments have been claimed significantly to improve outcome, or even bring about a 'cure' for autism. Among these are Holding Therapy, music therapy, Scotopic Sensitivity training, Facilitated Communication, Auditory Integration training, Conductive Education, Daily Life Therapy, Gentle Teaching, the Options Method, and the Waldon approach (see Howlin, 1998 for review). Reports on the extraordinary effects of other therapies, including swimming with dolphins, cranial osteopathy, or being swung around in nets, also make regular appearances in the press (Muller, 1993). Unfortunately, few of these methods have been subject to any form of experimental investigation. Amongst those that have, Facilitated Communication is now generally discredited (cf Bebko, Perry & Bryson, 1996; American Psychological Association, August 1994), and Auditory Integration therapy has been found to have no positive effects (Mudford et al., 2000).

Many different drug and vitamin interventions have also been claimed to produce significant improvements. However, again, adequate experimental research is limited and there is little, if any, information about long-term sequelae, especially when very young children are involved. Fenfluramine, for example, which throughout much of the 1980s was widely used as the drug treatment of choice for autism in the USA, has now been largely withdrawn because of concerns about serious side effects and potential long-term damage. Another recent treatment, extensively publicized on the Internet, involves the use of secretin infusions, which have been claimed to have almost 'miraculous' effects (Horvath et al., 1998; Rimland, 1998). However, an increasing number of parents are now beginning to report severe, adverse side-effects, and initial controlled trials (Sandler et al., 1999; Chez et al., 2000) indicate few differences in short-term outcome between children receiving secretin and those given placebo injections.

Why do families seek 'alternative' therapies?

Before simply dismissing 'alternative' approaches as unscientific nonsense, clinicians need to ask themselves why such diverse therapies appeal so strongly to some families. Firstly, most offer parents clear and explicit guidelines on what they themselves can do to help their child and they are encouraged to expect significant improvements (even though these expectations may some-times be unrealistic). In addition, parents are often given far more time, care and individual attention than is usually offered by hard pressed professionals working in state-run health, educational or social services. It is also important to recognize that most of these approaches use therapeutic strategies that will be of practical help for at least some of the children who undergo them. The emphasis on physical contact or exercise involved in Holding Therapy, Conductive Education or Daily Life Therapy may benefit many children. The focus on communication skills and the emphasis on augmentative forms of communication are positive features of Facilitated Communication. The use of ritualistic behaviours as rewards, or as a means of establishing the child's co-operation is an undoubted strength of the Options Method. Music therapy may be an excellent way of encouraging reciprocity, and programmes that emphasize more effective ways of integrating sensory input may be of value for others. Similarly, the avoidance of aversive procedures whenever possible and the emphasis on personal worth, as embodied in Gentle Teaching, are important factors in any intervention.

Crucially, however, it is evident that far too many families experience enormous difficulties in obtaining information about local facilities or schools (Howlin & Moore, 1997). It may be easier for parents to find out about 'exotic' therapies, such as swimming with dolphins (via the media or the Internet) than it is to access accurate information about appropriate nursery schools in their own neighbourhood. Better documented, and more readily available information about the benefits that local schools, units or therapy centres may be able to offer, could well prevent unnecessary wastage of parents' time and money.

Pre-school interventions

Studies of home-based interventions, specifically designed for young children with autism (Lovaas, 1987; Howlin & Rutter, 1987), indicated that if parents can be helped to develop appropriately structured and consistent management strategies from the outset this can enhance social, cognitive and linguistic development and minimize later behavioural problems. Specialist school programmes also have positive effects (see Rogers, 1996). The most successful interventions appear to involve intensive support (of 15 or more hours per week), tend to last at least 6 months, and require a high adult:child ratio. However, because of problems in methodology and research design, conclusions about their effectiveness, especially in the longer term, remain limited. Progress appears to be enhanced if intervention begins before the child is 5 years of age but there is no information on exactly how early programmes should begin. Similarly, although some research indicates that IQ and language are important predictive variables, with the most handicapped children making least progress, other studies have found no relationship between pre-treatment level and outcome.

Intensive home-based behavioural programmes

One of the most controversial approaches to early intervention has been the home-based behavioural programme of Lovaas (1987). Therapy, which is provided on a 1:1 basis for 40 or more hours a week and lasts for at least 2 years, is claimed to bring about 'recovery' from autism (Perry, Cohen & DeCarlo, 1995). Children involved are reported to have shown large and significant gains in IQ (of 30 points or more), rates of integration into mainstream school are high and around 40% are said to have achieved 'normal functioning', with the improvements persisting into early adolescence (McEachin, Smith & Lovaas, 1993). Although methodologically stronger than other early intervention projects, there have been criticisms concerning the experimental design and particular controversy over the use of terms such as 'recovery' or 'normal functioning' (see Mesibov, 1993; Gresham & MacMillan, 1998). The few 'replication' studies that have been conducted have generally used a modified design, with smaller numbers of children (e.g. Sheinkopf & Siegel, 1998), and although progress seems to have been accelerated by these interventions, few children are reported as achieving normal functioning. It is also evident that not all children respond equally favourably to intervention. In particular, progress tends to be more limited in children with an IQ in the severe-profound range, and in those who fail to acquire verbal imitation within the first 4–6 months of intervention (Smith & Lovaas, 1997).

Longer term evaluations, covering many different aspects of functioning are required if the true cost-effectiveness of the time, effort and energy expended by families in these programmes is to be adequately assessed. Future research also needs to concentrate on developing appropriate strategies to compare different intervention models, and to examine more closely the differential effects of treatment techniques, intensity, structure and setting on different subgroups of children within the autistic spectrum.

The importance of appropriate education

Whatever the controversy over other forms of treatment, the importance of specialized educational programmes for children with autism and other forms of severe intellectual impairment is extensively documented (Burack, Root & Zigler, 1997). The TEACCH programme (Schopler, Mesibov & Hearsey, 1995) was originally developed in North Carolina (USA) but is now widely used throughout the US and many parts of Europe. It is an educational approach that is founded on the need for structure, and emphasizes the need for appropriate environmental organization and the use of clear visual cues to circumvent communication difficulties. The programme takes account of developmental levels and the importance of individually-based teaching, as well as incorporating behavioural and cognitive strategies.

Many other approaches to education have been described, often focusing specifically on the fundamental impairments associated with autism. These include non-verbal programmes designed to improve social and communication functioning, such as the Picture Exchange Communication System (PECS; Bondy & Frost, 1996; see also Quill, 1995); the use of typically developing peers to encourage social interactions and play (Wolfberg & Schuler, 1993; Lord, 1995); interventions to develop cognitive and meta-cognitive abilities (e.g. the 'Bright Start Programme' of Butera & Haywood, 1995) and strategies to enhance learning more generally (Jordan & Powell, 1995; Koegel & Koegel, 1995; Powell & Jordan, 1997). However, few (including the TEACCH programme) have been independently evaluated (Campbell et al., 1996) and there are no studies of their longer term effectiveness.

Interventions in adolescence and adulthood

In comparison with the vast amount of research on interventions for children with autism, there are very few studies of special therapeutic programmes for older individuals. Much of the literature pertaining to this age group focuses on the modification of very challenging behaviours or the acquisition of basic life skills by those with severe or profound intellectual disabilities. However, outcome studies suggest that most individuals tend to improve with age and for some (particularly those who become more aware of their difficulties) adolescence can often be a period of remarkable improvement and change (Kanner, 1973). Programmes to enhance social understanding and improve interpersonal behaviours have been found to have positive, if somewhat circumscribed effects (Mesibov, 1984; Howlin & Yates, 1999; Attwood, 2000). Thus, wider provision of social skills programmes for adolescents and young adults could help to minimize the many problems they face in daily social interactions at school and work. Many others might profit from cognitive–behavioural programmes to help them cope more effectively with emotional or practical difficulties (Hare, Jones & Paine, 1999; Stoddart, 1999). Success in the job market can also be significantly improved by supported employment schemes that focus on teaching appropriate work and social skills. Even individuals with moderate to severe intellectual impairments have been helped to find and maintain employment by these means (Smith, Belcher & Juhrs, 1995; Keel, Mesibov & Woods, 1997). For those who are more able such schemes can significantly increase the chances of individuals' finding employment, and lead to much higher and better paid levels of work (Mawhood & Howlin, 1999).

Finding the appropriate treatment for depression and anxiety-related disorders can also prove difficult, and although medication can be helpful this rarely works in isolation. Psychoanalytically-based interventions may be considered (Maratos, 1996) but there is little evidence of their effectiveness (Campbell et al., 1996). Individual psychotherapy or counselling may assist higher functioning people to deal with anxiety or depression, and the pain that comes from recognizing their difficulties and differences. However, clinical experience suggests that this *must* be combined with direct practical advice on how to deal with problems, otherwise many individuals become obsessed with the past, or with other possible explanations for their difficulties, making it almost impossible for them to 'move on' in a positive way. If appropriately adapted, cognitive behavioural approaches seem to be of potential benefit (Hare et al., 1999; Stoddart, 1999), although there is very little systematic research in this area and even single case studies are rare.

The principal components of effective intervention

On the whole, the most effective treatments do not espouse the view that one approach is successful for all. Instead, whether the basic approach is developmental, educational, behaviourist or a combination of all these, there is recognition of the need for individually designed programmes. These will need to take account of the underlying deficits that are fundamental to the disorder, as well as the individual's profile of skills and difficulties. Interventions may involve a wide range of different techniques and the choice of these will depend not only on individual characteristics but also on family factors that can affect the ways in which intervention strategies can be used.

In general, the most successful programmes, whether they involve children or adults, have the following components in common:

- A combination of behaviourally oriented strategies with developmental and educational approaches that are relevant to the individual's pattern of skills and deficits (Koegel & Koegel, 1995; Schopler et al., 1995; Howlin, 1998).

- Acceptance that the profound communication deficits in autism, which are found at all levels of intellectual ability, may never be fundamentally altered. However, much can be done by fostering a more 'autism friendly' environment. Ensuring that the language used by parents and other carers is appropriate for the individual's *comprehension* level; that 'words mean what words say' (i.e. avoiding metaphor, abstract and hypothetical concepts, and the need to interpret non-verbal cues); and that verbal messages are augmented as much as possible by visual means, can sometimes result in much greater progress than direct attempts to increase spoken vocabulary (Howlin, 1998).

- Recognition of the need for structured educational/daily living programmes, with a particular emphasis on visually based cues. These provide the individual who has autism with a predictable and readily understandable environment, which helps to minimize confusion and distress (Jordan & Powell, 1995; Quill, 1995; Schopler & Mesibov, 1995).

- Acknowledgement that many so-called undesirable or challenging behaviours are frequently a reflection of limited behavioural repertoires or poor communication skills. A focus on skill enhancement and the establishment of more effective communication strategies are therefore often the most successful means of reducing difficult or disruptive behaviours (Schuler et al., 1989; Durand & Carr, 1991; Prizant et al., 1996).

- Awareness of the fundamental inability in autism to interpret and respond appropriately to normal social cues. Behaviours that are tolerable in young children (stripping off clothing, sniffing people's ears, stroking women's tights, etc) may become totally unacceptable if they persist into adulthood. It is therefore essential to develop simple but firm rules in childhood to avoid the emergence of later social problems (Howlin, 1998). Clear and direct feedback is also necessary – people with autism do *not* recognise subtle or unspoken signs of disapproval.

- A focus on the development of social-communication and play activities, especially with peers (Wolfberg & Schuler, 1993; Lord, 1995; Quill, 1995) and, if possible, the implementation of specialist training programmes, for example to improve 'mind-reading' skills (Ozonoff & Miller, 1995; Swettenham, 1995; Howlin et al., 1998) or social understanding (Mesibov, 1984; Williams, 1989; Gray, 1995).

- Understanding the importance of obsessions and rituals (Howlin & Rutter, 1987; Schopler, 1995; Howlin, 1998). These may be the underlying cause of many behaviour problems and, again, often become progressively more unacceptable with age. However, rituals, routines or special interests can also play a vital role in reducing anxiety or distress; they are powerful sources of motivation and reinforcement, and may also open the door to social contacts. From early childhood, it is important to set clear limits so that the individual is fully aware when, where, with whom, and how often these behaviours are allowed, so they do not disrupt other activities but can, at the same time, be used effectively.

- The implementation of treatment approaches that are family centred, rather than exclusively child oriented is most likely to ensure effective generalization and maintenance of skills (Marcus, Kunce & Schopler, 1997). Establishing successful management strategies that can be implemented consistently but in ways that do not demand extensive sacrifice in terms of time, money or other aspects of family life, seems most likely to offer benefits for all involved.

Lastly, but perhaps most importantly, there is a crucial need for early diagnosis and the provision of appropriate advice and support for parents. Although this can do much to help minimize or avoid later problems, delays in diagnosis are still common. In a large scale survey Howlin & Ashgarian (1999) found that despite the fact that the majority of parents became concerned in the first months or year of the child's life, they faced many delays and frustrations in obtaining a diagnosis. Many children were not diagnosed until 5 years of age or later, well after the optimal period for the onset of intervention. In the case of more able children and for those with Asperger syndrome, the average age of diagnosis was around 11 years. Such delays can result in the development of ineffective management strategies at home, unnecessary escalation of behaviour problems, exclusion from appropriate educational provision, severe limitations on employment and residential opportunities in adulthood, and consequently high rates of psychiatric and emotional problems.

Conclusions

Almost three decades ago, Kanner (1973) noted that in the 30 years since he had first described children with autism:

'There has been a hodge-podge of theories, hypotheses and explanations ... yet no-one has succeeded in finding a therapeutic setting, drug, method or technique that has yielded the same or lasting results for all children. It is expected that a next 30 or 20 year follow-up will be able to present a report of ... more hopeful prognosis'.

Despite sometimes extravagant claims for the effectiveness of various therapies there is no evidence to suggest that *long-term outcome* can be dramatically improved following the implementation of any particular intervention programme (Howlin, 1998). It is true that early intervention and support for parents can help to minimize secondary behavioural problems and to ensure that individuals develop their existing skills to the full. Moreover, improvements in educational provision for children with autism over the past 50 years have also resulted in steady increases in academic attainments (Rutter & Bartak, 1973; Venter, Lord & Schopler, 1992). Nevertheless, for the majority of individuals with autism their associated learning disabilities will severely limit their ability to live independently. Provision for this group has undoubtedly improved over the last few decades although there is still much scope for further progress. Specialist education has become increasingly available, and supported employment and living schemes have enabled many to attain a level of functioning that would never have been envisaged 50 years ago. Paradoxically, however, it can be far more difficult for higher functioning individuals to obtain the help and support they need. Their parents often experience considerable difficulties in obtaining a diagnosis and the choice of appropriate educational provision is very limited. Psychiatric and emotional difficulties seem to be a particular risk as these individuals grow older and become more aware of their social difficulties and differences. Nevertheless, very few have access to counselling or cognitive–behavioural interventions from professionals who understand the nature of their difficulties. Support throughout further education is in short supply and help for adults to find and maintain work or to live independently of their families is almost non-existent. Although some adults are able to live alone, find work, make relationships, even get married, outcome within this more able group remains highly variable. To some extent prognosis is related to innate cognitive and linguistic abilities but the adequacy of local provision also has a significant impact on prognosis. For example, access to appropriately structured educational programmes may have a crucial

Table 6.3. Autism: implications for intervention

- Claims of cures for autism remain unsubstantiated, but much can be done to prevent the escalation of problems over time by ensuring families have access to early diagnosis, adequate advice about management and to appropriate educational provision
- Although very many specialist educational and psychological programmes have been developed for use with children with autism, relatively few clinical or research studies have focused on ways of helping adolescents or adults. More effective interventions to minimize the social and emotional difficulties that they face are urgently required
- Outcome generally will depend on innate factors, such as language ability and IQ. However, for individuals of higher ability (IQ 70 +) the ultimate level of independence achieved will be largely determined by the availability of appropriate support at school, throughout higher education, in employment and in finding suitable accommodation
- Although provision for children and adults with autism has improved greatly over the past few decades, the level of support available for those who are more able is often very limited. Educational, social and mental health services need to be more aware of the needs of this group and to offer a much wider range of suitable provision
- There are no epidemiological data on the incidence of psychiatric disorders in people with autism but case reports suggest that while schizophrenia is relatively rare, health professionals need to be alert to the increased risk of affective disorders in adulthood. Differential diagnosis will require detailed developmental history from parents or other family members
- Whatever the autistic individual's level of functioning, professionals involved in education, placement or therapy should accept the need to work in close collaboration with parents. Their advice and knowledge can be crucial in ensuring that the support offered is appropriate and adequate.

influence on later academic and occupational attainments. Similarly, the provision of supported employment schemes can significantly improve the chances of individuals' finding and maintaining suitable employment. Specialist social skills groups, also, may help to improve social competence and to develop peer relationships. The challenge now is to ensure that access to support of this kind becomes far more widely available.

It is also essential to ensure that professionals responsible for the care of adults with autism continue to involve families as closely as possible. Parents may often be excluded from decisions relating to therapy or placement on the grounds of 'confidentiality', or the mistaken belief that individuals with autism are capable of making informed choices about hypothetical or abstract situations. It can be also very difficult for some professionals to accept the need for the direct involvement of parents in diagnosing or treating psychiatric illness.

However, family members are likely to know far more about the autistic person's needs, skills and disabilities than anyone else, and their input can be invaluable, both in making a differential diagnosis and in assessing the effects of intervention.

Finally, whatever improvements are made in therapy or service provision, it is also clear that diagnostic provision needs to improve considerably if individuals with autism are to receive the help they need. The average age at which children are diagnosed is still far too high (Howlin & Ashgarian, 1999) especially in the case of more able individuals. Late diagnosis can result in inadequate support for parents and teachers, an escalation of behavioural problems, increasing exclusion and isolation, and perhaps severe emotional and psychiatric problems in later life.

For a summary of the clinical implications of autistic disorders, see Table 6.3.

REFERENCES

Abramson, R.K., Wright. H.H, Cuccara. M.L., Lawrence. L.G., Babb. S., Pencarinha. D., Marstellar. F. & Harris. E.C. (1992). Biological liability in families with autism. *Journal of the American Academy of Child and Adolescent Psychiatry*, **31**: 370–1.

American Psychiatric Association (1994). *Diagnostic and Statistical Manual of Mental Disorders. (DSM-IV)*. 4th edn. Washington DC: American Psychiatric Association.

Asperger, H. (1944). Autistic psychopathy in childhood. [Translated and annotated by U. Frith] Cited in *Autism and Asperger Syndrome*, ed. U. Frith (1991), pp. 37–62. Cambridge: Cambridge University Press.

Attwood, A. (2000). Strategies for improving the social integration of children with Asperger syndrome. *Autism: International Journal of Research and Practice*, **4**: 85–100.

Baron-Cohen, S. (1988). Assessment of violence in a young man with Asperger's Syndrome. *Journal of Child Psychology and Psychiatry*, **29**: 351–60.

Baron-Cohen, S. (1995). *Mindblindness: An Essay on Autism and Theory of Mind*. Cambridge, MA: The MIT Press.

Bailey, A., Phillips, W. & Rutter, M. (1996). Autism: towards an integration of clinical, genetic and neurobiological perspectives. *Journal of Child Psychiatry and Psychology*, **37**: 89–126.

Bebko, J.M., Perry, A. & Bryson, S. (1996). Multiple method validation study of facilitated communication. II. Individual differences and subgroup results. *Journal of Autism and Developmental Disorders*, **26**: 19–42.

Bondy, A. & Frost, L. (1996). Educational approaches in pre-school: behavior techniques in a public school setting. In *Learning and Cognition in Autism*, ed. E. Schopler & G.B. Mesibov, pp. 311–34. New York: Plenum Press.

Burack, J.A., Root, R. & Zigler, E. (1997). Inclusive education for children with autism: reviewing ideological, empirical and community considerations. In *Handbook of Autism and Pervasive Developmental Disorders*, 2nd edn, ed. D. Cohen & F. Volkmar, pp. 796–807. New York: Wiley.

Butera, G. & Haywood, H.C. (1995). Cognitive education of young children with autism: an application of Bright Start. In *Learning and Cognition in Autism*, ed. E. Schopler & G. B. Mesibov, pp. 227–56. New York: Plenum Press.

Campbell, M., Schopler, E., Cueva. J.E. & Hallin, A. (1996). Treatment of autistic disorder. *Journal of the American Academy of Child and Adolescent Psychiatry*, **35**: 134–43.

Chesterman, P. & Rutter, S.C. (1994). A case report: Asperger's syndrome and sexual offending. *Journal of Forensic Psychiatry*, **4**: 555–62.

Chez, M.G., Buchanan, C.P., Bagan, B.T., Hammer, M.S., McCarthy, K.S., Ovrutskaya, I., Nowinski, C.V. & Cohen, Z.S. (2000). Secretin and autism: a two-part clinical investigation. *Journal of Autism and Developmental Disorders*, **30**: 87–94.

Chung, S.Y., Luk, F.L. & Lee, E.W.H. (1990). A follow-up study of infantile autism in Hong Kong. *Journal of Autism and Developmental Disorders*, **20**: 221–32.

Clarke, D.J., Baxter, M., Perry, D. & Prasher, V. (1999). Autism, affective disorders and psychoses. *Autism: International Journal of Research and Practice*, **3**: 149–64.

Clarke, D.J., Littlejohns, C.S., Corbett, J.A. & Joseph, S. (1989). Pervasive developmental disorders and psychoses in adult life. *British Journal of Psychiatry*, **155**: 692–9.

De Giacomo, A. & Fombonne, E. (1998). Parental recognition of developmental abnormalities in autism. *European Child and Adolescent Psychiatry*, **7**: 131–6.

DeMeyer, M.K., Barton, S., DeMyer, W.E., Norton, J.A., Allan, J. & Steele, R. (1973). Prognosis in autism: a follow-up study. *Journal of Autism and Childhood Schizophrenia*, **3**: 199–246.

Durand, B.M. & Carr, E.G. (1991). Functional communication training to reduce challenging behaviour: maintenance and application in new settings. *Journal of Applied Behavior Analysis*, **24**: 251–4.

Everall, I.P. & Le Couteur, A. (1990). Fire-setting in an adolescent boy with Asperger's syndrome. *British Journal of Psychiatry*, **157**: 284–7.

Folstein, S., Bisson, E., Santangelo, S.L. & Piven, J. (1998). Finding specific genes that cause autism; a combination of approaches will be needed to maximise power. *Journal of Autism and Developmental Disorders*, **28**: 439–46.

Fombonne, E. (1999). The epidemiology of autism: a review. *Psychological Medicine*, **29**: 769–86.

Frith, U. (1991). *Autism and Asperger Syndrome*. Cambridge: Cambridge University Press.

Frith, U., Soares, I. & Wing, L. (1993). Research into the earliest detectable signs of autism: what parents say. *Communication*, **27**: 17–18.

Ghaziuddin, M., Tsai, L.Y. & Ghaziuddin, N. (1991). Brief report. Violence in Asperger syndrome: A critique. *Journal of Autism and Developmental Disorders*, **21**: 349–54.

Ghaziuddin, M., Tsai, L.Y. & Ghaziuddin, N. (1992). Co-morbidity of autistic disorder in children and adolescents. *European Journal of Child and Adolescent Psychiatry*, **1**: 209–13.

Gillberg, C. (1991). Outcome in autism and autistic-like conditions. *Journal of the American Academy of Child and Adolescent Psychiatry*, **30**: 375–82.

Gillberg, C. (1992). Epilepsy. In *The Biology of the Autistic Syndromes*, 2nd edn, ed. C. Gillberg & M. Coleman, pp. 60–73. Oxford: MacKeith Press.

Gillberg, C. (1998). Chromosomal disorders and autism. *Journal of Autism and Developmental Disorders*, **28**: 415–26.

Gillberg, C., Ehlers, S., Schaumann, H., Jakobsson, G., Dahlgren, S.O., Lindblom, R., Bagen-holm, A., Tjus, T. & Blidner, E. (1990). Autism under age 3 years: a clinical study of 28 cases referred for autistic symptoms in infancy. *Journal of Child Psychology and Psychiatry*, **31**: 921–34.

Gillberg, C. & Steffenberg, S. (1987). Outcome and prognostic factors in infantile autism and similar conditions: a population-based study of 46 cases followed through puberty. *Journal of Autism and Developmental Disorders*, **17**: 272–88.

Goode, S., Rutter, M. & Howlin, P. (1994). A twenty-year follow-up of children with autism. Paper presented at the 13th biennial meeting of the International Society for the Study of Behavioral Development, Amsterdam, The Netherlands.

Gray, C.A. (1995). Teaching children with autism to 'read' social situations. In *Teaching Children with Autism: Strategies to Enhance Communication and Socialization*, ed. A. Quill, pp. 219–42. New York: Delmar.

Gresham, F.M. & MacMillan, D.L. (1998). Early Intervention Project: can its claims be substantiated and replicated. *Journal of Autism and Developmental Disorders*, **28**: 5–13.

Hall, S. (1997). *The development of stereotyped and self injurious behaviours*. Unpublished PhD thesis, University of London.

Hare, D., Jones, J.P.R. & Paine, C. (1999). Approaching reality: the use of personal construct assessment in working with people with Asperger syndrome. *Autism: International Journal of Research and Practice*, **3**: 165–76.

Horvath, K., Stefanotos, G., Sokolski, K.N., Wachtel, R., Nabors, L. & Tildon, T. (1998). Improved social and language skills after Secretin administration in patients with autistic spectrum disorders. *Journal of the Association of the Academy of Minority Physicians*, **9**: 9–15.

Howlin, P. (1997a). *Autism: Preparing for Adulthood*. London: Routledge.

Howlin, P. (1998). *Treating Children with Autism and Asperger Syndrome: A Guide for Parents and Professionals*. Chichester: Wiley.

Howlin, P. & Ashgarian, A. (1999). The diagnosis of autism and Asperger syndrome: findings from a survey of 770 families. *Developmental Medicine and Child Neurology*, **41**: 834–9.

Howlin, P., Baron-Cohen, S., Hadwin, J. & Swettenham, J. (1998). *Teaching Children with Autism to Mindread. A Practical Manual for Parents and Teachers*. Chichester: Wiley.

Howlin, P. & Goode, S. (1998). Outcome in adult life for individuals with autism. In *Autism and Developmental Disorders*, ed. F. Volkmar, pp. 209–41. New York: Cambridge University Press.

Howlin, P., Mawhood, L.M. & Rutter, M. (2000). Autism and developmental receptive language disorder. A follow-up comparison in early adult life. II. Social, behavioural and psychiatric outcomes. *Journal of Child Psychology and Psychiatry*, **41**: 561–76.

Howlin, P. & Moore, A. (1997). Diagnosis in autism: a survey of over 1,200 parents. *Autism: International Journal of Research and Practice*, **2**: 135–62.

Howlin, P. & Rutter, M. (1987). *Treatment of Autistic Children*. Chichester: Wiley.

Howlin, P. & Yates, P. (1999). The potential effectiveness of social skills groups for adults with autism. *Autism: International Journal of Research and Practice*, **3**: 299–307.

International Molecular Genetic Study of Autism Consortium (1998). A full genome screen for autism with evidence for linkage to a region on chromosome 7q. *Human Molecular Genetics*, **7**: 571–8.

International Molecular Genetic Study of Autism Consortium (2001). A genome screen for autism: strong evidence for linkage to chromosomes 2q, 7q, and 16p. *American Journal of Human Genetics* **69**: 570–81.

Isager, T., Mouridsen, S.E. & Rich, B. (1999). Mortality and causes of death in pervasive developmental disorders. *Autism: International Journal of Research and Practice*, **3**: 7–16.

Jordan, R. & Powell, S. (1995). *Understanding and Teaching Children with Autism*. Chichester: Wiley.

Kanner, L. (1943). Autistic disturbances of affective contact. *Nervous Child*, **2**: 217–50.

Kanner, L. (1949). Problems of nosology and psychodynamics of early infantile autism. *American Journal of Orthopsychiatry*, **19**: 416–26.

Kanner, L. (1973). *Childhood Psychosis: Initial Studies and New Insights*. New York: Winston/Wiley.

Keel, J.H., Mesibov, G. & Woods, A.V. (1997). TEACCH – Supported employment programme. *Journal of Autism and Developmental Disorders*, **27**: 3–10.

Klin, A. & Volkmar, F.R. (1997). Asperger's syndrome In *Handbook of Autism and Pervasive Developmental Disorders*, 2nd edn, ed. D. Cohen & F. Volkmar, pp. 94–125. New York: Wiley.

Kobayashi, R., Murata, T. & Yashinaga, K. (1992). A follow-up study of 201 children with autism in Kyushu and Yamguchia, Japan. *Journal of Autism and Developmental Disorders*, **22**: 395–411.

Koegel, R.L. & Koegel, L.K. (1995). *Teaching Children with Autism: Strategies for Initiating Positive Interactions and Improving Learning Opportunities*. Baltimore: Brookes.

Lainhart, J.E. & Folstein, S.E. (1994). Affective disorders in people with autism: a review of published cases. *Journal of Autism and Developmental Disorders*, **24**: 587–601.

Larsen, F.W. & Mouridsen, S.E. (1997). The outcome in children with childhood autism and Asperger syndrome originally diagnosed as psychotic. A 30-year follow-up study of subjects hospitalized as children. *European Child and Adolescent Psychiatry*, **6**: 181–90.

Lauritsen, M., Mors, O., Mortensen, P.B. & Ewald, H. (1999). Infantile autism and associated autosomal chromosome abnormalities: a register based study and a literature survey. *Journal of Child Psychology and Psychiatry*, **40**: 335–46.

Lockyer, L. & Rutter, M. (1969). A five to fifteen year follow-up study of infantile psychosis. III. Psychological aspects. *British Journal of Psychiatry*, **115**: 865–82.

Lockyer, L. & Rutter, M. (1970). A five to fifteen year follow-up study of infantile psychosis. IV. Patterns of cognitive abilities. *British Journal of Social and Clinical Psychology*, **9**: 152–63.

Lord, C. (1995). Facilitating social inclusion: examples from peer intervention Programs. In *Learning and Cognition in Autism*, ed. E. Schopler & G.B. Mesibov, pp. 221–39. New York: Plenum Press.

Lord, C. & Bailey, A. (2001). Autism and pervasive developmental disorders. In *Child and Adolescent Psychiatry: Modern Approaches*, 4th edn., ed. M. Rutter & E. Taylor, pp. 569–91. Oxford: Blackwell.

Lord, C. & Rutter, M. (1994). Autism and pervasive developmental disorders. In *Child and*

Adolescent Psychiatry: Modern Approaches, ed. M. Rutter, E. Taylor & L. Hersov, 3rd edn, pp. 569–93. Oxford: Blackwell.

Lord, C., Rutter, M. & Le Couteur, A. (1994). Autism Diagnostic Interview-Revised: a revised version of a diagnostic interview for caregivers of individuals with possible pervasive developmental disorders. *Journal of Autism and Developmental Disorders*, **24**: 659–85.

Lord, C. & Schopler, E. (1985). Differences in sex ratios in autism as a function of measured intelligence. *Journal of Autism and Development Disorders*, **15**: 185–93.

Lord, C. & Venter, A. (1992). Outcome and follow-up studies of high functioning autistic individuals. In *High Functioning Individuals with Autism*, ed. E. Schopler & G.B. Mesibov, pp. 187–200, New York: Plenum.

Lotter, V. (1974a). Factors related to outcome in autistic children. *Journal of Autism and Childhood Schizophrenia*, **4**: 263–77.

Lotter, V. (1974b). Social adjustment and placement of autistic children in Middlesex: a follow-up study. *Journal of Autism and Childhood Schizophrenia*, **4**: 11–32.

Lovaas, O.I. (1987). Behavioral treatment and normal educational and intellectual functioning in young autistic children. *Journal of Consulting and Clinical Psychology*, **55**: 3–9.

Maestrini, E., Marlow, A.J., Weeks, D.E. & Monaco, A.P. (1998). Molecular genetic investigations of autism. *Journal of Autism and Developmental Disorders*, **28**: 427–37.

Maratos, O. (1996). Psychoanalysis and the management of pervasive developmental disorders, including autism. In *Children with Autism: Diagnosis and Interventions to Meet Their Needs*, ed. C. Trevarthen, K. Aitken, D. Papoudi & J. Robarts, pp. 161–71. London: Jessica Kingsley.

Marcus, L.M., Kunce, L.J. & Schopler, E. (1997). Working with families. In *Handbook of Autism and Pervasive Developmental Disorders*, 2nd edn, ed. D. Cohen & F. Volkmar, pp. 631–49. New York: Wiley.

Mawhood, L. & Howlin, P. (1999). The effectiveness of a supported employment scheme for high functioning adults with autism. *Autism: International Journal of Research and Practice*, **3**: 229–54.

Mawhood, L.M., Howlin, P. & Rutter M. (2000). Autism and developmental receptive language disorder – a follow-up comparison in early adult life. I. Cognitive and language outcomes *Journal of Child Psychology and Psychiatry*, **41**: 547–59.

Mawson, D., Grounds, A. & Tantam, D. (1985). Violence in Asperger's syndrome: a case study. *British Journal of Psychiatry*, **147**: 566–9.

McEachin, J.J., Smith, T. & Lovaas, O.I. (1993). Long-term outcome for children with autism who received early intensive behavioral treatment. *American Journal of Mental Retardation*, **97**: 359–72.

Mesibov, G.B. (1984). Social skills training with verbal autistic adolescents and adults: a program model. *Journal of Autism and Developmental Disorders*, **14**: 395–404.

Mesibov, G.B. (1993). Treatment outcome is encouraging: comments on McEachin et al. *American Journal of Mental Retardation*, **97**: 379–80.

Mudford, O.C., Cross, B.A., Breen, S., Cullen, C., Reeves, D., Gould, J. & Douglas, J. (2000). Auditory integration training for children with autism: no behavioral benefits detected. *American Journal of Mental Retardation*, **105**: 118–29.

Muller, J. (1993). Swimming against the tide. *Communication*, **27**: 6.

National Autistic Society (1997). Statistics sheet 1. *How many people have autistic spectrum disorders?* London: National Autistic Society Publications.

Nordin, V. & Gillberg, C. (1998). The long-term course of autistic disorders: update on follow-up studies. *Acta Psychiatrica Scandinavica*, **97**: 99–108.

Ozonoff, S. & Miller, J. (1995). Teaching Theory of Mind: a new approach to social skills training for individuals with autism. *Journal of Autism and Developmental Disorders*, **25**: 415–34.

Perry, R., Cohen, I. & DeCarlo, R. (1995). Case study: deterioration, autism and recovery in two siblings. *Journal of the American Academy of Child and Adolescent Psychiatry*, **34**: 233–37.

Petty, L.K., Ornitz, E.M., Michelman, J.D. & Zimmerman, E.G. (1984). Autistic children who become schizophrenic. *Archives of General Psychiatry*, **41**: 129–35.

Pickles, A., Bolton, P., Macdonald, H., Bailey, A., Le Couteur, A., Sim, L. & Rutter, M. (1995). Latent class analysis of recurrence risk for complex phenotypes with selection and measurement error: a twin and family history study of autism. *American Journal of Human Genetics*, **57**: 717–26.

Piven, J., Harper, J., Palmer, P. & Arndt, S. (1995). Course of behavioral change in autism: a retrospective study of high-IQ adolescents and adults. *Journal of the American Academy of Child and Adolescent Psychiatry*, **35**: 523–9.

Powell, S. & Jordan, R. (Eds) (1997). *Autism and Learning: A Guide to Good Practice*. London: David Fulton.

Prizant, B.M., Schuler, A.L., Wetherby, A.M. & Rydell, P. (1996). Enhancing language and communication development: Language approaches. In *Handbook of Autism and Pervasive Developmental Disorders*, 2nd edn, ed. D. Cohen & F. Volkmar, pp. 572–605. New York: Wiley.

Quill, K. A. (1995). *Teaching Children with Autism: Strategies to Enhance Communication and Socialization*. New York: Delmar.

Rimland, B. (1998). The use of secretin in autism: some preliminary answers. *Autism Research Review International*, **12**, 3.

Rogers, S.J. (1996). Brief report: early intervention in autism. *Journal of Autism and Developmental Disorders*, **26**: 243–6.

Rumsey, J.M., Rapoport, J.L. & Sceery, W.R. (1985). Autistic children as adults: psychiatric social and behavioural outcomes. *Journal of the American Academy of Child Psychiatry*, **24**: 465–73.

Rutter, M. (1972). Childhood schizophrenia reconsidered. *Journal of Autism and Childhood Schizophrenia*, **2**: 315–37.

Rutter, M., Anderson-Wood, L., Beckett, C., Bredenkampf, D., Castle, J., Groothues, J., Kreppner, J., Keaveney, L., Lord, C., O'Connor, T.G. & the ERA Study Team (1999). Quasi-autistic patterns following severe early global privation. *Journal of Child Psychology and Psychiatry*, **40**: 537–50.

Rutter, M., Bailey, A., Bolton, P. & Le Couteur, A. (1994). Autism and known medical conditions: myth and substance. *Journal of Child Psychology and Psychiatry*, **35**: 311–22.

Rutter, M. & Bartak, L. (1973). Special educational treatment of autistic children: a comparative study. II. Follow-up findings and implications for services. *Journal of Child Psychology and Psychiatry*, **14**: 241–70.

Rutter, M., Greenfield, D. & Lockyer, L. (1967). A five to fifteen year follow-up study of infantile psychosis. II. Social and behavioural outcome. *British Journal of Psychiatry*, **113**: 1183–99.

Rutter, M. & Lockyer, L. (1967). A five to fifteen year follow-up study of infantile psychosis. I. Description of Sample. *British Journal of Psychiatry*, **113**: 1169–82.

Sandler, A.D., Sutton, K., De Weese, J., Girardi, M.A. Sheppard, V. & Bodfish, J.W. (1999). A double blind placebo controlled trial of synthetic human secretin in the treatment of autism and pervasive developmental disorder. *The New England Journal of Medicine*, **341**: 1801–6.

Schopler, E. (Ed.) (1995). *Parent Survival Manual: A Guide to Crisis Resolution in Autism and Related Developmental Disorders*. New York: Plenum.

Schopler, E. & Mesibov, G.B. (Eds) (1995). *Learning and Cognition in Autism*. New York: Plenum Press.

Schopler, E., Mesibov, G.B. & Hearsey, K. (1995). Structured teaching in the TEACCH system. In *Learning and Cognition in Autism*, ed. E. Schopler & G.B. Mesibov, pp. 243–67. New York: Plenum Press.

Schopler, E., Mesibov. G.B. & Kunce. L.J. (1998), *Asperger Syndrome or High Functioning Autism?* New York: Plenum.

Schuler, A.L., Peck, C.A., Willard, C. & Theimer, K. (1989). Assessment of communicative means and functions through interview: assessing the communicative capabilities of individuals with limited language. *Seminars in Speech and Language*, **10**: 51–61.

Scragg, P. & Shah. A. (1994). Prevalence of Asperger's syndrome in a secure hospital. *British Journal of Psychiatry*, **165**: 679–82.

Sheinkopf, S.J. & Siegel, B. (1998). Home-based behavioral treatment for young children with autism. *Journal of Autism and Developmental Disorders*, **28**: 15–23.

Smalley, S. (1998). Autism and tuberous sclerosis. *Journal of Developmental Disorders*, **28**: 407–14.

Smith, B., Chung, M.C. & Vostanis, P. (1994). The path to care in autism: is it better now? *Journal of Autism and Developmental Disorders*, **24**: 551–64.

Smith, M., Belcher, R. & Juhrs, P. (1995). *A Guide to Successful Employment for Individuals with Autism*. Baltimore: Paul H. Brookes.

Smith, T. & Lovaas, O.I. (1997). The UCLA young autism project: a reply to Gresham and MacMillan. *Behavioral Disorders,* **22**: 203–15.

Stoddart, K. (1999). Adolescents with Asperger syndrome: 3 cases studies of individual and family therapy. *Autism: International Journal of Research and Practice*, **3**: 255–72.

Sverd, J., Montero, G. & Gurevich, N. (1993). Brief report: cases for an association between Tourette's syndrome, autistic disorder and schizophrenia-like disorder. *Journal of Autism and Developmental Disorders*, **23**: 407–14.

Swettenham, J. (1995). Can children with autism be taught to understand false beliefs using computers? *Journal of Child Psychology and Psychiatry*, **37**: 157–66.

Szatmari, P., Bartolucci, G. & Bremner, R.S. (1989a). Asperger's syndrome and autism: a comparison of early history and outcome. *Developmental Medicine and Child Neurology*, **31**: 709–20.

Szatmari, P., Bartolucci, G., Bremner, R.S., Bond, S. & Rich, S. (1989b). A follow-up study of high functioning autistic children. *Journal of Autism and Developmental Disorders*, **19**: 213–26.

Szatmari, P., Bartolucci, G., Finlayson, A. & Krames, L. (1986). A vote for Asperger's syndrome. *Journal of Autism and Developmental Disorders*, **16**: 515–17.

Szatmari, P., Jones, M.B., Zwaigenbaum, L. & MacLean, J.E. (1998). Genetics of autism: overview and new directions. *Journal of Autism and Developmental Disorders*, **28**: 363–80.

Tantam, D. (1991). Asperger's Syndrome in adulthood. In *Autism and Asperger Syndrome*, ed. U. Frith, pp. 147–83. Cambridge: Cambridge University Press.

Taylor, B., Miller, E., Farrington, C.P. Petropoulos, M-C., Favot-Mayaud, I., Li, J. & Wright, P. (1999). Autism and measles, mumps, and rubella vaccine: no epidemiological evidence for a causal association. *The Lancet,* **353**: 2026–9.

Venter, A., Lord, C. & Schopler, E. (1992). A follow-up study of high functioning autistic children. *Journal of Child Psychology and Psychiatry*, **33**: 489–507.

Volkmar, F.R. & Cohen, D.J. (1991). Comorbid association of autism and schizophrenia. *American Journal of Psychiatry*, **148**: 1705–7.

Volkmar, F., Klin, A. & Cohen, D. (1997). Diagnosis and classification of autism and related disorders. In *Handbook of Autism and Pervasive Developmental Disorders*, 2nd edn, ed. D. Cohen & F. Volkmar, pp. 5–40. New York, Wiley.

Volkmar, F., Stier, D. & Cohen, D. (1985). Age of recognition of pervasive developmental disorders. *American Journal of Psychiatry*, **142**: 1450–2.

Williams, T.I. (1989). A social skills group for autistic children. *Journal of Autism and Developmental Disorders*, **19**: 143–56.

Wing, L. (1981). Asperger's syndrome: a clinical account. *Psychological Medicine*, **11**: 115–29.

Wing, L. (1986). Clarification on Asperger's syndrome. Letter to the Editor. *Journal of Autism and Developmental Disorders*, **16**: 513–15.

Wing, L. & Gould, J. (1979). Severe impairments of social interaction and associated abnormalities in children: epidemiology and classification. *Journal of Autism and Developmental Disorders,* **9**: 11–29.

Wolfberg, P.J. & Schuler, A.L. (1993). Integrated play groups: a model for promoting the social and cognitive dimensions of play. *Journal of Autism and Developmental Disorders*, **23**: 1–23.

Wolff, S. & McGuire, R.J. (1995). Schizoid personality in girls: a follow-up study. What are the links with Asperger's syndrome? *Journal of Child Psychology and Psychiatry*, **36**: 793–818.

World Health Organization (1992). *International Classification of Diseases*. ICD-10 (10th edn). *Diagnostic Criteria for Research*. Geneva: WHO.

7

Down syndrome

Janet Carr

Introduction

Down syndrome, the single most common condition causing learning disability, was first systematically described in 1866 by John Langdon Down. He named the condition 'mongolism' a term that was in use until the early 1970s, when it was superseded by 'Down's (now Down) syndrome'. A variety of physical features occurs in people with Down syndrome although usually not all are present in any one individual. They include short stature, a rounded head, characteristic folds at the inner corners of the eyes, broad hands with a single palmar crease and a short incurved little finger. About half of all infants with Down syndrome are born with a heart defect (Hallidie-Smith, 1996). A major defining feature is intellectual disability, though its degree varies widely. No consistent relationship has been shown between the number of physical features present and severity of disability (Cunningham et al., 1991). Women with Down syndrome are potentially fertile and 32 pregnancies (one of twins) have been noted in the literature worldwide (Rani et al., 1990). Of these infants, about one-third themselves had the Down syndrome karyotype, about one-fifth had disabilities other than Down syndrome and about two-fifths were normal. None of the 25 surviving infants appears to have been brought up by his or her own mother. Men are generally subfertile and only one authenticated case of a man with Down syndrome fathering a child has been reported (Sheridan et al., 1989). In this case the mother miscarried at 17 weeks, the fetus having no observable abnormalities.

In 1959 there was a major breakthrough in the understanding of Down syndrome when Lejeune, Gautier and Turpin showed that, while the cells of human subjects normally contain 46 chromosomes (23 pairs) those of people with Down syndrome contain 47 (22 pairs and one triplet), the extra chromosome being one of group G, or 21. The majority of people with Down syndrome (about 94%) has what is referred to as standard trisomy 21. There are also the translocation and the mosaic forms (about 3% each; Fryers, 1984). In the translocation form the extra chromosome is attached to part of another chromosome. This form, although rare, is important because, unlike the other two, it occurs independently of maternal age, and the condition may be inherited, generally from the mother. If this is the case the chance of any future pregnancy involving a child with Down syndrome is greatly increased, rising to about one in six (Kessling & Sawtell, 1996). In the mosaic form both normal and abnormal cells are found. While the three groups are not obviously distinguishable one from another, those with the mosaic form have been found to have higher average IQs (Fishler & Koch, 1991). There is, however, great variation between individuals and the prognosis for a person with the mosaic form is not necessarily better than for those with other forms of the condition.

Prevalence (the number of people with Down syndrome alive in the community at any one time) varies according to age group and is always highest at the earliest ages, declining as some infants and young children, and smaller numbers of adolescents and young adults, die. In whole populations, prevalence has been calculated to be of the order of 4.63 per 10 000 (Stratford & Steele, 1985). Males outnumber females by about 1.3 : 1, possibly due to higher mortality in females, especially in infancy (Gibson, 1978).

The belief that people with Down syndrome have a short life span is still commonly held, but the position has changed significantly over the last half century. In 1929, average life expectancy was 9 years and by 1947 this had increased only to 12 years (Penrose, 1949). More recently, thanks mainly to surgery to correct common heart defects, and to the use of antibiotics in the management of respiratory infections, life expectancy has risen to 'at least 45' (A. Holland, pers. comm.). Similarly, while in the study of Penrose (1949) the oldest living person known was 44 years old, by 1975 the oldest traced was 63 (Carr, 1975) and by 1990 three people, aged 74, 75 and 86, were known to be alive and well (Dalton & Wisniewski, 1990). This quadrupling of life expectancy over half a century is obviously a matter for celebration. It leads, however, to two concerns. First, parents, who previously had felt confident that at least they would be able to look after their child throughout his or her life, are now faced with the probability that their offspring with Down syndrome will outlive them, with all the anxieties about future care that this may entail. Second, it has made clear the particular vulnerability of the group to Alzheimer's disease.

Despite their intellectual disabilities, people with Down syndrome have popularly been viewed as particularly loving and lovable people. Dissenting voices have been heard (Blacketer-Simmonds, 1953), but there has been some research support for the stereotype – children and adults with Down syndrome being more positively rated than were people with other kinds of learning disability (Johnson & Abelson, 1969; Silverstein et al., 1985). Since the stereotype is so well known the question arises as to whether it might have influenced the research responders, especially if they had not had much firsthand experience of people with Down syndrome. Support for this proposition came from Wishart & Johnston (1990) who showed that the more experience raters had with children with Down syndrome the less they adhered to the stereotype. Silverstein et al. (1985) also put forward the intriguing suggestion that research supporting the stereotype may simply demonstrate its influence on the behaviour of the carer-raters: carers who expect pleasant behaviours may behave in such a way that pleasant behaviours are forthcoming. If this suggestion could be substantiated, it would have considerable implications for advice for parents and training for carers.

Causation

Many different environmental conditions have been considered as possibly causing Down syndrome. Radiation, either from nuclear plants or X-rays of the mother, fluoride, viruses and maternal thyroid antibodies have all been investigated but no association with Down syndrome has been established (Fryers, 1984). Major exposure to radiation, for example from an atomic explosion, may actually result in fewer babies with Down syndrome, probably because of an increased miscarriage rate (Steele, 1996). The most firmly established cause of the birth of a child with Down syndrome is age of the mother. The risks increase from about 1 in 1500 for 20-year-old mothers to 1 in 400 at age 35 and about 1 in 30 at age 45 (Cuckle, Wald & Thompson, 1987). In one study women under 25 years were responsible for 50% of all births but only 15% of babies with Down syndrome; women aged 35 and older accounted for 10% of births but 47% of those with Down syndrome (Fryers, 1984). Nevertheless, because far more babies are born to younger than to older mothers, the great majority of children with Down syndrome are born to younger women and only about 30% to women aged 35 or older (Steele, 1996). The importance of paternal age in causing Down syndrome has been disputed, but the consensus now is that it is not significant once maternal age has been allowed for (Zaremba, 1985). Birth order has no effect when the mother's age has been allowed for (Penrose & Smith, 1966). Why some women, of any age, have a child with Down syndrome, when others of a similar age do not, is still unknown.

General health

Although Down syndrome used to be associated with a very high, early mortality rate, good general physical health is now reported in 80% or more of young adults (Holmes, 1988; Shepperdson, 1992). Amongst 21-year-olds, serious illnesses were no more frequent than in a non-disabled comparison group, and the people with Down syndrome had suffered fewer serious accidents than had the comparison group (Carr, 1995). Surgical interventions for congenital heart disorders are now much more common and more successful than formerly (Hallidie-Smith, 1996). Epilepsy is generally reported in fewer than 15%, but late onset seizures can occur in middle-age, possibly as an early sign of Alzheimer's disease (Prasher, 1995a). Thyroid dysfunction (almost invariably hypothyroidism) has been estimated to occur in nearly 40% of adults with Down syndrome (Anneren & Pueschel, 1996). The condition has particular significance in this population as the presenting signs can mimic the early stages of Alzheimer's disease (Thase, 1982; Prasher & Krishnan, 1993).

Skin disorders are common, affecting about 25% of 21- to 35-year-olds (Carr, 1995 and unpub. data) and 40% of an older group (mean age 42 years; Prasher, 1994a). People with Down syndrome have a high incidence of periodontal disease (Barden, 1985) – in Carr's 30- and 35-year-olds, 10 and 20% respectively had loose, few or no teeth. Reports of visual problems vary widely, from less than a third of some adult groups (Holmes, 1988; Myers & Pueschel, 1991; Prasher, 1994b) to 52% and 62% of 30- and 35-year-olds who at least needed spectacles (J. Carr unpub. data). Estimates of hearing problems also vary from 10–20% (Myers & Pueschel, 1991) to 21% for 30- and 35-year-olds (J. Carr unpub. data) and 31% for a sample with a mean age of 42 years (Prasher, 1995c). About three-quarters of all adults with Down syndrome are overweight or obese (Bell & Bhate, 1992; Prasher, 1995b). Obesity bears no relation to degree of learning disability, is more frequent in those living in the community than in institutions and declines in frequency with age (Prasher, 1995b). Women with Down syndrome tend to go through the menopause earlier (median age 47 years) than do women with other learning disabilities (median age 49 years) (Carr & Hollins, 1995; Schupf et al., 1997; Cosgrave et al., 1999).

In summary, most people with Down syndrome enjoy reasonably good health, although heart, skin and sensory problems may be troublesome.

Lifestyles

The majority of children with Down syndrome grow up in their own homes, and have done so for at least the last four decades. In the late 1950s, two-thirds of children and adults with Down syndrome lived at home (Tizard & Grad, 1961). In Carr's (1995) study, 79% of 11-year-olds and 61% of 21-year-olds lived at home, as did 60% of 30-year-olds (Carr, 2000). Individuals in Carr's (1995) study, who were at school between 1971 and 1985, with only three exceptions, attended schools for children with severe learning disabilities, but in 1990 nearly 20% were reported to be in mainstream schools (Sloper et al., 1990) and the number is almost certainly higher now. Results from a postal survey suggest that it has become increasingly possible over the last few years for a child with Down syndrome to gain a primary school place, although secondary school is more difficult (Lorenz, 1999).

More than 80% of adults with Down syndrome attend adult day centres, some also going to classes at colleges of further education. A small number – 5–15% – is without any day placement. Several studies (e.g. Holmes, 1988; Shepperdson, 1992) have shown fewer than 5% in paid (part-time) employment. Jobs held may be in supermarkets – shelf stacking, filling customers' bags, etc. – or in hotels or restaurants, serving, cleaning, and so on, while some have held clerical jobs or have worked in the arts. It is likely that many more people with Down syndrome could work if job opportunities and training were more available.

In terms of sexual relationships, 17% of adolescents (Pueschel & Scola, 1988) and 39% of young adults are reported as having a boy- or girl-friend (Holmes, 1988; Carr, 1995). Three-quarters of these relationships in Carr's (1995) study were said not to be serious; two of the young people had gone as far as getting engaged, but over half of the serious relationships were discouraged by parents or carers. Fewer than a third had had any sex education and none had married, although there are occasional reports of people with Down syndrome who have married (Cunningham, 1982; Brown, 1996).

Effect on families

The birth of a baby with Down syndrome usually comes as a tremendous shock to the family, but much can be done to help them cope. In numerous research studies parents have said that what they wanted of this difficult occasion was that they should be told early and truthfully – they were resentful when they felt they had been kept in the dark – and sympathetically, not brushed off with a brusque delivery of the information. In a study in which these guidelines were followed parents had no complaints of how they were told, compared with 80% of a control group who expressed dissatisfaction (Cunningham, Morgan & McGucken, 1984). As the child grows older most families adjust and are not seriously distressed. Mothers have been found to be no more anxious and depressed than mothers of non-disabled children (Ryde-Brandt, 1988) nor is family functioning significantly impaired (Van Riper, Ryff & Pridham, 1992). Despite some gloomy pronouncements on the likelihood of marital discord following the birth of a child with Down syndrome, there is little evidence of this (Byrne, Cunningham & Sloper, 1988). Carr (1995) found no differences in marriage ratings between families with a non-disabled 21-year-old or one with Down syndrome, and although fewer marriages had ended in divorce in the Down syndrome families, the difference was not significant.

Some studies have suggested that family functioning is *better* when a child has Down syndrome rather than another disabling condition. Cahill & Glidden (1996) carefully matched two groups of families, one group with children with Down syndrome, the other with children with various other types of developmental disability. There were no differences between the two groups but all the families were functioning well and close to the norms for families in general. What does emerge from many researches is the greater 'burden of care' (Tizard & Grad, 1961) borne, especially by the mother. For example, in families with a child with Down syndrome, parents spent more time in child care and less in social activities or paid employment than did parents of comparable children without Down syndrome, although in other areas, such as sleep, shopping and educational activities the groups did not differ (Barnett & Boyce, 1995). This was confirmed by Carr (1995), especially amongst families with a 21-year-old, where five times as many mothers of controls worked full-time compared with the Down syndrome group. Two-thirds of those mothers of people with Down syndrome who were working felt that their ability to do so had been affected by the restriction on the hours they could work (largely governed by the hours of the day centre the young person attended), and thus on the kind of work they could take. Others had given up work because of the needs of the young person. On the other hand, only 20% of the mothers said they had been made lonely by having the child, and an equal number felt that they had gained friends. Scores on Rutter's Malaise Scale (Rutter, Tizard & Whitmore, 1970) were higher at both 11 and 21 years for mothers of people with Down syndrome and more stress was reported by both mothers and fathers in the study by Cuskelly, Chant & Hayes (1998), although the stress levels reported were well within the normal range. In Carr's (1995) study higher Malaise scores were found in mothers who described themselves as depressed and by those from manual workers' families. Scores were also higher for those mothers whose offspring were more dependent (unable to go out beyond the garden) and lower where he or she was a good reader. No other significant factors, relating either to the mothers themselves or to the abilities or personalities of the people with Down syndrome, could be identified.

Turning to brothers and sisters, a source of distress for many parents is the worry that their other children will suffer from the presence of a sibling with Down syndrome. Early reports suggested that this was the case, but more recent research has shown few adverse effects. Siblings neither are reported nor report themselves as overburdened by caregiving (or other) tasks (Boyce, Barnett & Miller, 1991; Holmes & Carr, 1991; Boyce & Barnett, 1993). They get on well with the disabled sibling, and are no more jealous than siblings of non-disabled children (Byrne et al., 1988). Neither age nor sex has been shown to have a major effect. In two studies more disturbance was found in sisters (Gath, 1973; Cuskelly & Gunn, 1993), especially older sisters (Gath, 1974), but later studies could detect no disadvantage to brothers or sisters (Gath & Gumley, 1987; Cuskelly et al., 1998).

Overall the main finding of research concerned with the effect on families has been of 'an overwhelming impression of family "normality", variety and strength' (Byrne et al., 1988: p. 135). With all the extra difficulties they face, families of children and adults with Down syndrome cope, survive, and are 'more comparable to than different from families of non-disabled children' (Van Riper et al., 1992).

Progress from child- to adulthood

The development of people with Down syndrome can be considered from three main perspectives: the development of intellectual abilities; of motor ability; and of temperament and behaviour.

Intellectual abilities

Infants with Down syndrome have mean scores on standardized developmental measures that are somewhat, but not very far, below those achieved by infants generally. A number of studies of babies aged 6 months has found mean developmental quotients of 70–80 (Share, Webb & Koch, 1961; Carr, 1975; Ramsay & Piper, 1980). However, as they grow older, average scores decline, resulting in mean IQs of around 50 at the age of 4 years (Carr, 1985) and between 37 and 41 at 11 years old (Melyn & White, 1973; Kostrzewski, 1974; Carr & Hewett, 1982). There are few studies of adolescents but in Carr's longitudinal study of adults up to the age of 35 years (Carr, 2000) mean IQs, for the 37 people tested on all three occasions, were 43.1 at age 21, 41.7 at age 30, and 41.2 at age 35 years. Other cross-sectional studies of non-institutionalized people aged 30–60 + years have shown mean IQs fluctuating between 46 and 53 (Devenny et al., 1996), and similar though slightly lower figures for a comparably aged institutionalized group (Roeden & Zitman, 1997). These results are derived from somewhat disparate studies, but it is apparent that decline in IQ between age 21 and 35 years is minimal, and there is little evidence of consistent decline even well into the sixth decade. One study indeed reported that people tested first at an average age of 21 years and then again 6 years later showed an *increase* of 2 years' mental age over the period (Berry et al., 1984). This result is attributed to the regime the participants were engaged in, but no details of this are given and the findings have yet to be replicated.

Until now the discussion has concerned average scores, but anyone familiar with people with Down syndrome will be aware of the great range and variety in ability and achievement that occur within this population. On tests of intellectual ability, IQ scores of people with Down syndrome may range from around 15 to 75 or above. At the upper end of the range it is possible to meet a person with Down syndrome who can hold a lively conversation, is self-reliant, travels independently and has a job. Some people with Down syndrome have worked in offices, written books, shown marked artistic skill and had major roles in TV films. At the lower end of the range an individual may have little ability to communicate and will require a great deal of day-to-day care. The majority falls between these two extremes. Thus, although diagnosis of Down syndrome indicates the likelihood of an upper limit to ability, the differences *between* individuals are as striking as those found in any population.

Academic attainments

Many people with Down syndrome are able to learn to read, some achieving considerable proficiency. Children with Down syndrome, with an average age of 8 years (mean IQ 59), had a mean reading age of 7.2 years (Pieterse & Treloar, 1981). However, subsequent progress tends to be limited and the mean reading age for a group of 21-year-olds (mean IQ 54), was only 7.8 years, with a few obtaining reading ages of 9 and 12 years (Carr, 1995). These scores were for reading accuracy, and reading comprehension, where this has been studied, has usually been lower. Reading is highly correlated with IQ (Carr, 1995) (although other factors such as family background and gender are also involved). In Carr's (1995) study no 21-year-old with a mental age below 5 years 8 months was able to score on the reading test, and only four young men, who could not read at all, had mental ages higher than this.

Arithmetic is known to be more difficult than reading for people with Down syndrome. Children scored more highly on reading than on arithmetic tests (Irwin, 1989) and mean reading age surpassed mean arithmetic age by almost 4 years (Dunsdon, Carter & Huntley, 1960). In adulthood, average reading age was more than 2 years above average arithmetic age (Carr, 1995). Sixty-three per cent of the 21-year-olds in this study could do no more than recognize numbers and count; 25% could add two digits (4 + 3), and only 15% could subtract one number from another (5 − 2). Only two of the most able could do any two-figure adding or subtraction; none succeeded with multiplication or division. The highest arithmetic age gained was just under 8 years compared with the highest reading age of 12 years.

Motor performance

Infants with Down syndrome are markedly hypotonic and, although this hypotonia diminishes with age, muscle tone remains poor throughout life. Motor development of children with Down syndrome parallels quite closely that for mental development (see Carr, 1975: p. 34). Motor milestones are reached later than in non-disabled children but reports vary as to how much later. For example, walking alone, which is attained by non-disabled children at about 12 months, is reported to be achieved by children with Down syndrome at average ages of between 19 and 29 months (Share & French, 1974; Carr, 1975; Cunningham, 1982; Champion, 1987). In adolescence, motor development was related more to mental than to chronological age; proficiency in running speed, agility, balance and co-ordination increased, though slowly, and fine motor co-ordination and balance were poor even at 16 years of age (Jobling, 1998). Difficulties with balance are probably responsible for the wide stance and unsteady gait commonly seen in adults with Down syndrome (Penrose & Smith, 1966).

Temperament and behaviour

While the stereotype already described is not entirely substantiated, infants with Down syndrome were rated by their mothers as becoming easier in temperament as they grew older (Gunn, Berry & Andrews, 1981, 1983). In adolescence, mothers rated the children as being less active and persistent, more predictable, positive and distractible than mothers of the normative sample (Gunn & Cuskelly, 1991). In Carr's (1995) study of 11-year-olds with and without Down syndrome, more than half in each group were said to be easy, and this increased at 21 years of age to about three-quarters. In those with Down syndrome, specific behaviour problems – aggression, tantrums, etc. – were less marked at 21 than at 11 years of age, apart from rebelliousness, which increased from 50% at 11 to 67% at 21 years of age. The number rated as generally co-operative also increased from 11 to 21 years of age, a finding corroborated in a somewhat older group (average 28 years) by Holmes (1988).

In general then, people with Down syndrome are as variable in personality as they are in their abilities; there is a certain amount of support for the 'amiable' stereotype; and difficulties of temperament and behaviour tend to diminish as they grow from child- to adulthood.

Mental health

People with Down syndrome appear to be less vulnerable to a number of psychiatric disorders – neuroses, schizophrenia, paranoia – than are individuals with other learning disabilities (Myers & Pueschel, 1991; Collacott, Cooper & McGrother, 1992). In one study overall prevalence of psychiatric disorders was 22%, increasing with age from 17.6% in those under the age of 20 to 30.6% in those over the age of 28 years (Myers & Pueschel, 1991). Psychiatric disorders were more common in those with a severe learning disability, and increased in frequency with age in this group. However, in general there were fewer psychiatric disorders in people with Down syndrome than in those with other forms of learning disability (Myers & Pueschel, 1991; Haveman et al., 1994). Autism – once thought to be very rare in Down Syndrome – has been reported in a number of studies (Howlin, Wing & Gould, 1995). In older people with Down syndrome, psychological problems were associated with dementia (Haveman et al., 1994), and dementia itself accounted for nearly half the disorders noted (Prasher, 1995d). Depression is more common in people with Down syndrome than in individuals with other forms of learning disability, occurring in 5–10%, with a mean age of onset of 29–30 years (Collacott et al., 1992; Prasher & Hall, 1996). Obsessive–compulsive disorder, with the emphasis on the compulsive aspect, also seems to occur more frequently in Down syndrome than in other intellectual disability disorders (rates are estimated as 4.5%; Prasher & Day, 1995). Reported rates of conduct disorders vary from very low (Collacott et al., 1992) to relatively common (Prasher, 1995d). Mania, manic-depression and anorexia have been reported on isolated occasions (Cottrell & Crisp, 1984; Cook & Leventhal, 1987; Holt, Bouras & Watson, 1988; Haeger, 1990). Self-injury occurs only rarely in people with Down syndrome (Myers & Pueschel, 1991), and in only one of the 30- and 35-year-old group (the same one at each age) did it constitute a serious problem (J. Carr, unpub. data).

Effects of ageing and Alzheimer's disease

That ageing occurs early in people with Down syndrome was first noted by Fraser & Mitchell (1876), who described the deaths of a number of people as apparently having had no specific cause but being precipitated by 'a sort of premature senility'. Fifty years later the characteristic indicators of Alzheimer's disease were identified post-mortem in the brains of people with Down syndrome (Struwe, 1929) and have been adjudged to appear in the brains of all people with Down syndrome who died over the age of 40 (Thase, 1982) or even earlier (Heston, 1977). While these neuropathological indicators can be identified only post-mortem, clinical signs of the disease in people with Down syndrome have been summarized by Oliver & Holland (1986) as: behavioural (becoming 'unmanageable' or withdrawn); loss of self-care skills; deterioration in the use or understanding of language; apathy; and later complete helplessness. In some people these signs show clearly but in others they may be less obvious, especially if the person is already severely disabled.

The reports that Alzheimer's disease occurred universally in adults with Down syndrome caused considerable distress to carers, especially parents. More recently it has become apparent that, while the neurological indicators are found more frequently and earlier than in the general population, the clinical signs described above are much less inevitable, cross-sectional studies suggesting they are seen in only 10–45% of older people with Down syndrome. As in the general population they occur in increasing numbers of people as they get older but not in substantial numbers until after the age of 50 years, and more so after 60 years (Zigman et al., 1987). Even at the oldest ages the rate is well below 100% (Zigman et al., 1995), upper figures of 45% (Thase, 1988) and 54.5% (Prasher, 1995e) being given. Mean age at onset has been given as between 44 and 54 years, and mean duration of the disease as between 3.7 and 6 years (Dalton and Crapper-McLachlan, 1986, cited by Prasher, 1995e; Thase, 1988; Prasher, 1995e). People with Down syndrome at all levels of learning disability are affected.

Exploration of the indicators of Alzheimer's disease in people with Down syndrome have focused on three main areas: general ability (IQ); memory; and daily living skills such as dressing and toileting. Most studies of intelligence in old age have used a variety of tests – Stanford Binet; Peabody Picture Vocabulary test; and WISC – and have been cross-sectional, although clearly longitudinal research would be preferable. Most studies agree that the raw scores, on which IQs for people with learning disabilities are based, decline with age in people with Down syndrome (as they do in non-disabled people). Declines occurred more frequently in those aged over 45 years but were mainly small and of doubtful significance (Fenner, Hewitt & Torpy, 1987; Haxby, 1989; Devenny et al., 1996). Small declines in IQ in people with Down syndrome should be regarded as part of the normal ageing process and any decline needs to be considerable to be indicative of dementia.

Using tests of memory, the scores of people with Down syndrome have been found to decrease with increasing age (Thase, 1988). Failure of memory function began at an average of 49 years (Dalton & Crapper-McLaughlan, 1984) and affected tests of both auditory and visual skills (Marcell & Weeks, 1988). Longitudinal studies have shown decline in memory function to be an early sign of deterioration in people with Down syndrome, occurring before aphasia, apraxia or agnosia become evident (Oliver et al., 1998; Dalton et al., 1999).

Practical and daily living skills also decline as people become older. However, few differences have emerged between people with Down syndrome and those with other forms of learning disabilities apart from greater loss of eating skills and mobility for those with Down syndrome, and then only for those over 60 years (Silverstein et al., 1986). Later studies have suggested that the greater decline in the skills of people with Down syndrome is seen after 50 years of age but becomes more pronounced after 60 years of age (Zigman et al., 1987, 1989, 1995; Silverstein et al., 1988). These studies showed that the decline occurred in people living both in institutions and in the community. It was found in individuals with mild/moderate disabilities but not in those with severe disabilities (presumably because of floor effects) and occurred before cognitive decline was apparent, thus suggesting that changes in daily living skills may be a sensitive indicator of the ageing process.

In summary, most research reveals little evidence of deterioration in IQ, memory or practical skills in the majority of people with Down syndrome before the age of 50 years, or in some cases 60 years, well beyond the age at which the neuropathological signs of Alzheimer's disease are seen in this population. Moreover, in most studies fewer than 50%, even in the oldest age groups, showed clear signs of dementia. A variety of reasons has been proposed to account for the lack of association between neuropathological signs and cognitive performance: inadequate test procedures; the 'floor effect' (i.e. low scores in severely and profoundly learning disabled people may prevent decline being observable); or the possibility of a prolonged 'incubation period' before symptoms become apparent. Certainly before any individual is diagnosed with the disease other possible explanations for changes in behaviour, especially the possibility of sensory problems, depressive illness or thyroid dysfunction, should be considered, particularly if the person concerned is young. Despite the publicity given to the link between Down syndrome and Alzheimer's disease, families and carers may be reassured to know that 'the association of DS [Down syndrome] and the full clinical-neurological condition of (Alzheimer's) is far from absolute' (Thase, 1988: p. 361).

Treatment and remediation

Over the years much effort has gone into attempts to find physically-based treatments for people with Down syndrome. These have included the administration of dried thyroid gland, pituitary, thymus and cellular extracts, glutamic acid, dehydroepiandosterone and vitamin–mineral preparations. Almost without exception these were initially hailed as effective treatments but when tested in controlled studies none could be shown to be beneficial (Penrose & Smith, 1966: pp. 172–3). A later study suggested that a vitamin and mineral supplement could enhance IQ (Harrell et al., 1981). Again, well designed trials failed to substantiate these claims (Rolland & Spiker, 1985). Facial plastic surgery has been advocated, mainly with the aim of making the child less identifiable as having Down syndrome, but also, in the case of tongue reduction, to improve articulation. All these operations are likely to cause the child some degree of pain and are of doubtful benefit (Hayes, 1996). In a carefully controlled study, Cunningham et al. (1991) found no relationship between child appearance and any of the measures used, including child development, social and independent functioning, parental stress and quality of family life. Tongue reduction, which if it resulted in improved articulation could offer a real benefit to the children, has not been shown to have any significant effect (Parsons, Iacona & Rozner, 1987). Hayes (1996) points out the appeal of these treatments for parents, when conventional therapies do not offer the possibility of a cure, and stresses that professionals need to tread a fine line between answering questions honestly about the treatments, and being unduly discouraging of parents' understandable hopes.

Interventions have been focused on children, with the expectation that advances achieved in early years would benefit the person throughout his or her life. Those currently on offer fall into three main groups:

- Antenatal screening, with the option of termination of the pregnancy if the fetus is found to be affected by Down syndrome.
- Early intervention/intensive programming.
- Educational approaches.

Antenatal screening

Towards the end of the 1960s it became possible to screen pregnant women for a number of disabling conditions, including Down syndrome. Commonly, screening is available only to older women (i.e. aged 35 years or over) or to those at special risk because a close relative has Down syndrome. Even with this limited availability it was expected that the incidence of Down syndrome would fall. However, there is little evidence that this has occurred, due probably to the unavailability of screening to younger mothers (to whom about 70% of babies with Down syndrome are born), the low take-up of screening by some mothers, and the refusal of it by others, on moral or religious grounds, or because of possible health risks.

Although it is theoretically possible, by the use of screening and termination procedures, to prevent most children with Down syndrome from being born it is highly questionable whether this could ever be acceptable in practice. People with physical disabilities have argued that 'a disabled identity is one to be valued just like gender or ethnic identity' (Williams, 1995) and the same can be argued for a learning disability identity. Proponents of screening believe it will reduce human suffering, opponents that it is primarily aimed at economic benefit in reducing the cost of life-long care for people with Down syndrome, and that it demeans those already in the community. Fears are expressed that, because of economic factors, mothers are pressured into having the tests and then pressured to accept termination if the fetus is found to be affected. If this is the case it is also true that other parents have been equally distressed when the possibility of detection of abnormality was not discussed or offered to them in the antenatal period, and the baby was subsequently born with Down syndrome. Unless in the long-term it is seen as entirely unacceptable to countenance screening in any circumstances, the principle should surely be that it should be offered, with a balanced account of the full range of the characteristics and capabilities of people with Down syndrome, and the parents allowed to make their own decision (Quinn, 1996).

Early intervention

Early studies of the development of infants with Down syndrome focused on comparisons of the rates of progress in groups of children reared either in their own homes for at least some years, or entirely in institutions (mainly long-term 'subnormality hospitals'). All found the abilities of the home-reared children to be superior to those of the institution-reared groups (e.g. Centerwall & Centerwall, 1960; Shotwell & Shipe, 1964). However, when special programmes of individual attention and stimulation were introduced into the regimes of the institution reared children, the gap between them and their home-reared contemporaries was considerably reduced (Lyle, 1960; Bayley, Rhodes & Gooch, 1966). There followed a spate of studies in which infants and young children with Down syndrome were given extra teaching and stimulation. The earliest concerned children in institutions, (Bayley et al., 1966; Aronson & Fallstrom, 1977). Later, mothers and their babies attended developmental clinics and were coached in remedial activities (Connolly & Russell, 1976; Ludlow & Allen, 1979; Connolly et al., 1980; Piper & Pless, 1980), or families were visited and advised at home (Brinkworth, 1973; Hanson & Schwarz, 1978; Cunningham, 1982) or attended group training sessions (Bidder, Bryant & Gray, 1975). Some studies had their own controls but three (Connolly & Russell, 1976; Hanson & Schwarz, 1978; Connolly et al., 1980; Cunningham, 1982) relied on 'untreated' children from earlier studies. All but one of the 'intervention' studies reported significant IQ advantage for the trained groups over the period of the study. The exception was the study by Piper & Pless (1980); here the scores of both groups declined, rather more in the experimental than in the control group, though differences were not significant. Apart from this unusual result, the outstanding feature of this study is that all the assessments were done blind – the assessor was not one of those concerned with the intervention and did not know which group, experimental or control, the children were in. This was clearly not the case in most of the other studies, while in others no information is given on this point.

Nevertheless, the generally positive results led to a wave of optimism that the intellectual disabilities of people with Down syndrome were capable of considerable amelioration. Programmes to help parents stimulate their own children, based mainly on the Portage model (Shearer & Shearer, 1972) proliferated, and since it was felt to be unethical not to offer this service to any child or family, untreated comparison groups were rarely used. Subsequently some workers have expressed doubts about the, by now widely accepted, premise that early intervention programmes confer lasting benefit on people with Down syndrome. Gibson & Harris (1988) examined the overall findings from 21 intervention studies. They concluded that, first, the studies provided good evidence of short-term gains in IQ, eye–hand and fine motor co-ordination for the children concerned, especially where the programmes were parent oriented. Second, over time these gains were dissipated, the usual outcome being a gradual return to the level of the comparison groups. Cunningham (1987) and his colleagues have carried out one of the largest studies and explored many facets of intervention, including intensity, frequency and age at which the intervention began. Early results showed the expected superiority of the experimental group over Carr's (1975) cohort who had not received intervention. By the time Cunningham's group were 5 years old, however, compared with a contemporaneous comparison group no significant effects of the intervention on the children's development, nor on behaviour problems, nor on family characteristics such as stress or cohesion, could be seen. Significant effects that remained were that the intervention children were more likely to have attended mixed or mainstream pre-school facilities, their mothers were more likely to be employed and more likely to be prepared to leave the child unsupervised for longer periods.

Considering the high hopes surrounding the proliferation of early intervention programmes these are disappointing conclusions. Nevertheless it is not suggested that the programmes be abandoned, rather that they should be tailored to take account of the research findings and to attempt to provide help in the most appropriate way. Gibson & Harris (1988) point out that much is known about the ways in which children with Down syndrome learn; that this knowledge should be incorporated into the curriculum and, controversially perhaps, that it might be more fruitful to concentrate the teaching in late rather than early childhood, and in early adulthood. Cunningham (1987) concurs with Gibson and Harris' view that ordinarily sensible parents are probably all a child with Down syndrome needs in the first two years. He stresses the importance of social-interactive models of intervention and, especially, that of enhanced support for parents. These are as yet untried strategies and, as Gibson & Harris (1988) emphasize, if they were to be adopted they should be scrutinized in 'well-designed longitudinal comparison studies'. It has to be said that there is little sign of these alternative strategies being implemented, and the Portage model of early intervention continues to be provided, in the UK at least, as if the more recent research discussed here had never been conducted.

Educational approaches

It is sometimes suggested that it is more important to teach daily life skills to people with Down syndrome than reading and numbers. However, both for the pleasure of the people themselves, and to enable them to manage their lives effectively, a case can be made for the teaching of basic educational skills to be emphasized in the school years and continued into adult life. Programmes have been devised for teaching both reading (Buckley, Bird & Byrne, 1996; Farrell, 1996) and numbers (Kramer & Krug, 1973; Hanrahan & Newman, 1996) to children with Down syndrome. These incorporate innovative teaching strategies that may well be useful, although there is no research evidence for their effectiveness.

It has come to be increasingly accepted that children with Down syndrome should be taught in mainstream schools and that, educationally and socially, this constitutes the optimum educational setting for them. There is, however, little research to support this view, and what evidence there is, is conflicting. For example, the positive findings regarding educational attainment reported by Sloper and co-workers (1990) were not supported by Fewell & Oelwein

(1990). Where social integration is concerned, several studies have shown that real integration, and the development of close friendships between those with and without Down syndrome, are limited (Sinson & Wetherick, 1981; Ashman & Elkins, 1996). Nor did pupils with Down syndrome at mainstream schools experience increased social contacts in out-of-school hours (Sloper et al., 1990). These findings may only show that the best ways in which to include children with Down syndrome in ordinary schools have yet to be established. There is as yet no evidence concerning long-term effects of mainstream schooling on the adult life of people with Down syndrome.

Looking to the future

Many changes have taken place during the twentieth century in the lives of people with Down syndrome: life expectancy has quadrupled; attitudes have moved towards greater acceptance of people with learning disabilities in society; babies with Down syndrome whose parents feel unable to bring them up are no longer consigned to institutions but are popular candidates for adoption; and older people who have to move out of the family now go to small homes within the community. Further developments will certainly take place. Here we will consider those likely to occur in education and employment, and in the medical and psychiatric fields.

Further education and employment

People with Down syndrome can benefit from education that continues well beyond school-leaving age. Farrell (1996) presents a strong case for this continuation and offers suggestions for its implementation – for example, the inclusion of at least some phonics in the teaching of reading to people more usually taught by a whole-word approach, and an emphasis on reading for pleasure. It is doubtful whether many adults with Down syndrome receive such teaching to any substantial degree. In Carr's (1995) study, some 12% of 21-year-olds attended colleges of further education, usually for one to three days a week, and this proportion increased to 27% at 35 years of age (Carr, unpub. data). However, reports from parents and carers indicated that much of the time there was spent in activities such as drama, cooking, arts and crafts, gardening and so on. Fewer than a third of those at all three ages attended classes in literacy and numeracy, again usually for an hour a week. Valuable as are the other activities mentioned, the figures suggest that important literacy and numeracy skills are neglected in this group. Indeed, reading and number age ability barely altered between ages 21 and 35 years, being around 8 years for reading and 5 years for number (Carr, 1995 and unpub. data). People with Down syndrome are able to read for pleasure, and some do, and basic numeracy skills are important for people wishing to live independently. More people with Down syndrome should be given the opportunity to increase their mastery of these skills, although this may require 'concerted action at central and local levels' (Riches, 1996).

Many people with Down syndrome are capable of paid employment, many wish for it, and those who obtain it experience immense pride and satisfaction. Perera (1996) states that 'people with Down syndrome of any age and condition can work', given sufficient support and attention to their particular needs. It is certainly true that many more could work than currently do. In a number of studies fewer than 5% of adults with Down syndrome were employed, most of these part-time (Carr, 1994). Of 30- and 35-year-olds, 10 and 8% respectively had part-time jobs and nominal wages; just one woman in each age group was working almost full-time, and was paid the normal rate for the job (Carr, unpub. data). Perera (1996) believes that, for people with Down syndrome to succeed in the job market, attention must be paid to the personality and aptitudes of each person and an individualized training programme instituted, and gives examples of how this could be done. While recognizing the magnitude of the task, and present limitations on the job market, this is still a worthwhile aim to which to aspire.

Medical and psychiatric aspects

Medical progress is likely to involve greater sophistication in surgical techniques, new and more effective antibiotics, and more effective ways of treating hearing and thyroid problems. Much research is currently underway into Alzheimer's disease. Important discoveries are being made regarding genetic aspects (Hodes, 1994) and a number of treatment possibilities, for example dietary modifications, vitamins and other medicational remedies, are seen as deserving thorough evaluation (Holland, 1997).

Meanwhile it is clear that, given the medical problems to which they are prone, people with Down syndrome need to have routine medical checks throughout their lives (Prasher, 1994a). Anneren and Pueschel (1996) outline a programme of preventive medicine for children which could be adapted and extended for adults. They recommend that people with Down syndrome should have regular assessments of their sight and hearing (at least every 2 years for the latter). Wax in the ears is a common cause of poor hearing, and there is an increased risk of cataracts in this group. In addition, both hearing and visual problems are associated with poorer adaptive skills in the whole population, and, for those under 40 years of age, with a higher level of behaviour problems (Prasher, 1994b, 1995c). The prevention of sensory problems could have valuable side benefits. Epilepsy, however, has been found not to be related either to poorer adaptive skills or to behavioural problems, although this is contrary to some previous findings (Prasher, 1995a). Thyroid status also should be reviewed regularly, although it is encouraging that those with hypothyroidism seem no more likely to become demented than are those without the condition (Prasher, 1995e). Despite the frequency of heart defects in this population, heart rate and blood pressure have been found to be low in adults, and they may be at lower risk for coronary heart disease although, with a greater prevalence of cardiac valve defects, at higher risk for some other cardiac problems (Prasher, 1994a). Nevertheless because of the possibility of subclinical conditions, prophylactic antibiotics are advised before surgery or dental treatment, and this becomes essential where the person has mitral valve insufficiency (Anneren & Pueschel, 1996).

Regular screening is recommended for many common health problems of people with Down syndrome. In addition there is a growing awareness that more should be done to promote a healthier lifestyle. As they grow older, there is a tendency for people with Down syndrome to become sedentary and obese, this last being particularly marked in women (Bell & Bhate, 1992). Dieting is difficult for anyone, not least for those with Down syndrome, so prevention, starting in childhood, should be the aim. (A simple booklet is available, written especially for people with Down syndrome, by Sawtell, 1993). An active lifestyle not only helps weight control but may also promote muscle strength and cardiovascular fitness, both vulnerable areas for this population. Participation in many activities could be encouraged – swimming and horse riding are popular, and others such as football, bowling, aerobics, weight lifting and skiing are possible (Reid & Block, 1996). Attention to all these aspects of their lives could lead to better health and perhaps further increases in the lifespan of people with Down syndrome.

Where mental health is considered, the two main areas of concern are depression and dementia/Alzheimer's disease. In the manifestation of depression, where psychotic features are absent, the major signs noted are biological, such as sleeping and eating disorders, and psychomotor retardation and depressed mood (Anneren & Pueschel, 1996). Reports of the course of the illness vary. Follow-up after a year of a group treated with antidepressants showed that mood, energy and sleep had improved but not psychomotor retardation or poor concentration and only one of the 10 people had recovered to pre-episode level (Prasher & Hall, 1996). Another group with a history of depression, at

7-year follow-up showed no depressive symptoms but their adaptive skills were lower than in those with no history of depression (Collacott et al., 1992). Among the reasons put forward for this is that these skill deficits may indicate the first signs of dementia, and it is suggested that individuals with Down syndrome who develop depression in early life may be at greater risk for Alzheimer's disease subsequently. Two studies report the use of ECT with five severely depressed people with Down syndrome who had previously been treated with antidepressant medication. Between five and 14 treatments were given, without serious side-effects. Marked improvements were seen in all five, with a return to normal life, and this was maintained in follow-ups of between 6 months and 2 years (Warren, Holroyd & Folstein, 1989; Lazarus, Jaffe & Dubin, 1990).

As in the general population, dementia is seen in increasing numbers of people with Down syndrome as they age, affecting about half over the age of 60 years (Prasher, 1995e). Where the condition is suspected in a person with Down syndrome the first necessity is to determine whether the signs are in fact due to this disease or to some other process. Hypothyroidism can be revealed by a blood test (although taking blood from a person with Down syndrome is not always straight forward – in 20% of the sample in Prasher's (1995e) study it proved impossible) and can resolve when treated with thyroxine. The condition can be mistaken for dementia (Prasher & Krishnan, 1993) with a full return to normality with treatment. People with sensory problems may display some of the signs of dementia, such as loss of skills and increase in challenging behaviours (Prasher, 1994b, 1995c). Some signs of depression – for example, disturbed sleep and eating patterns, leading to loss of weight – are also similar to those of dementia, with the added complication that depression is in itself often one of the indicators of dementia (Prasher, 1995e).

Once other conditions have been ruled out, and it is established that a person with Down syndrome is suffering with Alzheimer's disease, there is little information as to how this should be handled. Brown (1996) calls for increased support for people with Down syndrome as they age. More specifically, Prasher (1995e) considers whether the care of people with Down syndrome and dementia should be provided by general services for the elderly, by services already available for people with learning disabilities, or – this author's preferred option – by a sub-speciality of the latter. On how best to care, day-to-day, for such people, the scientific literature is silent. However, Kerr (1997) offers a wealth of suggestions on the topic, and on how to help people maintain skills and interests for as long as possible. This includes: making communication meaningful; creating an environment suitable for people with particular deficits

Table 7.1. Practical and clinical implications of Down syndrome

- Life expectancy for people with Down syndrome has increased dramatically. Most now will be likely to outlive their parents
- Individuals with Down syndrome vary in personality and abilities as much as do people in the population generally
- Although they have a somewhat shorter life span than average, by no means all will suffer from dementia, and few before the age of 60
- The possibility of a thyroid deficiency, depression or sensory loss should always be investigated when a diagnosis of dementia is under consideration
- Families of people with Down syndrome generally adjust and cope, and 'are more comparable to than different from' families of non-disabled people (Van Riper et al., 1992).

such as confusion, or visual or hearing difficulties; and specific interventions, for example, Reality Orientation, reminiscence, and music. The publication by Kerr (1997) should be a welcome resource to professionals, parents and carers, while the research advocated by Prasher (1995e), on the best way to care for people with Down syndrome and Alzheimer's disease, is awaited.

For a summary of the practical and clinical implications of Down syndrome see Table 7.1.

REFERENCES

Anneren, G. & Pueschel, S. (1996). Preventive medical care. In *New Approaches to Down Syndrome*, ed. B. Stratford & P. Gunn, pp. 143–53. London: Cassell.

Aronson, M. & Fallstrom, K. (1977). Immediate and long term effects of developmental training in children with Down's syndrome. *Developmental Medicine and Child Neurology*, **19**: 489–94.

Ashman, A.E. & Elkins, J. (1996). School and integration. In *New Approaches to Down Syndrome*, ed. B. Stratford & P. Gunn, pp. 341–57. London: Cassell.

Barden, H.S. (1985). Dentition and other aspects of growth and development. In *Current Approaches to Down's syndrome*, ed. D. Lane & B. Stratford, pp. 71–84. London: Holt, Rinehart & Winston.

Barnett, W.S. & Boyce, G.C. (1995). Effects of children with Down syndrome on parent activities. *American Journal on Mental Retardation*, **100**(2): 1115–27.

Bayley, N., Rhodes, L. & Gooch, B. (1966). A comparison of the development of institutionalized and home reared mongoloids. A follow up study. *California Mental Health Research Digest*, **4**: 104–5.

Bell, A.J. & Bhate, M.S. (1992). Prevalence of overweight and obesity in Down's syndrome and other mentally handicapped adults living in the community. *Journal of Intellectual Disability Research*, **36**: 359–64.

Berry, P., Groenweg, G., Gibson, D. & Brown, R.I. (1984). Mental development of adults with Down syndrome. *American Journal of Mental Deficiency*, **89**: 252–6.

Bidder, R.T., Bryant, G. & Gray, O.P. (1975). Benefits to Down's syndrome children through training their mothers. *Archives of Diseases in Childhood*, **50**: 383–6.

Blacketer-Simmonds, D.A. (1953). An investigation into the supposed difference existing between mongols and other mentally defective subjects with regard to certain psychological traits. *Journal of Mental Science*, **99**: 702–19.

Boyce, G.C. & Barnett, W.S. (1993). Siblings of persons with mental retardation: a historical perspective and recent findings. In *The Effects of Mental Retardation, Disability and Illness*, ed. Z. Stoneman & P.W. Berman, pp. 145–84. Baltimore: P.H. Brookes.

Boyce, G.C., Barnett, W.S. & Miller, B.C. (1991). Time use and attitudes among siblings: a comparison in families of children with and without Down syndrome. Poster presented at the *Biennial Meeting of the Society for Research in Child Development*, Seattle, WA.

Brinkworth, R. (1973). The unfinished child. Effects of early home training on the mongol infant. In *Mental Retardation and Behavioural Research*, ed. A.D.B. Clarke. London: Churchill Livingstone.

Brown, R.I. (1996). Growing older: challenges and opportunities. In *New Approaches to Down Syndrome*, ed. B. Stratford & P. Gunn, pp. 436–50. London: Cassell.

Buckley, S., Bird, G. & Byrne, A. (1996). Reading acquisition by young children. In *New Approaches to Down Syndrome*, ed. B. Stratford & P. Gunn, pp. 268–79. London: Cassell.

Byrne, E.A., Cunningham, C.C. & Sloper, P. (1988). *Families and their Children with Down's Syndrome*. London: Routledge.

Cahill, B.M. & Glidden, L.M. (1996). Influence of child diagnosis on family and parental functioning: Down's syndrome versus other disabilities. *American Journal on Mental Retardation*, **101**: 149–60.

Carr, J. (1975). *Young Children with Down's syndrome*. London: Butterworths.

Carr, J. (1985). The development of intelligence. In *Current Approaches to Down's syndrome*, ed. D. Lane & B. Stratford, pp. 315–43. London: Holt, Rinehart & Winston.

Carr, J. (1994). Annotation: long term outcome for people with Down's syndrome. *Journal of Child Psychology and Psychiatry*, **35**: 425–39.

Carr, J. (1995). *Down's syndrome: Children Growing Up*. Cambridge: Cambridge University Press.

Carr, J. (2000). Intellectual and daily living skills of 30-year-olds with Down's syndrome: continuation of a longitudinal study. *Journal of Applied Research in Intellectual Disabilities*, **13**: 1–16.

Carr, J. & Hewett, S. (1982). Children with Down's syndrome growing up. *Association of Child Psychology and Psychiatry News*, Spring, 10–13.

Carr, J. & Hollins, S. (1995). Menopause in women with learning disabilities. *Journal of Intellectual Disability Research*, **39**: 137–9.

Centerwall, S.A. & Centerwall, W.R. (1960). A study of children with mongolism reared in the home compared to those reared away from home. *Pediatrics*, **25**: 678–85.

Champion, P. (1987). An investigation of the sensorimotor development of Down's syndrome infants involved in an ecologically based intervention programme: a longitudinal study. *British Journal of Mental Subnormality*, **33**(2): 88–99.

Collacott, R.A., Cooper, S.-A. & McGrother, C. (1992). Differential rates of psychiatric disorders in adults with Down's syndrome compared with other mentally handicapped adults. *British Journal of Psychiatry*, **161**: 671–4.

Connolly, B., Morgan, S., Russell, F. & Richardson, B. (1980). Early intervention with Down's syndrome children: a follow-up report. *Physical Therapy*, **60**: 1405–8.

Connolly, B. & Russell, F. (1976). Interdisciplinary early intervention program. *Physical Therapy*, **56**(2): 155–8.

Cook, E.H. & Leventhal, B.L. (1987). Down's syndrome and mania. *British Journal of Psychiatry*, **150**: 249–50.

Cosgrave, M.P., Tyrrell, J., McCarron, M. & Lawlor, B.A. (1999). Age at onset of dementia and age of menopause in women with learning disabilities. *Journal of Intellectual Disability Research*, **43**: 461–5.

Cottrell, D.J. & Crisp, A.H. (1984). Anorexia nervosa in Down's syndrome – a case report. *British Journal of Psychiatry*, **145**: 195–6.

Cuckle, H.S., Wald, N.J. & Thompson, S.G. (1987). Estimating a woman's risk of having a pregnancy associated with Down's syndrome using her age and serum alpha-fetoprotein level. *British Journal of Obstetrics and Gynaecology*, **102**: 387–402.

Cunningham, C.C. (1982). Psychological and educational aspects of handicap. In *Inborn Errors of Metabolism*, ed. F. Cockburn & R. Gitzelman, pp. 237–53. Lancaster: MTP Press.

Cunningham, C.C. (1987). Early intervention in Down's syndrome. In *Prevention of Mental Handicap: A World View* (RSM Services International Congress and Symposium Series No.112), ed. G. Hosking & G. Murphy, pp. 169–82. London: Royal Society of Medicine Services Ltd.

Cunningham, C.C., Morgan, P.A. & McGucken, R.B. (1984). Down's syndrome: is dissatisfaction with the diagnosis inevitable? *Developmental Medicine and Child Neurology*, **26**: 33–9.

Cunningham, C., Turner, S. Sloper, P. & Knussen, C. (1991). Is the appearance of children with Down's syndrome associated with their development and social functioning? *Developmental Medicine and Child Neurology*, **33**: 285–95.

Cuskelly, M., Chant, D. & Hayes, A. (1998). Behaviour problems in the siblings of children with Down's syndrome: association with family responsibilities and parental stress. *International Journal of Disability, Development and Education*, **45**: 295–311.

Cuskelly, M. & Gunn, P. (1993). Maternal reports of behavior of siblings of children with Down syndrome. *American Journal on Mental Retardation*, **97**: 521–9.

Dalton, A. & Crapper-McLachlan, D.R. (1984). Incidence of memory deterioration in ageing persons with Down's syndrome. In *Perspectives and progress in mental retardation*, vol. 2. ed. J.M. Berg, pp.55–62. Baltimore, MD: University Park Press.

Dalton, A. & Crapper-McLachlan, D.R. (1986). Clinical expression of Alzheimer's disease in Down's syndrome. *Psychiatric Perspectives in Mental Retardation*, **9**: 659–70.

Dalton, A.J., Mehta, P.D., Fedor, B.L. & Patti, P.J. (1999). Cognitive changes in memory precede those in praxis in persons with Down's syndrome. *Journal of Intellectual and Developmental Disability*, **24**: 169–87.

Dalton, A.J. & Wisniewski, H.M. (1990). Down's syndrome and the dementia of Alzheimer disease. *International Review of Psychiatry,* **2**: 43–52.

Devenny, D.A., Silverman, W.P., Hill, A.L., Jenkins, E., Sersen, E.A. & Wisniewski, K.E. (1996). Normal ageing in adults with Down's syndrome: a longitudinal study. *Journal of Intellectual Disability Research,* **40**(3): 208–21.

Down, J.L.H. (1866). Observations on an ethnic classification of idiots. *Clinical Lectures & Reports, London Hospital,* **3**: 259–62.

Dunsdon, M.I., Carter, C.O. & Huntley, R.M.C. (1960). Upper end of range of intelligence in mongolism. *Lancet,* **1**: 565–8.

Farrell, M. (1996). Continuing literacy development. In *New Approaches to Down Syndrome,* ed. B. Stratford & P. Gunn, pp. 280–9. London: Cassell.

Fenner, M.E., Hewitt, K.E. & Torpy, M. (1987). Down's syndrome: intellectual and behavioural functioning during adulthood. *Journal of Mental Deficiency Research,* **31**: 241–6.

Fewell, R.R. & Oelwein, P.L. (1990). The relationship between time in integrated environments and developmental gains in young children with special needs. *Topics in Early Childhood Special Education,* **10**: 104–16.

Fishler, K. & Koch, R. (1991). Mental development in Down syndrome mosaicism. *American Journal of Mental Deficiency,* **96**: 345–51.

Fraser, J. & Mitchell, A. (1876). Kalmuc idiocy: report of a case with autopsy with notes on 62 cases. *Journal of Mental Science,* **22**: 161.

Fryers, T. (1984). *The Epidemiology of Intellectual Impairment.* London: Academic Press.

Gath, A. (1973). The school age siblings of mongol children. *British Journal of Psychiatry,* **123**: 161–7.

Gath, A. (1974). Sibling reactions to mental handicap: a comparison of the brothers and sisters of mongol children. *Journal of Child Psychology and Psychiatry,* **15**: 187–98.

Gath, A. & Gumley, D. (1987). Retarded children and their siblings. *Journal of Child Psychology and Psychiatry,* **28**: 715–30.

Gibson, D. (1978). *Down's Syndrome: The Psychology of Mongolism.* Cambridge: Cambridge University Press.

Gibson, D. & Harris, A. (1988). Aggregated early intervention effects for Down Syndrome persons: patterning and longevity of benefits. *Journal of Mental Deficiency Research,* **32**: 1–17.

Gunn, P., Berry, P. & Andrews, R.J. (1981). The temperament of Down's syndrome infants: a research note. *Journal of Child Psychology and Psychiatry,* **22**: 189–94.

Gunn, P., Berry, P. & Andrews, R.J. (1983). The temperament of Down's syndrome toddlers. In *Approaches to Down Syndrome,* pp. 249–67. London: Cassell.

Gunn, P. & Cuskelly, M. (1991). Down syndrome temperament: the stereotype at middle childhood and adolescence. *International Journal of Disability, Development and Education,* **38**: 59–70.

Haeger, B. (1990). Mania in Down's syndrome (letter). *British Journal of Psychiatry,* **157**: 153.

Hallidie-Smith, K.A. (1985). The heart. In *Current Approaches to Down's syndrome,* ed. D. Lane & B. Stratford, pp. 52–70. London: Holt, Rinehart & Winston.

Hallidie-Smith, K.A. (1996). The heart. In *New Approaches to Down Syndrome,* ed. B. Stratford & P. Gunn, pp. 84–99. London: Cassell.

Hanrahan, J. & Newman, T. (1996). Teaching addition to children. In *New Approaches to Down Syndrome*, ed. B. Stratford & P. Gunn, pp. 300–8. London: Cassell.

Hanson, M.J. & Schwarz, R.H. (1978). Results of a longitudinal intervention program for Down's syndrome infants and their families. *Education and Training of the Mentally Retarded*, **13**: 403–7.

Harrell, H.F., Capp, R.H., Davis, D.R., Peerless, J. & Ravitz, L.R. (1981). Can nutritional supplements help mentally retarded children? *Proceedings of the National Academy of Science, USA*, **78**: 574–8.

Haveman, M.J., Maaskant, M.A., van Schrojenstein Lantman, H.M., Urlings, H.F.J. & Kessels, A.G.H. (1994). Mental health problems in elderly people with and without Down's syndrome. *Journal of Intellectual Disability Research*, **38**: 341–55.

Haxby, J.V. (1989). Neuropsychological evaluation of adults with Down's syndrome: patterns of selective impairment in non-demented old adults. *Journal of Mental Deficiency Research*, **33**: 193–210.

Hayes, A. (1996). Family life in community context. In *New Approaches to Down Syndrome*, ed. B. Stratford & P. Gunn, pp. 369–404. London: Cassell.

Heston, L.L. (1977). Alzheimer's disease, trisomy 21, and myeloproliferative disorders: associations suggesting a genetic diasthesis. *Science*, **196**: 322–3.

Hodes, R.J. (1994). Alzheimer's disease: treatment research finds new targets. *Journal of the American Geriatrics' Society*, **42**(6): 679–81.

Holland, A. (1997). Ageing and its consequences for people with Down's syndrome. *Down's Syndrome Association Newsletter*, **85**: 34–6.

Holmes, N. (1988). *The Quality of Life of Mentally Handicapped Adults and their Families*. Unpublished PhD thesis, University of London.

Holmes, N. & Carr, J. (1991). The pattern of care in families of adults with a mental handicap: a comparison between families of autistic adults and Down syndrome adults. *Journal of Autism and Developmental Disorders*, **12**: 159–76.

Holt, G.M., Bouras, N. & Watson, J.P. (1988). Down's syndrome and eating disorders. A case study. *British Journal of Psychiatry*, **152**: 847–8.

Howlin, P., Wing, L. & Gould, J. (1995). The recognition of autism in children with Down's syndrome – implications for intervention and some speculations about pathology. *Developmental Medicine and Child Neurology*, **37**: 398–414.

Irwin, K.C. (1989). The school achievement of children with Down's syndrome. *New Zealand Medical Journal*, **102**: 11–13.

Jobling, A. (1998). Motor development in school-aged children with Down's syndrome: a longitudinal perspective. *International Journal of Disability, Development and Education*, **45**: 283–93.

Johnson, A.W. & Abelson, R.W. (1969). The behavioral competence of mongoloid and non-mongoloid retardates. *American Journal of Mental Deficiency*, **73**: 856–7.

Kessling. A. & Sawtell, M. (1996). The genetics of Down's syndrome: a guide for carers. London: Down's Syndrome Association.

Kerr, D. (1997). *Down's Syndrome and Dementia*. Birmingham: Venture Press.

Kostrzewski, J. (1974). The dynamics of intellectual development in individuals with complete and incomplete trisomy of chromosome Group G in the karyotype. *Polish Psychological Bulletin*, **5**: 153–8.

Kramer, T. & Krug, D.A. (1973). A rationale and procedure for teaching addition. *Education and Training of the Mentally Retarded*, **8**: 140–5.

Lazarus, A., Jaffe, L. & Dubin, W.R. (1990). Electroconvulsive therapy and major depression in Down's syndrome. *Journal of Clinical Psychiatry*, **51**(10): 422–5.

Lejeune, J., Gautier, M. & Turpin, R. (1959). Les chromosome humaine en culture de tissus. *Compte rendu de l'Academie Science*, **248**: 602.

Lorenz, S. (1999). Experiences of inclusion for children with Down's syndrome in the UK. *Newsletter, Down's Syndrome Association*, **90**: 8.

Ludlow, J.R. & Allen, L.M. (1979). The effect of early intervention and pre-school stimulus on the development of the Down's syndrome child. *Journal of Mental Deficiency Research*, **23**: 29–44.

Lyle, J.G. (1960). The effect of an institution environment upon the verbal development of imbecile children. III: The Brooklands residential family unit. *Journal of Mental Deficiency Research*, **4**: 14–23.

Marcell, M.M. & Weeks, S.L. (1988). Short-term memory difficulties and Down's syndrome. *Journal of Mental Deficiency Research*, **32**: 153–62.

Melyn, M.A. & White, D.T. (1973). Mental and developmental milestones of non-institutionalised Down's syndrome children. *Pediatrics*, **52**: 542–5.

Myers, B.A. & Pueschel, S.M. (1991). Psychiatric disorders in persons with Down syndrome. *Journal of Nervous and Mental Disease*, **179**: 609–13.

Oliver, C., Crayton, L., Holland, A.J., Hall, S. & Bradbury, J. (1998). A four year prospective study of age-related cognitive change in adults with Down's syndrome. *Psychological Medicine*, **28**: 1365–77.

Oliver, C. & Holland, A.J. (1986). Down's syndrome and Alzheimer's disease: a review. *Psychological Medicine*, **16**: 307–22.

Parsons, C.L., Iacona, T.A. & Rozner, L. (1987). Effect of tongue reduction on articulation in children with Down's syndrome. *American Journal of Mental Deficiency*, **91**: 328–32.

Penrose, L.S. (1949). The incidence of mongolism in the general population. *Journal of Mental Science*, **95**: 685–8.

Penrose, L.S. & Smith, G.F. (1966). *Down's Anomaly*. London: J. & A. Churchill.

Perera, J. (1996). Social and labour integration of people with Down's syndrome. In *Down's Syndrome: Psychological, Psychobiological, and Socio-Educational Perspectives*, ed. J.A. Rondal, J. Perera, L. Nadel & A. Comblain, pp. 219–33. London: Whurr Publishers.

Pieterse, M. & Treloar, R. (1981). *The Down's Syndrome Program*. Progress Report, 1981, MacQuarie University. Cited by Buckley, S. (1985). Attaining basic educational skills: reading, writing and number. In *Current Approaches to Down's Syndrome*, ed. D. Lane & B. Stratford, pp. 315–43. London: Holt, Rinehart & Winston.

Piper, M.C. & Pless, I.B. (1980). Early intervention for infants with Down syndrome: a controlled trial. *Pediatrics*, **65**: 463–8.

Prasher, V.P. (1994a). Screening of medical problems in adults with Down syndrome. *Down's syndrome: Research and Practice*, **2**(2): 59–66.

Prasher, V.P. (1994b). Screening of opthalmic pathology and its associated effects on adaptive behaviour in adults with Down's syndrome. *The European Journal of Psychiatry*, **8**: 197–204.

Prasher, V.P. (1995a). Epilepsy and its associated effects on adaptive behaviour in adults with Down syndrome. *Seizure*, **4**: 53–6.

Prasher, V.P. (1995b). Overweight and obesity amongst Down's syndrome adults. *Journal of Intellectual Disability Research*, **39**: 437–41.

Prasher, V.P. (1995c). Screening of hearing impairment and its associated effects on adaptive behaviour in adults with Down's syndrome. *British Journal of Developmental Disabilities*, **61**(2): 126–32.

Prasher, V.P. (1995d). Prevalence of psychiatric disorders in adults with Down's syndrome. *The European Journal of Psychiatry*, **9**(2): 77–82.

Prasher, V.P. (1995e). End-stage dementia in adults with Down syndrome. *International Journal of Geriatric Psychiatry*, **10**: 1067–9.

Prasher, V.P. & Day, S. (1995). Brief report: obsessive-compulsive disorder in adults with Down's syndrome. *Journal of Autism and Developmental Disorders*, **25**(4): 453–8.

Prasher, V.P. & Hall, W. (1996). Short-term prognosis of depression in adults with Down's syndrome: association with thyroid status and effects on adaptive behaviour. *Journal of Intellectual Disability Research*, **40**: 32–8.

Prasher, V.P. & Krishnan, V.H.R. (1993). Hypothyroidism presenting as dementia in a person with Down's syndrome. *Mental Handicap*, **21**: 147–9.

Pueschel, S.M. & Scola, P.S. (1988). Parents' perceptions of social and sexual functions in adolescents with Down's syndrome. *Journal of Mental Deficiency Research*, **32**: 215–20.

Quinn, P. (1996). Should we prevent Down's syndrome? Letter. *British Journal of Learning Disabilities*, **24**: 88.

Ramsay, M. & Piper, M.C. (1980). A comparison of two developmental scales in evaluating infants with Down syndrome. *Early Human Development*, **4**: 89–95.

Rani, A.S., Jyothi, A., Reddy, P.P. & Reddy, O.S. (1990). Reproduction in Down's syndrome. *International Journal of Gynaecology and Obstetrics*, **31**: 81–6.

Reid, G. & Block, M.E. (1996). Motor development and physical education. In *New Approaches to Down Syndrome*, ed. B. Stratford & P. Gunn, pp. 309–40. London: Cassell.

Riches, V. (1996). Transition from school to community. In *New Approaches to Down Syndrome*, ed. B. Stratford & P. Gunn, pp. 143–53. London: Cassell.

Roeden, J.M. & Zitman, F.G. (1997). A longitudinal comparison of cognitive and adaptive changes in subjects with Down's syndrome and an intellectually disabled control group. *Journal of Applied Research in Intellectual Disabilities*, **10**(4): 289–302.

Rolland, C.P. & Spiker, D. (1985). Nutritional treatment for children. In *New Approaches to Down Syndrome*, ed. B. Stratford & P. Gunn, pp. 120–30. London: Cassell.

Rutter, M, Tizard, J. & Whitmore, K. (1970). *Education, Health and Behaviour*. London: Longman.

Ryde-Brandt, B. (1988). Mothers of primary school children with Down's syndrome: how do they experience their situation? *Acta Psychiatrica Scandinavia*, **78**: 102–8.

Sawtell, M. (1993). *Healthy Eating and Exercise: Information for Older Children and Adults with Down's Syndrome and their Carers*. London: Down's Syndrome Association.

Schupf, N., Zigman, W., Kapell, D., Lee, J.H. & Levin, B. (1997). Early menopause in women with Down's syndrome. *Journal of Intellectual Disability Research*, **41**: 264–7.

Share, J. & French, R.W. (1974). Early motor development in Down's syndrome children. *Mental Retardation*, **12**: 23–30.

Share, J., Webb, A. & Koch, R. (1961). A preliminary investigation of the early developmental status of mongoloid infants. *American Journal of Mental Deficiency*, **66**: 238–41.

Shearer, M. & Shearer, D. (1972). The Portage Project: a model for early childhood education. *Exceptional Children*, **36**: 172–8.

Shepperdson, B. (1992). *A longitudinal study of Down's syndrome adults*. End of Grant Award Report, Economic and Social Research Council, Swindon.

Sheridan, R., Llerena, J., Matkins, S., Debenham, P., Cawood, A. & Bobrow, M. (1989). Fertility in a male with trisomy 21. *Journal of Medical Genetics*, **26**: 294–8.

Shotwell, A.M. & Shipe, D. (1964). Effect of out-of-home care on the intellectual and social development of mongoloid children. *American Journal of Mental Deficiency*, **68**: 693–9.

Silverstein, A.B., Ageno, D., Alleman, K.T., Derecho, K.T., Gray, S.J. & White, J. (1985). Adaptive behavior of instutionalized individuals with Down syndrome. *American Journal of Mental Deficiency*, **89**: 555–8.

Silverstein, A.B., Herbs, D., Miller,T.J., Nasuta, R.,Williams, D.L. & White, J. (1988). Effects of age on the adaptive behavior of institutionalized and non-institutionalized individuals with Down's syndrome. *American Journal on Mental Retardation*, **92**: 455–60.

Silverstein, A.B., Herbs, D., Nasuta, R. & White, J.F. (1986). Effects of age on the adaptive behavior of institutionalized individuals with Down's syndrome. *American Journal of Mental Deficiency*, **90**: 659–62.

Sinson, J. & Wetherick, N.E. (1981). The behaviour of children with Down's syndrome in normal playgroups. *Journal of Mental Deficiency Research*, **25**: 113–20.

Sloper, P., Cunningham, C., Turner, S. & Knussen, C. (1990). Factors related to the academic attainments of children with Down's syndrome. *British Journal of Educational Psychology*, **60**: 284–98.

Steele, J. (1996). Epidemiology: incidence, prevalence and size of the Down's syndrome population. In *New Approaches to Down Syndrome*, ed. B. Stratford & P. Gunn, pp. 45–72. London: Cassell.

Stratford, B. & Steele, J. (1985). Incidence and prevalence of Down's syndrome – a discussion and report. *Journal of Mental Deficiency Research*, **29**: 95–107.

Struwe, F. (1929). Histopathologische Untersuchungen uber Enstehung und Wesen der senilen Plaques. *Zeitschrift fur die gesamte Neurologie und Psychiatrie*, **122**: 291.

Thase, M.E. (1982). Reversible dementia in Down's syndrome. *Journal of Mental Deficiency Research*, **26**: 177–92.

Thase, M.E. (1988). The relationship between Down syndrome and Alzheimer's disease. In *The Psychobiology of Down Syndrome*, ed. L. Nadel, pp. 345–68. Cambridge, MA: MIT Press.

Tizard, J. & Grad, J.C. (1961). *The Mentally Handicapped and their Families*. London: Oxford University Press.

Van Riper, M., Ryff, C. & Pridham, K. (1992). Parental and family well-being in families of children with Down's syndrome: a comparative study. *Research in Nursing and Health*, **15**: 227–35.

Warren, A.C., Holroyd, S. & Folstein, M.F. (1989). Major depression in Down's syndrome. *British Journal of Psychiatry*, **155**: 202–5.

Williams, P. (1995). Should we prevent Down's syndrome? *Learning Disabilities*, **23**: 46–50.

Wishart, J. & Johnston, F.H. (1990). The effects of experience on attribution of a stereotyped personality to children with Down's syndrome. *Journal of Mental Deficiency Research*, **34**: 409–20.

Zaremba, J. (1985). Recent medical research. In *Current Approaches to Down's syndrome*, ed. D. Lane & B. Stratford, pp. 27–54. London: Holt, Rinehart & Winston.

Zigman, W.B., Schupf, N., Lubin, R.A. & Silverman, W.A. (1987). Premature regression of adults with Down's syndrome. *American Journal of Mental Deficiency*, **92**: 161–8.

Zigman, W.B., Schupf, N., Silverman, W.P. & Sterling, R.C. (1989). Changes in adaptive functioning of adults with developmental disabilities. *Australian & New Zealand Journal of Developmental Disabilities*, **15**: 277–87.

Zigman, W.B., Schupf, N., Sersen, E. & Silverman, W.P. (1995). Prevalence of dementia in adults with and without Down's syndrome. *American Journal on Mental Retardation*, **100**: 403–12.

8

Fragile X syndrome

Randi J. Hagerman and Paul J. Hagerman

Introduction

Fragile X syndrome (FXS) is caused by a trinucleotide $(CGG)_n$ repeat expansion in the fragile X mental retardation 1 (FMR1) gene which is located near the end of the long arm of the X chromosome. Although by now over 200 genes have been identified on the X chromosome in which a mutation leads to learning disabilities, fragile X is the most common cause of X-linked learning disabilities, representing 30% of these disorders (Sherman, 1996). Fragile X also causes learning and emotional problems without mental retardation, indicating a very broad spectrum of involvement in this disorder.

Prevalence figures for FXS are complicated, as there have been new ways of diagnosing the syndrome, and different populations have been screened for this disorder. Before the FMR1 gene was discovered in 1991 (Verkerk et al., 1991), FXS was identified through cytogenetic testing, which revealed a fragile site near the end of the long arm of the X chromosome in affected individuals. However, other mutations besides the FMR1 mutation have been discovered which lead to a fragile site at this location. Although early cytogenetic studies suggested a prevalence figure of close to 1 per 1000 in the general population, more recent DNA studies of the CGG repeat element in the FMR1 gene have demonstrated that approximately 1 in 4000 males and 1 in 6000 females in the general population have learning disabilities caused by FXS (Turner et al., 1996; de Vries et al., 1997). These studies, however, have only screened individuals with global learning disabilities. A recent report by Crawford et al. (1999) assessed almost 3000 seven- to ten-year-old children in special education classes, which included children with global and other learning difficulties. They found that 1 in 362 white students and 1 in 422 black students in special education had the fragile X mutation. When these figures are extrapolated back to the general population, assuming that all children with fragile X would be in special education classes, the overall prevalence was determined to be 1 in 3460 (whites) and 1 in 4048 (blacks). It is important to realize, however, that some individuals, particularly females, with fragile X are relatively mildly affected, and they may not be identified as requiring special education. It is likely that approximately 1 in 2000 in the general population may be affected to some degree by the FMR1 mutation when individuals with mild learning difficulties and/or mild emotional problems are included.

Everyone carries the FMR1 gene, which produces a protein that is important for brain development. In the general population, the CGG repeat element in the FMR1 gene varies from approximately 6 to 54 repeats, with a mean of 29 to 30 repeats (Brown, 1996; Wells, Warren & Sarmiento, 1998). Individuals who have the premutation, defined as a small expansion of the CGG repeat number between 55 to 200 repeats, are carriers and are usually unaffected cognitively, although there are some exceptions to this rule as discussed below. The premutation occurs in approximately 1 in 250 females and 1 in 700 males in the general population (Rousseau et al., 1995, 1996). When the premutation is carried by a female and passed to the next generation, it will usually expand to a full mutation (more than 200 CGG repeats). The full mutation is usually methylated within the promoter region, including the CGG repeat, and is typically associated with a lack of activity of the gene, such that little or no FMR1 protein (FMRP) is produced.

Clinical involvement in fragile X is generally believed to result from a lack of FMRP. In the standard model for FMR1 expression, reduced levels of FMRP (or its absence) are thought to be due to transcriptional 'silencing' of the FMR1 gene, consequent to expansion of the CGG repeat into the full mutation range and accompanying methylation of the promoter region of the gene (Pieretti et al., 1991; Sutcliffe et al., 1992). Males with full mutation alleles that have escaped methylation generally possess detectable levels of FMRP (Smeets et al., 1995), and display a milder clinical phenotype, with specific learning disabilities in the absence of mental retardation (de Vries et al., 1996a; Hagerman, 1996b; Tassone et al., 1999). Women with full mutation alleles generally display milder clinical phenotypes, and possess higher levels of FMRP, due to the presence of some normal, active allele.

Clinical phenotype

Physical features

The physical phenotype of FXS is associated with a connective tissue disorder. Most individuals have soft velvet-like skin, hyperflexible joints, and somewhat prominent ears. The ear pinnae may have cupping, and the ears may appear to be prominent particularly at the tips. Finger joints can be hyperflexible, with thumbs that can be easily dislocated (double-jointed), and the fingers may bend back to greater than 90 degrees. Feet are often flat, and the ankles may pronate inward because of flexibility in the tendons around the joints.

Approximately 25% of young children with FXS may not show these typical physical features (Hagerman, 1999). As individuals age, the face may become long and narrow and the jaw may become prominent after puberty. Joint flexibility often decreases with age; approximately 30% of adults may have hyperextensibility of the finger joints. Macro-orchidism, or large testicles, are commonly seen in adolescence and adulthood, but are usually not present in the prepubertal child. Although the testicles are large, fertility appears to be normal. Males who have full mutation alleles in their blood will only transmit premutation alleles to the next generation. All of their daughters will be premutation carriers, but none of their sons will be carriers, because they receive the Y chromosome instead of the X. Females who have the premutation or the full mutation typically pass on the full mutation to their offspring when the abnormal X chromosome is transmitted. Females with the full mutation are less likely than males to show the typical physical features, because they have two X chromosomes, and the normal X chromosome is usually active in some cells (i.e. producing FMRP), which leads to less clinical involvement. The activation ratio (AR) is defined as the percentage of cells in which the normal X chromosome is active. The greater the activation ratio, the more FMRP produced, which leads to decreased clinical involvement (Mazzocco et al., 1997; Riddle et al., 1998; Tassone et al., 1999).

Additional physical features associated with fragile X include a high arched palate, a single or bridged palmar crease in the hand, a hallucal crease between the first and second toe on the sole of the foot, broad fingers and toes, and hypotonia in infancy (Hagerman, 1999).

Medical complications associated with the connective tissue abnormality in FXS include a higher incidence of inguinal or umbilical hernias, gastro-oesophageal reflux in infancy, an occasional joint dislocation, particularly at the shoulder, elbow or kneecap, and mitral valve prolapse secondary to a floppy mitral valve, which occurs in approximately 50% of adults with fragile X (Hagerman, 1996b). In childhood, recurrent otitis media infections, perhaps related to a collapsible eustachian tube, are a problem for over 60% of young children. Grommets (PE tubes) are often necessary to normalize hearing, which in turn leads to improvements in language and cognitive development. Ophthalmological problems including strabismus or refraction errors occur in 8–50% of affected children (King, Hagerman & Houghton, 1995; Hatton et al., 1998). These problems require treatment, and an evaluation by an ophthalmologist or optometrist is essential in early childhood. Seizures are seen in approximately 20% of children with FXS, but they usually improve or disappear in adolescence (Musumeci et al., 1999).

Cognitive features

Approximately 80% of males and 70% of females affected by FXS are intellectually impaired (IQ less than 70) (de Vries et al., 1996b; Hagerman, 1999). The degree of intellectual involvement can be correlated with the molecular measures, including the level of FMRP, the activation ratio, and whether the individual has a mosaic status (that is, some cells with the premutation and some cells with the full mutation, or some cells with a lack of methylation). The presence of mosaicism correlates with increased levels of FMRP, and the greater level of FMRP is correlated with higher IQ levels (Tassone et al., 1999). In a study assessing males with the FMR1 mutation, it was found that males with the full mutation in adulthood had a mean IQ of 41, whereas males with a mosaic pattern had a mean IQ of 60, and males who had more than 50% of their gene unmethylated had a mean IQ of 88 (Merenstein et al., 1996). The level of FMRP in peripheral blood leukocytes may be a useful prognostic indicator for the degree of cognitive involvement in adulthood. Recently developed measures of FMRP using immunocytochemical methods can document the percentage of lymphocytes that produce FMRP (Willemsen et al., 1997). Moreover, hair follicles have been used to detect the presence of FMRP in males and females (Willemsen et al., 1999). What is still needed, however, is a more accurate quantitative measure of actual FMRP levels in each leukocyte.

In a study of females, Performance IQ scores appeared to be more sensitive to the activity of the FMR1 gene than Verbal IQ (de Vries et al., 1996b; Riddle et al., 1998). Executive function deficits are common in females with FXS even when their IQ is in the normal range (Mazzocco, Pennington & Hagerman, 1993). Visual spatial perception problems, particularly difficulty on the Block Design and Object Assembly subtests of the Wechsler scales, are common in higher functioning females, and are also part of the global cognitive deficits found in more severely impaired males and females (Bennetto & Pennington, 1996). IQ decline is a common problem in both males and females who are significantly affected by FXS (Wright Talamante et al., 1996). Cognitive decline begins in middle childhood but becomes more significant in adolescence. If the fraction of FMRP-positive lymphocytes is greater than 50%, it is unlikely that cognitive decline will occur (Wright Talamante et al., 1996; Tassone et al., 1999).

Individuals with FXS have a number of areas of strength, including a good sense of humour, strong imitation skills, a good memory for events and directions, and intense interests in particular areas. They also learn from their environment to a greater extent than one would predict from their overall IQ. On the Kaufman Assessment Battery for Children (KABC), the Achievement scores are almost always higher than the Mental Processing Composite scores (MPC is an IQ equivalent), with the exception of the Arithmetic scores (Kemper et al., 1986). Maths is almost always a significant deficit area even in normal IQ individuals with FXS, perhaps because of the abstract reasoning necessary for maths concepts.

Neuropathology

Neuropathological studies in the knockout mouse and in three humans with FXS have demonstrated immature dendritic spines and a higher spine density compared with individuals without FXS (Comery et al., 1997; Irwin et al., 1999). These findings have lead to the hypothesis that FMRP is essential for the normal maturation of dendritic spines and for the normal pruning process of dendritic spine connections that occur in development. A deficiency of FMRP would therefore lead to an enhanced number of dendritic spines in FXS.

Neuroimaging studies in FXS have demonstrated an enlargement of the overall brain compared to controls (Schapiro et al., 1995) and enlargement of specific regions including the caudate and the hippocampus (Reiss, Lee & Freund, 1994; Reiss et al., 1995). In addition, the posterior cerebellar vermis is decreased in patients with FXS compared to controls (Reiss et al., 1991). The reason for these changes is unknown, although the consequences can be linked to the cognitive changes that are seen. The size of the posterior cerebellar vermis in females with FXS correlates with IQ measures and executive function deficits and inversely correlates with the number of schizotypal features seen (Mostofsky et al., 1998). Two recent autopsy studies of older men with FXS (age 67 and 87 years) have demonstrated focal Purkinje cell loss in the cerebellum (Sabaratnam, 2000).

Behaviour

Young children with fragile X usually present with language delay and hypotonia. Most children are not speaking in phrases by 2 years of age, although this usually appears between the ages of 3 and 5 years. Hyperactivity and a short attention span are typical in the pre-school period. Earlier in infancy, behaviour may be marked by irritability and a lack of typical cuddling. These problems may be related to sensory integration difficulties including avoidant behaviour to certain touch stimuli. Usually this sensitivity to touch is overcome in early childhood such that these children will hug, but intermittently they may demonstrate a sensitivity to touch, as when their fingernails are being cut, or their hair brushed.

The sensitivity that children with FXS demonstrate to visual, tactile, auditory and olfactory stimuli is described collectively as sensory integration dysfunction (Scharfenaker et al., 1996). Recent electrodermal studies, which measure sweat response to stimuli, have shown that children with FXS are over-reactive to a wide variety of sensory stimuli, with an enhanced amplitude and poor habituation compared to controls (Belser & Sudhalter, 1995; Miller et al., 1999). The sympathetic system controls the sweat response to stimuli, and these studies document an enhanced sympathetic response. This may be the physiological basis of the hyperarousal to sensory input in children with fragile X. This enhanced response may manifest clinically as an increase in anxiety in certain situations, particularly those that involve transitions or unfamiliar surroundings. Sometimes the anxiety may result in aggression or social withdrawal. Aggression is more common in adolescence and adulthood (Merenstein et al., 1996), and may be more difficult to handle at these ages. Many of the autistic-like features that have been described in FXS, including poor eye contact, hand flapping with excitement, hand biting when angry or anxious and tactile defensiveness, may be related to sensory integration dysfunction.

Most affected individuals are interested in social interactions, but shyness and social anxiety, along with sensory integration problems, may interfere with appropriate social behaviours (Freund, Reiss & Abrams, 1993; Hagerman, 1996b; Mazzocco et al., 1997; Franke et al., 1998). Emotional perception in facial expressions in boys with FXS was comparable to controls with a similar IQ (Turk & Cornish, 1998). However, approximately 15% of children and adults with FXS meet DSM-III or DSM-IV criteria for autism because of additional deficits in social relatedness (Hagerman et al., 1986; Baumgardner et al., 1995). When younger children with FXS are evaluated for autism, the rate may increase to 25 to 33% (Turk & Graham, 1997; Bailey et al., 1998b; Rogers, Wehner & Hagerman, 2000). The highest rate of 33% was reported for pre-school children with FXS aged between two and four years (Rogers et al., 2001). The autism of children with FXS was indistinguishable from that of children who had idiopathic autism using the ADOS and the ADI measures to assess autism. However, the autistic features of many children with FXS who are diagnosed in the pre-school period, will improve after intensive therapy focused on improving their social deficits and enhancing language and motor abilities. Those children whose autism persists into adulthood may have a core deficit in social relatedness which could reflect additional genetic factors superimposed on the FMR1 mutation. As their interest in social interactions evolves in early childhood, those with better linguistic, cognitive and imitation skills appear to do best in long-term follow-up. However, problems with shyness and social anxiety often persist, and in adulthood mild social withdrawal is very common (Kerby & Dawson, 1994).

Obsessive–compulsive behaviour is a common problem in both children and adults with FXS. In childhood, there may be intense interests in cars, sports or other objects. Perseverative behaviours and language are also common. Children often insist on watching the same video over and over again, or perseverate on certain themes seen in a video or movie. Well known phrases in films and television may be incorporated into a vocal routine that is often difficult to distinguish from a complex vocal tic. As an example, when the film *The Mask* became popular, many individuals with FXS adopted words and mannerisms taken from the main character, (e.g. 'smokin', said with a swing of the arm).

In adolescence, obsessional thinking may be focused on individuals of the opposite sex, with intense infatuations that, on occasion, lead to aggressive behaviour when that person is present. Sexual obsessions, such as a foot fetish, are not uncommon. Effeminate behaviour can be seen in approximately 20% of males with FXS. At first it was thought that this was related to enhanced imitation abilities and movements, such as flicking the hair or effeminate hand movements, which were demonstrated in a perseverative way by males who had female caretakers or females as case managers. However, the changes in neuroanatomical structure present in FXS, including enhanced dendritic connections and enhancement in the size of the hippocampus and caudate, may be a more likely cause for effeminate behaviour. Some adult males with FXS who are higher functioning and who have effeminate behaviour describe themselves as homosexuals in adulthood. For most males with FXS, the degree of intellectual deficit interferes with their sexual identity. The majority of males with FXS who have moderate learning disabilities or who are at the lower end of the mildly intellectual disabled range, are not sexually active. Males whose cognitive deficits fall within the very mild or borderline to normal range are usually sexually active and may have either a heterosexual or homosexual preference.

The most common behavioural problem in children with FXS is attention deficit hyperactivity disorder (ADHD). Approximately 70–80% of boys with FXS have some degree of ADHD, and most have hyperactivity combined with attention and concentration difficulties (Hagerman, 1996b). The hyperactivity tends to improve with age, and usually resolves by late adolescence or adulthood. However, the attentional difficulties, along with impulsivity and distractibility, often persist throughout adolescence and into adulthood. ADHD symptoms can be treated effectively with stimulant medications, as described below. Hyperactivity may also be associated with the problem of hyperarousal to sensory stimuli, and this can also be addressed with medication and psychological therapies.

Girls with FXS are less likely to be overtly hyperactive, although attention and concentration problems are common and are present in 30–50% of those with the full mutation (Hagerman et al., 1992; Freund et al., 1993). Girls with FXS who are not hyperactive or impulsive are at greater risk for selective mutism, which is associated with anxiety (Hagerman et al., 1999). The shyness and social anxiety problems may cause great difficulties in school, so it is usually in this environment that a child may become less and less talkative, whisper or become mute. Academic pressures to come up with an answer when questioned by a teacher in school may eventually lead to mutism in the classroom, and this problem usually continues in the medical clinic where the child is subsequently evaluated. Usually the parents indicate that communication at home among family members is normal. Selective mutism may also occur very rarely in higher functioning males with FXS.

In general, the communication of individuals with FXS usually includes perseverative and repetitive language with the frequent use of specific statements, such as 'let's get out of here' or 'I hate you' (Sudhalter et al., 1990; Sudhalter, Scarborough & Cohen, 1991). The use of these phrases and more automatic verbalizations is very common, in addition to mumbling with a lack of eye contact. Verbal dyspraxia is common in boys with FXS (Spinelli et al., 1995). Hand mannerisms such as hand flapping or other types of stereotypies may also occur during the communication process. Because of these oddities in communication and social interaction, some adolescent and adult individuals are described as having schizotypal features, features on the spectrum of pervasive developmental disorder (PDD) or Asperger-like features (Hagerman, 1996b). Because of the close association between FXS and autism spectrum disorders including Asperger syndrome, it is important that individuals who present with these diagnoses are also assessed using the FMR1 DNA test for FXS.

Involvement in individuals with the premutation

Most individuals who have the premutation (55-200 CGG repeats) have normal intellectual abilities (Reiss et al., 1993). However, they may have a limited number of physical features typical of the syndrome, when compared to controls, such as slightly prominent ears, a prominent jaw, or a high arched palate (Riddle et al., 1998). In addition, premature menopause is seen in approximately 25% of women who carry the premutation (Schwartz et al., 1994; Vianna-Morgante et al., 1996), and twinning occurs at a rate that is three times that of the normal population (Turner et al., 1994). Several studies have assessed emotional problems, and difficulties with anxiety, mood lability or depression can be seen in approximately 20–30% of women with the premutation (Franke et al., 1996; Sobesky et al., 1996; Franke et al., 1998).

More recently, a small number of individuals with the premutation have been detected with autism, or specific learning disabilities (including in maths), ADHD problems, or mood lability (Hagerman et al., 1996; Tassone et al., 2000b). In the standard model for FMR1 expression, individuals with premutation alleles are presumed to have normal levels of mRNA and protein, since such alleles are generally not methylated. However, FMR1 mRNA levels in premutation males were recently demonstrated to be elevated relative to those of normal controls, despite normal to moderately low FMRP levels (Tassone et al., 2000a). Furthermore, elevated mRNA levels persist in the full mutation range in the absence of methylation-coupled silencing (F. Tassone et al., unpub. data). These observations, coupled with the earlier observation that the efficiency of translation of the FMR1 mRNA is decreased in the full mutation range (Feng et al., 1995), suggest that elevated message levels may be a compensatory response to impaired translation. This implies that molecular-therapeutic strategies must consider means for enhancing/activating both transcription and translation, and that enhancement of translation alone may lead to clinical improvement.

Outcomes in adulthood

Cognitive abilities and attainments

Most males with FXS with the full mutation are moderately intellectually impaired (Merenstein et al., 1996), but they may show strengths relative to their IQ scores in adaptive behaviour and daily living skills (Dykens et al., 1996). There are various vocational endeavours in which they may excel; many do well in the catering or restaurant trades, particularly working in food preparation or washing dishes; they may also do well in laundry, gardening and janitorial work. However, vocational training is essential in secondary school, and in the United States (US) most special education programmes will continue job training until 21 years of age. The use of a job trainer after high school to develop specific skills in the job setting is also usually required. Individuals with moderate or severe learning disabilities will usually need a sheltered workshop setting with more limited vocational goals.

The memory skills of adults with FXS can be an advantage in the vocational setting. For instance, one adult we followed up did well at delivering mail inside of an office building, because he quickly learned the names of all of the people in the building, and he enjoyed the brief social interaction with these individuals as he delivered the mail.

Computer technology has been under-utilized in vocational training. Computer skills are typically emphasized in the US in elementary education, but not in high school or in vocational training. The ability to use computers can be a strength in many individuals with FXS and does not necessarily correlate with IQ (C. Bodine et al., unpub. data). Software programmes, such as Write Out Loud and Co:Writer, can help to improve written language output and computer technology can be used to enhance vocational endeavours. One example of this is a young man who works with his father selling plans via the computor for small construction projects, such as building a tool shed. He is able to handle the orders that come in, and can e-mail the appropriate plans to the customers. For those individuals with FXS who are socially very shy or have autistic features, interaction through e-mail is less intimidating.

Occasionally, behaviour problems such as mood instability, temper outbursts, aggression, or severe anxiety can interfere with vocational and social endeavours. Significant behavioural problems which interfere with daily living occur in approximately 50% of adults with FXS, and around one-third have problems with aggression (Hagerman, 1996b), although a longitudinal study showed that aggression was less of a problem after 7 years in follow-up (Einfeld, Tonge & Turner, 1999). A variety of psychopharmacological interventions can be helpful for these behaviour problems (see below). In addition, environmental modifications can significantly decrease excessive stimuli in a vocational setting, thereby decreasing hyperarousal, anxiety and subsequent aggression. In employment many individuals do well in settings without excessive stimuli or noise, such as janitorial work in an office building after hours, or working in a library or garden.

Social and emotional adjustment

Although the majority of adults with FXS do not have autism or severe social deficits, mild social interactional difficulties are common and are exacerbated by anxiety or hyperarousal. There is a tendency towards greater social withdrawal in adulthood, simply because many adults feel more comfortable watching their favourite television programmes or listening to the stereo in the quiet of their room, instead of interacting socially (Einfeld et al., 1999). It is important for adults with this tendency to have regularly scheduled and predictable social interactional activities to avoid increasing social isolation.

Higher functioning males and females with FXS are able to engage in more intense social interactions and sexual activity. Counselling can be helpful to deal with problems such as tactile defensiveness, and other difficulties associated with intimacy. Executive function deficits are typically seen in individuals with the full mutation who are higher functioning, or even in those with a normal IQ. These lead to problems in the ADHD spectrum, including impulsivity, attentional difficulties and organizational problems. In addition, features such as tangential language, poor topic maintenance and schizotypal features are commonly seen and are associated with the degree of executive function deficits that an individual manifests (Sobesky, 1996). It is unusual for a male with FXS to reproduce, but this occasionally occurs; in such cases all male children would be unaffected by FXS, but females would be premutation carriers. On the other hand, females with the full mutation more frequently reproduce than males, because their cognitive abilities are generally higher. Significant social and emotional problems occur, however, when the children of women with FXS are also significantly affected. We have seen several cases of child abuse when the mother herself has significant impulse control problems related to FXS and the children also have FXS. Significantly affected mothers, particularly those with mild learning disabilities, need high levels of support in their efforts to raise children with FXS, as well as unaffected children. Psychological intervention can be helpful, and can provide guidance to the parents in behavioural management and in sorting out the difficulties that they may be experiencing in their own lives (Sobesky, 1996).

In terms of psychiatric disorders, delusional behaviour (Silva, Ferrari & Leong, 1998) or even overt psychotic thinking may occasionally occur in adults with FXS (Hagerman, 1996a,b). These problems require treatment with antipsychotic medication as described below. Women with the premutation often experience significant levels of anxiety or depression, particularly if they are raising children with FXS (Franke et al., 1996; Franke et al., 1998). Supportive therapeutic work can provide guidance, behaviour management and further understanding and problem solving advice regarding their own psychopathology (Sobesky, 1996).

Physical problems

Connective tissue problems including loose joints and joint dislocations usually improve with age, perhaps related to changes in the tendons allowing for greater stability of the joint. Problems including hernia formation may persist into adulthood. On rare occasions, more significant orthopedic problems may occur in adulthood (Davids, Hagerman & Eilert, 1990), for example severe pes planus which requires orthopedic intervention, such as surgery, may occur in adulthood (Davids et al., 1990).

Approximately 50% of adults have mitral valve prolapse, presumably related to the elastin abnormalities associated with the connective tissue dysfunction in FXS (Waldstein et al., 1987). The mitral valve prolapse is usually benign, although on rare occasions it can lead to mitral regurgitation (Hagerman, 1996b). There have been a number of cases of sudden cardiac death in adults with FXS (Hagerman, 1996b; Sabaratnam, 2000; D.Z. Loesch, pers. comm.). It is possible that these deaths were caused by an arrhythmia associated with mitral valve prolapse, or a rare conduction problem which may be associated with the absence of FMRP. Further studies of cardiac pathology and sudden death are necessary. This problem may also explain the slightly increased rate of sudden infant death syndrome (SIDS) in infants with FXS (Fryns et al., 1988).

Hypertension is not uncommon in men with FXS, but it has not been studied. Perhaps the elevated blood pressure that is frequently seen relates to the anxiety that some individuals experience when they are seen in a clinic situation (Hagerman, 1996b). It is also possible that the connective tissue disorder and abnormal elastin fibres affect the resiliency of the blood vessel walls and predispose individuals to hypertension.

There are rare reports of patients who have also experienced dilated ureters and reflux associated with renal scaring and atrophy. There may be a predisposition for dilated ureters because of the connective tissue problems and elastin abnormalities seen in FXS (Hagerman, 1996b).

On occasion, seizures may persist into adulthood, although most disappear in adolescence or earlier (Musumeci et al., 1999).

Growth abnormalities can occur in individuals with FXS. These include an enhancement of growth in early childhood, and blunting of the adolescent growth spurt leading to a higher incidence of short stature in adulthood (Loesch, Huggins & Hoang, 1995). Hypothalamic dysfunction is probably related to these mild growth abnormalities, and it may also be the cause of macro-orchidism. The typical adult testicular size in men with FXS is approximately 50 ml, which is twice as large as normal, although sizes up to 100 ml have been reported (Butler et al., 1992). Macro-orchidism itself is not associated with medical problems, although it is possible that the weight of a significantly large testicle may predispose an individual to an inguinal hernia.

Interventions

Although no cure is yet available for FXS, there are various interventions that can be helpful. Usually a variety of interventions can work synergistically. For instance, the use of psychopharmacology, individual therapy in the language and motor area and psychological interventions can be quite helpful for the developmental and behavioural difficulties associated with FXS (Hagerman, 1996a; Scharfenaker et al., 1996; Sobesky, 1996).

Childhood

Young children present with hypotonia, language delays and motor problems (Bailey et al., 1998a). Behaviour difficulties such as irritability, tantrum behaviour or hyperactivity are also common. Early childhood intervention programmes that include language therapy and motor therapy are essential in the first 3 to 4 years of life. Many families find that working with a behavioural specialist to help with problems at home, including behavioural management techniques such as 'time out' and appropriate positive reinforcement, can be very beneficial. The use of sensory integration therapy through an occupational therapist has also been found to be helpful, although no controlled studies have been conducted (Scharfenaker et al., 1996). The occupational therapist can work on the development of fine and gross motor skills, in addition to motor planning and sensory integration.

Approximately 10% of children with FXS do not speak in short phrases by 5 years of age. Children with lower verbal abilities or those who are non-verbal require even more intensive speech and language therapy than those with mild delays. The combination of language therapy and occupational therapy can be beneficial, because the use of movement, rhythm, and even music can help to facilitate verbalizations. Augmentative communication techniques can also be helpful, including low-tech programmes such as the Picture Exchange Communication System (PECS) or high-tech aids such as a computer system that can be programmed for verbalizations (Hagerman, 1999).

Ongoing support with special education in elementary school is beneficial for the majority of children affected by FXS. Whenever possible, education in the mainstream situation should be sought, as most children with FXS will mimic the behaviours of other pupils in their class. If autism is present, then an intensive autism educational programme which includes behavioural strategies and the use of structured teaching programmes such as TEACCH, is helpful (Lovaas, 1987; Schopler, Mesibov & Hearsey, 1995; Rogers, 1998).

Medications can be beneficial for a variety of behavioural problems. Stimulants, including methylphenidate, dextroamphetamine, or Adderall, are generally used for the treatment of hyperactivity or ADHD symptoms (Hagerman, 1996a). If significant hyperarousal is present, then the use of clonidine or guanfacine can be helpful (Hagerman et al., 1995). Both of these agents have a calming effect and decrease the amount of noradrenaline at the synapse. This is clinically beneficial for many children with FXS, perhaps related to excessive sympathetic stimulation in FXS, although one of the side effects is significant sedation (Hagerman, Bregman & Tirosh, 1998). When clonidine is combined with stimulant medication then careful follow-up with electrocardiograms is needed to make sure that prolongation of cardiac conduction does not occur.

Treatment of excessive anxiety or obsessive–compulsive behaviour is frequently carried out with the use of a selective serotonin reuptake inhibitor (SSRI). Fluoxetine (Prozac) was one of the first SSRIs used clinically, and it is associated with significant social activation. Fluoxetine has been helpful in treating individuals with autism or pervasive developmental disorder (PDD-NOS) because of the beneficial effects on social activation and on enhancing language (DeLong et al., 1998). An SSRI such as fluoxetine may be considered in early childhood for those who have both FXS and autism. An SSRI such as fluoxetine, sertraline, paroxetine or fluvoxamine can also be given in middle childhood or adolescence if significant problems with anxiety or obsessive–compulsive behaviour develop. For mild degrees of moodiness, an SSRI may be helpful in smoothing out irritability or mild outbursts. More severe mood instability, however, requires the use of a mood stabilizer such as carbamazepine, valproic acid or lithium. The newer atypical antipsychotics such as risperidone, olanzapine or quetiapine (Seroquel) are also helpful in stabilizing mood and/or decreasing aggression when other agents are not effective. The atypical antipsychotics have a lower risk for tardive dyskinesias and are usually well tolerated (Kapur & Remington, 1996). An increase in appetite, which can lead to significant obesity, is a frequent problem with the use of risperidone and olanzapine. This problem is less likely with quetiapine but there has been very little paediatric experience with the use this drug. Risperidone has been used most commonly of all the atypical antipsychotics in childhood and it is usually well tolerated when the dose is kept low, i.e. 1–2 mg per day (Hagerman, 1999).

Medical intervention is important in the treatment of children with FXS.

Because recurrent otitis media infections are common and can interfere significantly with language development, it is important to treat recurrent infections aggressively with antibiotics and/or placement of PE tubes (grommets). In addition, children with FXS should be evaluated by an ophthalmologist or an optometrist to identify and treat problems such as strabismus and refraction errors, so that amblyopia does not develop. Normalization of both hearing and vision are essential for appropriate development and subsequent academic learning.

When there is a possible history of seizures, the person should receive an EEG, and if spike wave discharges are present, subsequent treatment with an anticonvulsant should be considered. Treatment with carbamazepine or valproic acid is usually sufficient to control the seizures (Wisniewski et al., 1991; Musumeci et al., 1999), although occasionally additional anticonvulsants such as gabapentin, lamotrigine or topiramate may be required. The newer anticonvulsants can be very beneficial as adjunctive agents in controlling seizures and may also be helpful in mood stabilization (Hagerman, 1999).

Adulthood

The transition from adolescence to adulthood may be difficult because of developmental problems including cognitive deficits and emotional difficulties. Some families have found that a gradual transition into living more independently can be helpful. For example, one family built an apartment attached to the family home to give their son with FXS some degree of independence, thus allowing for limited supervision from the family. Participation in adult programmes associated with supervised apartment living or group homes are more common alternatives. Most adult males with FXS require some degree of supervision in their living situation, but the supervision may be limited, such as daily or weekly visits. Adult programmes should involve some plans for enhancing social interaction, such as a bowling night or regularly scheduled group activities.

Behavioural problems that occur in adulthood include periodic outbursts with either verbal or physical aggression. These behaviour problems are often associated with anxiety and mood instability. Sometimes treatment with an SSRI alone will significantly decrease anxiety and obsessive–compulsive behaviour and smooth out minor problems with moodiness or aggression (Hagerman, 1999). In some instances, however, additional medication such as clonidine, a mood stabilizer, or an atypical antipsychotic, such as risperidone or quetiapine, is needed. Often an SSRI is combined with an atypical antipsychotic to decrease aggression and decrease anxiety. On occasion, sensory integration

Table 8.1. Clinical implications of fragile X syndrome (FXS)

- Counselling and cognitive-behavioural treatment with a psychologist or social worker can help individuals with FXS to recognize their emotional state and utilize self-calming techniques
- Counselling can also be helpful to treat interpersonal difficulties, and sexuality issues
- Anxiety and obsessive/compulsive behaviour is common in adult males and females with FXS and usually responds well to psychological interventions and medication
- Occasional excessive activation or mania may develop with the use of an SSRI, but this frequently responds to lowering the dose
- Social withdrawal is common in adulthood and requires efforts to plan and facilitate social interactions

therapy with an occupational therapist can be helpful to teach the adult calming techniques that can be carried out by the patients themselves or family members. Referral to a psychologist or social worker may also be beneficial to help the individual recognize his or her emotional state and to teach self-calming techniques such as visualization, counting or simply walking away from a situation that could cause a behavioural outburst. Counselling can also be helpful to sort out interpersonal difficulties or sexuality issues (Brown, Braden & Sobesky, 1991).

After an individual is diagnosed with FXS, genetic counselling is an essential part of the treatment programme (Cronister, 1996). The whole family tree needs to be reviewed, and individuals at risk for being carriers or affected by FXS should be tested with DNA studies to document the extent of the CGG repeat expansion. Genetic counselling can also be helpful in prenatal diagnostic studies that involve either chorionic villus sampling or amniocentesis. Decisions regarding continuation of a pregnancy or termination of an affected fetus are personal decisions made by the family and should be supported by the genetics counsellor and by the treatment team.

Families should also be referred to a parent support group where available and to the national and international support groups which have been set up to help families, to promote research and provide information and advice about the syndrome for families and professionals.

In the future, it can be expected that gene therapy or protein replacement therapy will be available for individuals with FXS. Until then a co-ordinated treatment programme that involves the input of a variety of professions, in addition to medical interventions, can lead to very productive lives and significant well being in those affected by FXS.

For a summary of the clinical implications of FXS see Table 8.1.

REFERENCES

Bailey, D.B., Hatton, D.D. & Skinner, M. (1998a). Early developmental trajectories of males with fragile X syndrome. *American Journal on Mental Retardation*, **103**: 29–39.

Bailey, D.B., Mesibov, G.B., Hatton, D.D., Clark, R.D., Roberts, J.E. & Mayhew, L. (1998b). Autistic behavior in young boys with fragile X syndrome. *Journal of Autism & Developmental Disorders*, **28**: 499–508.

Baumgardner, T.L., Reiss, A.L., Freund, L.S. & Abrams, M.T. (1995). Specification of the neurobehavioral phenotype in males with fragile X syndrome. *Pediatrics*, **95**: 744–52.

Belser, R.C. & Sudhalter, V. (1995). Arousal difficulties in males with Fragile X Syndrome: a preliminary report. *Developmental Brain Dysfunction*, **8**: 270–9.

Bennetto, L. & Pennington, B.F. (1996). The Neuropsychology of Fragile X Syndrome. In *Fragile X Syndrome: Diagnosis, Treatment and Research*, ed. R.J. Hagerman & A. Cronister, pp. 210–48. Baltimore: The Johns Hopkins University Press.

Brown, J., Braden, M. & Sobesky, W. (1991). The treatment of behavior and emotional problems. In *Fragile X syndrome: Diagnosis, Treatment, and Research*, ed. R.J. Hagerman & A.C. Silverman, pp. 311–326. Baltimore: The Johns Hopkins University Press.

Brown, W.T. (1996). The Molecular Biology of the Fragile X Mutation. In *Fragile X Syndrome: Diagnosis, Treatment, and Research*, ed. R.J. Hagerman & A. Cronister, pp. 88–113. Baltimore: The Johns Hopkins University Press.

Butler, M.G., Brunschwig, A., Miller, L.K. & Hagerman, R.J. (1992). Standards for selected anthropometric measurements in males with the fragile X syndrome. *Pediatrics*, **89**: 1059–62.

Comery, T.A., Harris, J.B., Willems, P.J., Oostra, B.A., Irwin, S.A., Weiler, I.J. & Greenough, W.T. (1997). Abnormal dendritic spines in fragile X knockout mouse: maturation and pruning deficits. *Proceedings of the National Academy of Sciences of the United States of America*, **94**: 5401–4.

Crawford, D.C., Meadows, I.L., Newman, J.L., Taft, L.F., Pettay, D.L., Gold, L.B., Hersey, S.U., Hinkle, E.F., Stanfield, M.L., Holmgreen, P., Yeargin-allsop, M., Boyle, C. & Sherman, S.L. (1999). Prevalence and phenotypic consequence of FRAXA and FRAXE alleles in a large, ethnically diverse, special education-needs population. *American Journal of Human Genetics*, **64**: 495–507.

Cronister, A.J. (1996). Genetic counseling. In *Fragile X Syndrome: Diagnosis, Treatment, and Research*, ed. R.J. Hagerman & A. Cronister, pp. 251–82. Baltimore: The Johns Hopkins University Press.

Davids, J.R., Hagerman, R.J. & Eilert, R.E. (1990). Orthopaedic aspects of fragile-X syndrome. *Journal of Bone & Joint Surgery – American Volume*, **72**: 889–96.

de Vries, B.B., Jansen, C.C., Duits, A.A., Verheij, C., Willemsen, R., van Hemel, J.O., van den Ouweland, A.M., Niermeijer, M.F., Oostra, B.A. & Halley, D.J. (1996a). Variable FMR1 gene methylation of large expansions leads to variable phenotype in three males from one fragile X family. *Journal of Medical Genetics*, **33**: 1007–10.

de Vries, B.B., van den Ouweland, A.M., Mohkamsing, S., Duivenvoorden, H.J., Mol, E., Gelsema, K., van Rijn, M., Halley, D.J., Sandkuijl, L.A., Oostra, B.A., Tibben, A. & Niermeijer, M.F. (1997). Screening and diagnosis for the fragile X syndrome among the mentally retarded:

an epidemiological and psychological survey. Collaborative Fragile X Study Group. *American Journal of Human Genetics*, **61**: 660–7.

de Vries, B.B., Wiegers, A.M., Smits, A.P., Mohkamsing, S., Duivenvoorden, H.J., Fryns, J.P., Curfs, L.M., Halley, D.J., Oostra, B.A., van den Ouweland, A.M. & Niermeijer, M.F. (1996b). Mental status of females with an FMR1 gene full mutation. *American Journal of Medical Genetics*, **58**: 1025–32.

DeLong, G.R., Teague, L.A. & McSwain Kamran, M. (1998). Effects of fluoxetine treatment in young children with idiopathic autism [see comments]. *Developmental Medicine & Child Neurology*, **40**: 551–62.

Dykens, E., Ort, S., Cohen, I., Finucane, B., Spiridigliozzi, G., Lachiewicz, A., Reiss, A., Freund, L., Hagerman, R. & O'Connor, R. (1996). Trajectories and profiles of adaptive behavior in males with fragile X syndrome: multicenter studies. *Journal of Autism and Developmental Disorders*, **26**: 287–301.

Einfeld, S., Tonge, B. & Turner, G. (1999). Longitudinal course of behavioral and emotional problems in fragile X syndrome. *American Journal of Medical Genetics*, **87**: 436–9.

Feng, Y., Zhang, F., Lokey, L.K., Chastain, J.L., Lakkis, L., Eberhart, D. & Warren, S.T. (1995). Translational suppression by trinucleotide repeat expansion at FMR1. *Science*, **268**: 731–4.

Franke, P., Leboyer, M., Gansicke, M., Weiffenbach, O., Biancalana, V., Cornillet-Lefebre, P., Croquette, M.F., Froster, U., Schwab, S.G., Poustka, F., Hautzinger, M. & Maier, W. (1998). Genotype–phenotype relationship in female carriers of the premutation and full mutation of FMR-1. *Psychiatry Research*, **80**: 113–27.

Franke, P., Maier, W., Hautzinger, M., Weiffenbach, O., Gansicke, M., Iwers, B., Poustka, F., Schwab, S.G. & Froster, U. (1996). Fragile-X carrier females: evidence for a distinct psycho-pathological phenotype? *American Journal of Medical Genetics*, **64**: 334–9.

Freund, L.S., Reiss, A.L. & Abrams, M.T. (1993). Psychiatric disorders associated with fragile X in the young female. *Pediatrics*, **91**: 321–9.

Fryns, J.P., Moerman, P., Gilis, F., d'Espallier, L. & Van den Berghe, H. (1988). Suggestively increased rate of infant death in children of fra(X) positive mothers. *American Journal of Medical Genetics*, **30**: 73–5.

Hagerman, R.J. (1996a). Medical Follow-up and Pharmacotherapy. In *Fragile X Syndrome: Diagnosis, Treatment, and Research*, ed. R.J. Hagerman & A. Cronister, pp. 283–331. Baltimore: The Johns Hopkins University Press.

Hagerman, R.J. (1996b). Physical and Behavioral Phenotype. In *Fragile X Syndrome: Diagnosis, Treatment and Research*, ed. R.J. Hagerman & A. Cronister, pp. 3–87. Baltimore: The Johns Hopkins University Press.

Hagerman, R.J. (1999). Fragile X Syndrome. In *Neurodevelopmental Disorders: Diagnosis and Treatment*, pp. 61–132. New York: Oxford University Press.

Hagerman, R.J., Bregman, J.D. & Tirosh, E. (1998). Clonidine. In *Psychotropic Medication and Developmental Disabilities: The International Consensus Handbook*, ed. S. Reiss & M.G. Aman, pp. 259–69. Columbus, Ohio: Ohio State University Nisonger Center.

Hagerman, R.J., Hills, J., Scharfenaker, S. & Lewis, H. (1999). Fragile X syndrome and selective mutism. *American Journal of Medical Genetics*, **83**: 313–17.

Hagerman, R.J., Jackson, A.W.D., Levitas, A., Rimland, B. & Braden, M. (1986). An analysis of autism in fifty males with the fragile X syndrome. *American Journal of Medical Genetics*, **23**: 359–74.

Hagerman, R.J., Jackson, C., Amiri, K., Silverman, A.C., O'Connor, R. & Sobesky, W. (1992). Girls with fragile X syndrome: physical and neurocognitive status and outcome. *Pediatrics*, **89**: 395–400.

Hagerman, R.J., Riddle, J.E., Roberts, L.S., Brease, K. & Fulton, M. (1995). A survey of the efficacy of clonidine in fragile X syndrome. *Developmental Brain Dysfunction*, **8**: 336–44.

Hagerman, R.J., Staley, L.W., O'Connor, R., Lugenbeel, K., Nelson, D., McLean, S.D. & Taylor, A. (1996). Learning-disabled males with a fragile X CGG expansion in the upper premutation size range. *Pediatrics*, **97**: 122–6.

Hatton, D.D., Buckley, E.G., Lachiewicz, A. & Roberts, J. (1998). Ocular status of young boys with fragile X syndrome: A prospective study. *Journal of the American Association for Pediatric Ophthalmology and Strabismus*, **2**: 298–301.

Irwin, S.A., Idupalapati, M., Mehta, A.B., Crisostomo, R.A., Rogers, E.J., Larsen, B.P., Alcantara, C.J., Harris, J.B., Patel, B.A., Gilbert, M.E., Chakravarti, A., Swain, R.A., Kooy, R.F., Kozlowski, P.B., Weiler, I.J. & Greenough, W.T. (1999). Abnormal dendritic and dendritic spine characteristics in fragile-X patients and the mouse model of fragile-X syndrome. Paper presented at the *Society for Neuroscience Annual Meeting, Miami Beach, Florida*, 1999.

Kapur, S. & Remington, G. (1996). Serotonin–dopamine interaction and its relevance to schizophrenia. *American Journal of Psychiatry*, **153**: 466–76.

Kemper, M.B., Hagerman, R.J., Ahmad, R.S. & Mariner, R. (1986). Cognitive profiles and the spectrum of clinical manifestations in heterozygous fragile (X) females. *American Journal of Medical Genetics*, **23**: 139–56.

Kerby, D.S. & Dawson, B.L. (1994). Autistic features, personality, and adaptive behavior in males with the fragile X syndrome and no autism. *American Journal of Mental Retardation*, **98**: 455–62.

King, R.A., Hagerman, R.J. & Houghton, M. (1995). Ocular findings in fragile X syndrome. *Developmental Brain Dysfunction*, **8**: 223–9.

Loesch, D.Z., Huggins, R.M. & Hoang, N.H. (1995). Growth in stature in fragile X families: a mixed longitudinal study. *American Journal of Medical Genetics*, **58**: 249–56.

Lovaas, O.I. (1987). Behavioral treatment and normal educational and intellectual functioning in young autistic children. *Journal of Consulting and Clinical Psychology*, **55**: 3–9.

Mazzocco, M.M., Kates, W.R., Baumgardner, T.L., Freund, L.S. & Reiss, A.L. (1997). Autistic behaviors among girls with fragile X syndrome. *Journal of Autism and Developmental Disorders*, **27**: 415–35.

Mazzocco, M.M., Pennington, B.F. & Hagerman, R.J. (1993). The neurocognitive phenotype of female carriers of fragile X: additional evidence for specificity. *Journal of Developmental and Behavioral Pediatrics*, **14**: 328–35.

Merenstein, S.A., Sobesky, W.E., Taylor, A.K., Riddle, J.E., Tran, H.X. & Hagerman, R.J. (1996). Molecular-clinical correlations in males with an expanded FMR1 mutation. *American Journal of Medical Genetics*, **64**: 388–94.

Miller, L.J., McIntosh, D.N., McGrath, J., Shyu, V., Lampe, M., Taylor, A.K., Tassone, F., Neitzel,

K., Stackhouse, T. & Hagerman, R.J. (1999). Electrodermal responses to sensory stimuli in individuals with Fragile X Syndrome: a preliminary report. *American Journal of Medical Genetics*, **83**: 268–79.

Mostofsky, S.H., Mazzocco, M.M.M., Aakalu, G., Warsofsky, I.S., Denckla, M.B. & Reiss, A. L. (1998). Decreased cerebellar posterior vermis size in fragile X syndrome. *American Academy of Neurology*, **50**: 121–30.

Musumeci, S.A., Hagerman, R.J., Ferri, R., Bosco, P., Dalla Bernardina, K., Tassinari, C.A., DeSarro, G.B. & Elia, M. (1999). Epilepsy and EEG findings in males with fragile X syndrome. *Epilepsia*, **40**: 1092–9.

Nolin, S.L., Lewis, F.A., 3rd, Ye, L.L., Houck, G.E., Jr., Glicksman, A.E., Limprasert, P., Li, S.Y., Zhong, N., Ashley, A.E., Feingold, E., Sherman, S.L. & Brown, W.T. (1996). Familial transmission of the FMR1 CGG repeat. *American Journal of Human Genetics*, **59**: 1252–61.

Pieretti, M., Zhang, F.P., Fu, Y.H., Warren, S.T., Oostra, B.A., Caskey, C.T. & Nelson, D.L. (1991). Absence of expression of the FMR-1 gene in fragile X syndrome. *Cell*, **66**: 817–22.

Reiss, A.L., Abrams, M.T., Greenlaw, R., Freund, L. & Denckla, M.B. (1995). Neurodevelopmental effects of the FMR-1 full mutation in humans. *Nature Medicine*, **1**: 159–67.

Reiss, A.L., Aylward, E., Freund, L.S., Joshi, P.K. & Bryan, R.N. (1991). Neuroanatomy of fragile X syndrome: the posterior fossa. *Annals of Neurology*, **29**: 26–32.

Reiss, A.L., Freund, L., Abrams, M.T., Boehm, C. & Kazazian, H. (1993). Neurobehavioral effects of the fragile X premutation in adult women: a controlled study. *American Journal of Human Genetics*, **52**: 884–94.

Reiss, A.L., Lee, J. & Freund, L. (1994). Neuroanatomy of fragile X syndrome: the temporal lobe. *Neurology*, **44**: 1317–24.

Riddle, J.E., Cheema, A., Sobesky, W.E., Gardner, S.C., Taylor, A.K., Pennington, B.F. & Hagerman, R.J. (1998). Phenotypic involvement in females with the FMR1 gene mutation. *American Journal on Mental Retardation*, **102**: 590–601.

Rogers, S.J. (1998). Empirically supported comprehensive treatments for young children with autism. *Journal of Clinical Child Psychology*, **27**: 168–79.

Rogers, S.J., Wehner, E.A. & Hagerman, R. (2001). The behavioral phenotype in fragile X syndrome: symptoms of autism in very young children with fragile X syndrome, idiopathic autism, and other developmental disorders. *Journal of Developmental and Behavioral Pediatrics*. (In press.)

Rousseau, F., Morel, M.-L., Rouillard, P., Khandjian, E.W. & Morgan, K. (1996). Surprisingly low prevalance of FMR1 premutation among males from the general population. *American Journal of Human Genetics*, **59**(A188): 1069.

Rousseau, F., Rouillard, P., Morel, M.L., Khandjian, E.W. & Morgan, K. (1995). Prevalence of carriers of premutation-size alleles of the FMRI gene – and implications for the population genetics of the fragile X syndrome. *American Journal of Human Genetics*, **57**: 1006–18.

Sabaratnam, M. (2000). Pathological and neuropathological findings in two males with fragile X syndrome. *Journal of Intellectual Disability Research*, **44**: 81–5.

Schapiro, M.B., Murphy, D.G., Hagerman, R.J. et al. (1995). Adult fragile X syndrome: neuropsychology, brain anatomy, and metabolism. *American Journal of Medical Genetics*, **60**: 480–93.

Scharfenaker, S., O'Connor, R., Stackhouse, T., Braden, M., Hickman, L. & Gray, K. (1996). An Integrated Approach to Intervention. In *Fragile X Syndrome: Diagnosis, Treatment, and Research*, ed. R.J. Hagerman & A. Cronister, pp. 349–411. Baltimore: The Johns Hopkins University Press.

Schopler, E., Mesibov, G.B. & Hearsey, K. (1995). Structured teaching in the TEACCH system. In *Learning and Cognition in Autism*, ed. E. Schopler & G.B. Mesibov, pp. 243–68. New York: Plenum Press.

Schwartz, C.E., Dean, J., Howard Peebles, P.N., Bugge, M., Mikkelsen, M., Tommerup, N., Hull, C., Hagerman, R., Holden, J.J. & Stevenson, R.E. (1994). Obstetrical and gynecological complications in fragile X carriers: a multicenter study. *American Journal of Medical Genetics*, **51**: 400–2.

Sherman, S. (1996). Epidemiology. In *Fragile X Syndrome: Diagnosis, Treatment, and Research*, ed. R.J. Hagerman & A. Cronister, pp. 165–92. Baltimore: The Johns Hopkins University Press.

Silva, J.A., Ferrari, M.M. & Leong, G.B. (1998). Erotomania in a case of fragile X syndrome. *General Hospital Psychiatry*, **20**: 126–7.

Smeets, H.J., Smits, A.P., Verheij, C.E., Theelen, J.P., Willemsen, R., van de Burgt, I., Hoogeveen, A.T., Oosterwijk, J.C. & Oostra, B.A. (1995). Normal phenotype in two brothers with a full FMR1 mutation. *Human Molecular Genetics*, **4**: 2103–8.

Sobesky, W.E. (1996). The Treatment of Emotional and Behavioral Problems. In *Fragile X Syndrome: Diagnosis, Treatment, and Research*, ed. R.J. Hagerman & A. Cronister, pp. 332–48. Baltimore: The Johns Hopkins University Press.

Sobesky, W.E., Taylor, A.K., Pennington, B.F., Bennetto, L., Porter, D., Riddle, J. & Hagerman, R.J. (1996). Molecular/clinical correlations in females with fragile X. *American Journal of Medical Genetics*, **64**: 340–5.

Spinelli, M., Rocha, A.C., Giacheti, C.M. & Richieri Costa, A. (1995). Word-finding difficulties, verbal paraphasias, and verbal dyspraxia in ten individuals with fragile X syndrome. *American Journal of Medical Genetics*, **60**: 39–43.

Sudhalter, V., Cohen, I.L., Silverman, W. & Wolf-Schein, E.G. (1990). Conversational analyses of males with fragile X, Down syndrome, and autism: comparison of the emergence of deviant language. *American Journal on Mental Retardation*, **94**: 431–41.

Sudhalter, V., Scarborough, H.S. & Cohen, I.L. (1991). Syntactic delay and pragmatic deviance in the language of fragile X males. *American Journal of Medical Genetics*, **38**: 493–7.

Sutcliffe, J.S., Nelson, D.L., Zhang, F., Pieretti, M., Caskey, C.T., Saxe, D. & Warren, S.T. (1992). DNA methylation represses FMR-1 transcription in fragile X syndrome. *Human Molecular Genetics*, **1**: 397–400.

Tassone, F., Hagerman, R.J., Ikle, D., Dyer, P.N., Lampe, M., Willemsen, R., Oostra, B.A. & Taylor, A.K. (1999). FMRP expression as a potential prognostic indicator in fragile X syndrome. *American Journal of Medical Genetics*, **84**: 250–61.

Tassone, F., Hagerman, R.J., Taylor, A.K., Gane, L.W., Godfrey, T.E. & Hagerman, P.J. (2000a). Elevated levels of *FMR1* mRNA in carrier males: a new mechanism of involvement in fragile X syndrome. *American Journal of Human Genetics*, **66**: 6–15.

Tassone, F., Hagerman, R.J., Taylor, A.K., Mills, J.B., Harris, S.W., Gane, L.W. & Hagerman, P.J.

(2000b). Clinical involvement and protein expression in individuals with the *FMR1* premutation. *American Journal of Medical Genetics*, **91**: 144–152.

Turk, J. & Cornish, K. (1998). Face recognition and emotion perception in boys with fragile-X syndrome. *Journal of Intellectual Disability Research*, **42**: 490–9.

Turk, J. & Graham, P. (1997). Fragile X syndrome, autism, and autistic features. *Autism*, **1**: 175–97.

Turner, G., Robinson, H., Wake, S. & Martin, N. (1994). Dizygous twinning and premature menopause in fragile X syndrome [letter] [see comments]. *Lancet*, **344**: 1500.

Turner, G., Webb, T., Wake, S. & Robinson, H. (1996). Prevalence of fragile X syndrome. *American Journal of Medical Genetics*, **64**: 196–7.

Verkerk, A.J., Pieretti, M., Sutcliffe, J.S. et al. (1991). Identification of a gene (FMR-1) containing a CGG repeat coincident with a breakpoint cluster region exhibiting length variation in fragile X syndrome. *Cell*, **65**: 905–14.

Vianna-Morgante, A.M., Costa, S.S., Pares, A.S. & Verreschi, I.T. (1996). FRAXA premutation associated with premature ovarian failure. *American Journal of Medical Genetics*, **64**: 373–5.

Waldstein, G., Mierau, G., Ahmad, R., Thibodeau, S.N., Hagerman, R.J. & Caldwell, S. (1987). Fragile X syndrome: Skin elastin abnormalities. *Birth Defects: Original Article Series*, **23**: 103–14.

Wells, R.D., Warren, S.T. & Sarmiento, M. (1998). *Genetic Instabilities and Hereditary Neurological Diseases*, San Diego: Academic Press.

Willemsen, R., Anar, B., Otero, Y.D., de Vries, B.B., Hilhorst-Hofstee, Y., Smits, A., van Looveren, E., Willems, P.J., Galjaard, H. & Oostra, B.A. (1999). Noninvasive test for fragile X syndrome, using hair root analysis. *American Journal of Human Genetics*, **65**: 98–103.

Willemsen, R., Smits, A., Mohkamsing, S., van Beerendonk, H., de Haan, A., de Vries, B., van den Ouweland, A., Sistermans, E., Galjaard, H. & Oostra, B.A. (1997). Rapid antibody test for diagnosing fragile X syndrome: a validation of the technique. *Human Genetics*, **99**: 308–11.

Wisniewski, K.E., Segan, S.M., Miezejeski, C.M., Sersen, E.A. & Rudelli, R.D. (1991). The Fra(X) syndrome: neurological, electrophysiological, and neuropathological abnormalities. *American Journal of Medical Genetics*, **38**: 476–80.

Wright Talamante, C., Cheema, A., Riddle, J.E., Luckey, D.W., Taylor, A.K. & Hagerman, R.J. (1996). A controlled study of longitudinal IQ changes in females and males with fragile X syndrome. *American Journal of Medical Genetics*, **64**: 350–5.

9

Prader–Willi and Angelman syndromes: from childhood to adult life

Anthony Holland, Joyce Whittington and Jill Butler

Introduction

The Prader–Willi (PWS) and Angelman syndromes (AS) are two distinct syndromes that have in common either a deletion at the locus 15q11.2 or the presence of other genetic abnormalities of chromosome 15. PWS was the first to be described by Swiss paediatricians in 1956 (Prader, 1956). The main features noted at that time were neonatal hypotonia, impaired sexual development, a propensity to severe obesity and intellectual disabilities (mental retardation). In 1961 Prader and Willi reported on a total of 14 Swiss children with similar characteristics. In the same year in the English literature, Laurance (1961) described six children with the same pattern of phenotypic characteristics. Other reports, from elsewhere in the world, soon appeared (Forssman & Hagberg, 1964; Dunn, 1968). In a paper describing nine children, together with a review of other papers, Laurance (1967) listed the main features as: neuromuscular (neonatal hypotonia); 'mental disorders' (i.e., IQs in the low 2% of the population); abnormalities in body configuration (obesity and poor growth); skeletal disorders (mainly scoliosis); characteristic facial appearance (almond-shaped eyes, high cranial vault); endocrine abnormalities (risk of diabetes mellitus); and delayed gonadal development. Other features, such as an apparent high pain threshold, were also noted. Although possible chromosome abnormalities were described at that time, the genetic abnormality most commonly associated with the syndrome was not established for over a decade. In 1981, Ledbetter et al. confirmed the presence of a chromosomal deletion on the proximal part of the long arm of chromosome 15 and subsequently the genetic basis for PWS has been further clarified.

In 1965, Angelman described three unrelated children with similar phenotypes. The main features included flattening of the head antero-posteriorly, jerky movements, protruding tongues and periods of intense laughter. The now unacceptable names of 'puppet children' or 'happy puppet syndrome' were used at that time. Angelman also noted the presence of primary optic atrophy, incomplete development of the choroid in the eyes, frequent fits (similar to hypsarrythmia), ataxia with weakness of the limbs, similar to that found with cerebellar disorders, and profound 'mental retardation'. The clinical characteristics were subsequently further refined, and the relatively low recurrence risk of 4% in families of affected children argued against earlier suggestions of an autosomal recessive disorder. Magenis et al. (1987) found evidence of a chromosomal deletion on chromosome 15 and Pembury et al. (1989) reported two unrelated people with AS with small deletions on the proximal part of the long arm of chromosome 15. Among 10 further individuals who were investigated, five were karyotypically normal, four had deletions within 15q11-13 and one had a pericentric inversion involving the same chromosome region. The authors surmized that a combination of chromosomal deletions and autosomal recessive inheritance combined to give a recurrence risk of less than 25%.

The genetic basis of PWS and AS

In the late 1980s, geneticists were faced with the conundrum that a chromosomal deletion on an apparently similar part of chromosome 15 could give rise to two phenotypically different syndromes. Using high resolution and fluorescent banding techniques, as well as investigating the parental origin of the chromosome 15 with the deletion, Magenis et al. (1990) were able to demonstrate that the sizes of the deletions were generally different (AS being larger) and, more importantly, the gender of the parent of origin of the deleted chromosome 15 was different in the two syndromes (Nicholls, 1993). In all those with AS and chromosome 15 deletions, the deletions were on the chromosome 15 of maternal origin. In the case of PWS, deletions were on the paternal chromosome 15. The potential importance of gender specific 'genomic imprinting' was therefore considered a possible explanation for the observation that two radically different syndromes had an apparently similar chromosomal basis. The final confirmation of this hypothesis was the observation that non-deletion cases of PWS were almost invariably due to the inheritance of both copies of chromosome 15 from the mother (maternal hetero- or iso-disomy) In AS, both came from the father (Nicholls et al., 1989; Nicholls, 1993). Thus, when uniparental disomies occurred, both copies of particular genes, which were either maternally or paternally imprinted, would have been switched off. This is illustrated in Figure 9.1.

The size of the chromosomal deletion for both PWS and AS is usually approximately 4 megabases (Mb). Within this region there is an imprinted region of approximately 2Mb that contains the genes whose expressions

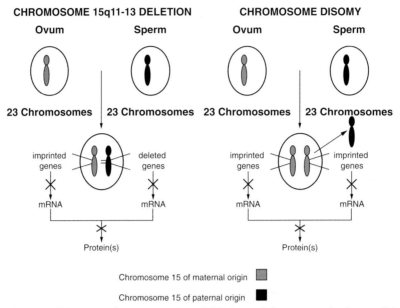

Figure 9.1. Diagrammatic representation of deletion and disomy genetic abnormalities leading to Prader–Willi syndrome.

depend on the gender of the parent of origin (see Cassidy & Schwartz, 1998 for review). The loss of expression of one gene (UBE3A) is known to cause AS (Matsuura et al., 1997) but no specific gene(s) has been definitely identified as the cause of PWS. At one time the gene coding for a small nuclear ribonucleo-protein (SNRPN) which controls gene splicing, was considered the most likely candidate (Reed & Leff, 1994; Glenn et al., 1996) but there have been two cases of PWS in which this gene was preserved (Schulze et al., 1996; Conroy et al., 1997). Microdeletions of what is referred to as the 'imprinting centre' (IC) at 15q11-q13 have also been identified in families with PWS or AS (Ohta et al., 1999). The IC is thought to control the re-setting of parental imprints in that chromosomal region during gametogenesis. The authors suggest that their findings indicate that promoter elements of the SNRPN gene may play a key role in the initiation of imprint switching during spermatogenesis. They also reported three people with sporadic PWS and imprinting mutations outside the IC. Thus, it would appear that there is an epigenetic effect of this imprinting mutation on the process of switching from the maternal to the paternal imprint during spermatogenesis. Seven genes or expressed sequences (ESTs) have been potentially implicated in PWS in that they are maternally imprinted and expressed from the paternal chromosome 15 only (Nicholls, Saitoh & Hors-themke, 1998). Other potentially important genes include necdin (Nakada et

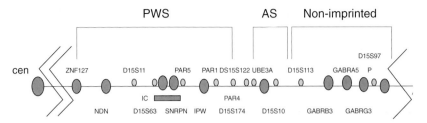

Figure 9.2. Chromosomal map of 15q11-q13. PWS, Prader–Willi syndrome; AS, Angelman syndrome.

al., 1998), and the gene for the zinc-finger protein – ZNF127 (Jong et al., 1999).

In essence it is important to consider these two syndromes as being both genotypically and phenotypically distinct. PWS is likely to be a 'contiguous gene syndrome' in which the failure of expression of specific maternally imprinted genes is of aetiological significance. In contrast, AS has been shown to be due to the loss of expression of a single paternally imprinted gene. This may occur because of a mutation affecting UB3EA, the deletion of the maternal copy of that gene (in the presence of the normal imprinted paternal copy), or the presence of a paternal chromosome 15 disomy. This genetic map is given in Figure 9.2.

Clinical features of PWS

Since the original description of this syndrome there have been advances in the following clinical areas of study. First, the diagnostic criteria have been more clearly defined and the major and minor criteria identified separately for infants, children and adults (Holm et al., 1992, 1993). Secondly, there have been more detailed investigations of the cognitive and behavioural characteristics of the syndrome, and attempts to delineate the underlying mechanisms that lead to the main behavioural phenotypic characteristic – over-eating and resultant obesity (see review by Holland, 1998). Thirdly, the relationship between the two main chromosomal types of PWS and the physical and behavioural phenotype have been investigated (e.g., Gillessen-Kaesbach et al., 1995; Dykens, Cassidy & King, 1999).

Diagnostic criteria at different ages

The consensus diagnostic criteria were initially proposed by a group of experts and field tested by the examination of 113 people with PWS (Holm et al., 1993). Differences were noted in those below and above 3 years of age and for this reason the major and minor criteria proposed for each age group are different.

From birth to 3 years of age, the main characteristics found in all cases were hypotonia, feeding problems (often requiring use of naso-gastric tubes or other augmented feeding methods), dysmorphic appearance, genital hypoplasia and developmental delay. Excessive weight gain could also occur towards the end of this period. In addition, poor fetal activity, weak cry, lethargy and temperature instability were observed in 10–60% of affected infants.

After 3 years of age, the following characteristics were found in 75% or more of those seen and these are considered major criteria: hypotonia, obesity, learning disabilities, behaviour problems, short stature, dysmorphism and hypogonadism. The minor criteria identified included those listed as above in infancy, hyperphagia, decreased vomiting, sleep disturbance, skin picking, articulation problems, small hands and feet and viscous saliva. Additional supportive diagnostic findings were also suggested: hypopigmentation, eye abnormalities, high pain threshold, abnormal temperature regulation, scoliosis, osteoporosis, straight ulnar border to the hands and special skills at jigsaws (Holm et al., 1992). These were retained in the 1993 classification (Holm et al., 1993), but the order of importance, especially of minor and supportive criteria, was changed. A further revision is currently proposed.

In summary, the most striking changes over time are poor feeding becoming excessive feeding (leading to obesity), increasing severity of developmental delays and intellectual disabilities becoming more apparent, and delays in sexual development and growth becoming more obvious. Behaviour problems may also emerge as development progresses.

The behavioural and cognitive phenotype of PWS

Since the original description of PWS, increasing attention has been paid to delineating and understanding the pattern of cognitive development and behavioural profiles associated with the syndrome. Many of the initial reports described early developmental delay, the need for special help at school and, in addition to the over-eating, temper tantrums, a tendency to repetitive behaviours and skin picking. Subsequent studies have attempted to investigate more systematically whether such observations are indicative of a specific behavioural phenotype.

Eating behaviour and obesity

A striking feature of the syndrome is the low birth weight and extreme floppiness at birth. Feeding is a cause of major concern, as the baby cannot suckle normally. However, often as early as 2 years of age, the picture changes and a child previously in the lower percentiles for weight frequently crosses the 50th percentile and is soon recognized as being obese (Ehara, Ohno & Takeshita, 1993). Over-eating and the very severe obesity that follows become a central feature of the syndrome. The likely reasons for this would appear to be a failure of the normal satiety response following food intake (Zipf et al., 1983; Holland et al., 1993). When faced with food the vast majority (but not all) of individuals with PWS eat continuously and show no slowing down of their eating behaviour. Treatment with pancreatic polypeptide infusion (Berntson et al., 1993) and naloxone (Zipf & Bernston, 1987) has been tried experimentally but with limited effect. Holland et al. (1993) used visual ana-logue scales to assess feelings of hunger and fullness before, during and after food intake, and showed that people with PWS did eventually satiate but only after eating three times more in calories than a control group. Feelings of hunger also returned shortly after food was no longer available. Measures of blood levels of glucose, insulin and cholecystokinin conducted at the same time indicated that eventual satiation was associated with a rise in blood glucose levels into the diabetic range. Blood levels of cholecystokinin were also very high but did not correlate with hunger or fullness. It would appear that the normal feedback mechanism, which results in loss of feelings of hunger and increased feelings of fullness and, in turn, to cessation of eating, is faulty. The likely pathophysiological mechanism is at the level of the hypothalamus. As yet there have been limited investigations of this area of the brain in people with PWS; the main one being that of Swaab, Purba & Hofman (1995). In this study a reduction in the oxytocin-containing neurones in the paraventricular nucleus was found and the authors proposed that this might account for the failure of satiation following food intake. The hormone leptin, which has been shown to influence body weight through its influence on eating behaviour, has also been investigated in PWS. Leptin is produced by fat cells, and the blood levels in people with PWS have been shown to relate to body fat content (Butler et al., 1998). Thus a failure to produce leptin does not explain the over-eating behaviour.

There have been attempts to control the obesity through surgical interven-tion or by the use of medication. In the case of the former the risks may be high and it does not resolve the fundamental problem – the desire to keep eating. Fenfluramine has been used but was found not to affect eating behav-iour (Selikowitz et al., 1990) and has now been discontinued because of its effects on the heart. At present the only effective way of preventing obesity is strict control over access to food (Holland, 1998). This approach has led to debate as to the legal and ethical basis for such control, particularly in adult life (Holland & Wong, 1999).

Increasingly the diagnosis of PWS is made shortly after birth and parents are advised to monitor food intake and weight, and therefore obesity can be prevented. The extent to which enforced dieting in early life affects weight management and prognosis in later life is unknown.

Cognitive abilities

Curfs et al. (1991) studied the cognitive profile of 26 children and adolescents with PWS using the WISC-R. The mean full-scale score was 62.3 with scores ranging from 36 to 96. In 15 children there was a significant verbal/performance difference with 10 having higher performance scores. When scores on individual sub-tests were considered, there was a general strength (in comparison to other sub-tests) in block design. No relative weaknesses were reported. Overall the authors concluded that those with PWS perform better on visual motor discrimination tasks than on auditory processing tasks. A later study confirmed this finding for those with deletions, but suggested that chromosome 15 disomy results in higher verbal than performance scores (Roof et al., 2000).

Speech

Akefeldt, Akefeldt & Gillberg (1997) studied voice, speech and language characteristics in a group of 11 children and young adults with PWS. Oral motor dysfunction and specific abnormalities in pitch and resonance were reported. The authors proposed that both cerebral dysfunction and the anatomy of the mouth and pharynx may have accounted for this.

Sleep abnormalities

Abnormalities of the upper airway have also been investigated as part of a sleep study (Richards et al., 1994). This study found evidence of pharyngeal abnormalities that, along with the complications of obesity, might account for the obstructive component of sleep apnoea that is commonly observed. Excessive daytime sleepiness has also been frequently reported and may sometimes be due to the lack of or poor quality sleep at night. However, the fact that this is not always the case suggests that there may be a central component contributing to an abnormal pattern of sleep. It seems likely that sleep apnoea may be central in origin although obesity may aggravate it further (Clift, Dahlitz & Parkes, 1994; Richdale, Cotton & Hibbit, 1999).

Behaviour problems persisting into adulthood

Maladaptive behaviours

Greenswag (1987) conducted one of the largest scale follow-up investigations of adults with PWS. In an informant based questionnaire study of 232 individuals she found that a very high proportion of informants reported problems such as stubbornness, sleepiness, antisocial and belligerent behaviours, as well as describing the person with PWS as slow-moving and good-natured. The most prominent physical characteristic was obesity and this was so severe in 11 people that gastric bypass operations had been undertaken. High blood pressure, diabetes mellitus and respiratory problems were commonly reported complications of the obesity. Nearly half the group had been hospitalized after the age of 16 years for severe physical problems and 25 had been hospitalized for psychiatric disorders. Nearly all were described as being 'below average intellectually' with 75% having received special education. Ninety-five per cent of this adult group had no financial resources of their own, the great majority was living in supported settings and very few were fully independent. A similar picture with respect to educational history and general functioning in adult life was found by Waters, Clarke & Corbett (1990). Although approximately half of the 61 adults with PWS surveyed had attended mainstream primary school, the majority required special help in secondary school and only just over 10% left school with at least one Certificate of Secondary Education (CSE).

A distinct pattern of maladaptive behaviour was reported by Clarke et al. (1996). Using the Aberrant Behaviour Checklist, they compared 30 adults with PWS with 30 with non-specific learning disabilities. Scores on Factors (I) and (V) were high. These included ratings of temper, impulsivity, non-compliance, mood disorder, inactivity and repetitive speech. There were no significant differences according to gender, age or Body Mass Index (BMI). However, the most overweight individuals scored highest on Factors (I) and (IV) compared to those with the lowest BMI. Dykens & Cassidy (1995) investigated some of the potential correlates of maladaptive behaviour in 86 children and adults with PWS. Temper tantrums and impatience were the two most commonly reported problems in children, and temper tantrums and eating problems in adults. The severity of behaviour problems tended to increase with age, as did social withdrawal, negative self-image and depressive symptoms. In the adults, contrary to expectation, lower BMI was associated with greater problems. Males showed more severe depressive symptoms than females. Generally, many of the maladaptive behaviours and mood problems were described as waxing and waning throughout adult life. Symons et al. (1999) found skin picking, especially on the front of the legs and head, to be a particularly common form of self-injurious behaviour, occurring in 81% of the individuals studied. Other forms of self-injury, including nose picking and self-biting, were much rarer (17% to 29%). All these behaviours were less marked when children were very young but emerged in later childhood. Akefeldt & Gillberg (1999) found no correlation between the severity of self-injurious behaviours and IQ.

Obsessions and compulsions

A consistent finding emerging from both questionnaire studies and anecdotal reports has been the observation that people with PWS characteristically engage in repetitive behaviours, appear to dislike change in routine and engage in repetitive questioning. Dykens, Leckman & Cassidy (1996) used the Yale–Brown Obsessive Compulsive Scale to investigate the extent of obsessive–compulsive disorder in individuals with PWS. Parents and caregivers of 91 people with reported PWS between the ages of 9 years and 47 years completed this and other questionnaires. In over half the participant group, hoarding and the need to know, tell or ask were present. Ideas of symmetry, and arranging according to certain rules were present in between 30 and 40%, and 25% showed excessive showering, toileting and grooming. The limitation of the study was that it was an informant-based postal questionnaire study (with some telephone contact) and therefore the precise nature of and best way to conceptualize such symptomatology is unclear. Many of these symptoms are present relatively early in life, which suggests that the obsessional characteristics might best be conceptualized as part of a syndrome of arrested development rather than as an acquired obsessive–compulsive disorder. This issue requires further research.

Psychiatric disorder

Case reports of people with PWS have raised the possibility of an increased risk for psychiatric illness. Verhoeven, Curfs & Tuinier (1998) described six people with PWS and psychotic illness and concluded that cycloid psychosis was the most common and appropriate diagnosis. Clarke (1998), using a checklist for psychopathology with a group of 95 individuals aged 16 years or over, reported that 6.3% had had a possible psychotic disorder in the previous month. The possibility of an increased risk of psychiatric illness in PWS was supported by recent research by Boer et al. (2001). In a population-based study they found that approximately 25% of all those over the age of 16 years had had a serious psychiatric illness, usually an affective psychosis.

Comparisons between deletion and disomy in PWS

Whilst both chromosome 15 deletions of the PWS critical region and the inheritance of chromosome 15 disomy have similar genetic outcomes (the failure of expression of specific maternally imprinted genes), there is a theoretical difference between the two chromosome types. It has been estimated that the classical 4 megabase deletion of the PWS critical region contains approximately 100 genes. Those with the disomy will have two copies of these genes (both from a chromosome 15 of maternal origin), whereas those with the deletion will only have one copy. It is possible that the expression of only one copy of specific genes may have an affect on the phenotype that would only be apparent in those with PWS due to a chromosome 15 deletion, not those with the disomy.

Gillessen-Kaesbach et al. (1995) undertook a phenotype study of 167 people with PWS (116 with, and 51 without, a deletion). The focus of the study was primarily on the diagnostic criteria and physical phenotype, not the behaviour. No differences were found for the early diagnostic markers, or for feeding problems, eye abnormalities, congenital anomalies, thick saliva, scoliosis, sexual development, or diabetes mellitus. The only differences were that the mean birth weights for males and females were lower in those with the deletion. Hypo-pigmentation was also more common in this group (52% vs 23%) and is considered to be due to the presence of the gene for the type II oculo-cutaneous albinism (the P locus) which is located in the PWS critical region and is thought not to be imprinted (Rinchik et al., 1993).

In a similar comparison, Cassidy et al. (1997) found that those with disomy had been born to mothers with a higher mean maternal age and there were higher rates of hypo-pigmentation among those with deletions. Rates of skin picking and high pain perception were also lower in those with disomy, and facial characteristics were less marked, but the differences were not significant. Dykens et al. (1999) compared 23 people with PWS due to a deletion and 23 people with PWS due to disomy. The severity of the characteristic behaviours associated with PWS (measured using the Child Behaviour Checklist) appeared reduced in those with disomy (controlling for IQ differences) compared to those with the deletion. In particular, those with disomy scored lower on both internalizing and externalizing scores, repetitive behaviours (skin picking, nail biting) and obsessive–compulsive behaviours. The authors suggest that the mechanism described above may account for such differences or the observation that imprinting of genes may not be absolute, but could be 'leaky', particularly in those with disomy since both alleles of specific genes are imprinted. Thus there may be some expression of 'PWS genes' even though they are imprinted.

Linking gene expression to brain function and behaviour in PWS

A major research challenge is to establish the basic mechanisms that might link the failure of gene(s) expression in PWS and the observed phenotype characteristic of the syndrome. Hypothalamic dysfunction is likely to be central but it would seem unlikely that this might account for the intellectual impairment that is present. Anecdotally, the effects of the use of growth hormone in childhood suggest that some of the physical features (facial appearance, small hands and feet) may be secondary to growth hormone deficiency. Magnetic resonance studies of the posterior pituitary (Miller et al., 1996) and post-mortem studies (Gabreels et al., 1998) support the view that there may be a processing deficit of vasopressin due to the absence of the neuroendocrine polypeptide 7B2, the gene which is close to the PWS critical region on chromosome 15. Thus, specific hypotheses about the underlying abnormality that might lead to an abnormal satiety response to food intake can begin to be constructed and tested. As the genetic basis of the syndrome is elucidated, a combination of mRNA expression studies on post-mortem brain tissue, structural and functional brain scanning studies and clearer characterization of the behavioural phenotype may enable connections to be made.

Clinical features of AS

There has been considerably less investigation of the clinical features of AS compared to those of PWS. Clayton-Smith et al. (1993) described 82 people with AS between the ages of 17 months and 26 years. In three families there were two affected siblings and in one family, three. The most striking features were the severe developmental delay and marked absence of speech development together with 'attacks' of giggling. Severe sleep disturbance and epilepsy were also noticeable. One-third had no speech and none spoke more than six recognizable words. However, the majority were able to communicate in other ways – 20% used Makaton and many were developing their own personal signs or gestures. Some could point to pictures to indicate need. Distinctive patterns of behaviour and play were also noted. There was a particular love of water, which could include jumping into swimming pools and lakes at every opportunity. There was also a fascination with mirrors, reflections and plastic, and favourite toys included balloons, musical toys and anything that made a loud noise. Contrary to the original report by Angelman (1965), visual impairment was not common. Older individuals were said to be able to undertake simple household tasks, and the hyperactivity of childhood diminished in adult life. None was considered capable of independent living.

Diagnostic criteria for AS

The findings from the study by Clayton-Smith et al. (1993), together with others, became incorporated into more formal diagnostic criteria by the Scientific and Research Advisory Board of the AS Foundation in the United States, which established consensus diagnostic criteria for the syndrome (Williams et al., 1995). The criteria covered all the three major genetic sub-types: deletions on chromosome 15 of maternal origin involving the AS critical region; uniparental disomy (UPD); and those with neither a deletion nor UPD.

There is usually a normal prenatal and birth history. At birth, head circumference is normal and there are no major birth defects. Developmental delays become apparent between 6 and 12 months and may increase over time but there is no evidence of regression. Metabolic, haematological and biochemical investigations are normal. There may be some evidence of cortical atrophy on a CT or MRI brain scan.

The clinical characteristics have been divided into: (1) those always present; (2) those that are frequent – more than 80%; and (3) associated characteristics – 20–80%. Those in group 1 include developmental delay associated with severe functional disabilities, no or minimal use of spoken words (receptive and non-verbal communication said to be better than verbal skills), evidence of a movement or balance disorder, usually leading to ataxia of gait and/or tremulous movement of the hands, and a combination of frequent laughing, apparent happy demeanor and excitability with hand-flapping movements and short attention span.

In group 2 the features include a delayed and disproportionate growth of the head (such as flat occiput) leading to microcephaly by age 2 years, the onset of severe seizures before the age of 3 years, and an abnormal EEG with large amplitude slow waves facilitated by eye closure. The associated features of group 3 include flat occiput, the presence of an occipital groove, protruding tongue, sucking/swallowing disorders and feeding problems in infancy, protruding jaw (prognathia), wide mouth and widely spaced teeth, excessive chewing and mouth movements, hyperactive lower limbs with deep tendon responses, hypo-pigmentation (in those with chromosome deletion only), increased sensitivity to heat, sleep disturbance and attraction to, and fascination with, water.

Behavioural and cognitive phenotype of AS

These areas have only recently begun to be investigated systematically and early reports were primarily descriptive (Hersh et al., 1981; Zori et al., 1992). Two striking findings are the marked impairment in spoken language, which is usually limited to none or very few words, and the occurrence of uncontrollable bursts of laughter (Summers et al., 1995). Anecdotally, the laughter is said to relate to some possible event and in the paper by Clayton-Smith et al. (1993) almost all were described as 'happy' and were said to enjoy slapstick humour but not cartoons. Given the limited language development, it is very difficult to be certain to what extent the 'laughter' is an external representation of finding something funny or whether it may be some reflex response to environmental stimulation. More formal assessments of cognitive ability and the precise nature of the language deficit are still needed.

Summers et al. (1995) in their extensive literature review identified a total of 34 studies on the nature and frequency of behaviour problems in people with AS. Eighty-four per cent of individuals reported had marked speech deficits and 83% episodes of uncontrollable laughter. The latter was considered to be pathognomonic of the syndrome because of the low threshold for its occurrence (Robb et al., 1989). Early feeding problems, resolving by one year, and hyperactivity persisting into later life, were also common. Repetitive behaviours and aggression were cited as being present in approximately 10% of cases reviewed.

In the same authors' own study of 11 children (mean age 5.4 years) moderate to profound levels of developmental disability were found, with evidence of developmental problems being recognized by parents very early in life (Summers et al., 1995). Again, inappropriate laughter and speech delay were the most striking features. Expressive language was most obviously affected with no babbling or no use of words being common. However, gestures were often present. All 11 children had problems with concentration and excessive activity, and poor sleep was reported to occur in the majority.

In a later study, Summers & Feldman (1999) systematically assessed 27 people (age 2.08 to 25.33 years, mean 9.08 years) with genetically or clinically confirmed AS, identified through an advert in the AS newsletter. They were compared with two groups, IQ, chronological age and gender matched from a 'behaviour' clinic and a 'non-referred' group in the community. Behaviour ratings were obtained using the Aberrant Behaviour Checklist. The AS group scores were significantly lower on the 'irritability' and 'lethargy' scales. People with AS were less likely to display temper tantrums and outbursts, and had fewer 'mood' related problems. The authors suggest that people with AS may in fact be more resilient to emotional and behavioural problems compared to others with intellectual disabilities.

Comparison between deletion and disomy AS

Such studies that have been done have been descriptive in nature and there has been no systematic evaluation of the extent of intellectual and functional impairments or of behaviour in the different genetic forms. Smith, Buchholz & Robson (1997) described two boys and two girls with AS due to chromosome 15 disomy. Along with other data, they proposed that people with this genetic form of AS tended to have less severe developmental brain abnormalities, as some of the associated characteristics such as epilepsy, microcephaly and the motor abnormalities, seemed less marked. For example, two of the four cases reported by Smith et al. (1997) had never had epilepsy and were not on anticonvulsants. Head circumference was normal for three of the four. Dan et al. (2000) describe two people meeting the diagnostic criteria for AS but whom they considered to be atypical in presentation. One was thought to have an imprinting defect and the other uniparental disomy. In both cases speech and motor skills were better developed than would normally be expected; epilepsy was of later onset and the EEG pattern was atypical.

Conclusions

These two syndromes are considered together only because of the similar chromosomal deletion on chromosome 15 reported to be present in a significant proportion of those with either of the syndromes. The only phenotypic similarity between the two is the fact that, in both conditions, individuals with chromosome 15 deletions have higher rates of hypo-pigmentation due to the presence of the gene for the type II oculo-cutaneous albinism (the P locus) which is located in the PWS/AS critical region and is not imprinted (Rinchik et al., 1993). It is now clearly established that they are both genotypically and phenotypically distinct and separate syndromes.

Their importance, however, has been to establish vividly the role of gender specific genomic imprinting and how this mechanism has a very specific effect on brain development and therefore on intellectual, social and emotional development and behaviour. Failure of expression (for whatever genetic reason) of the paternally imprinted UBE3A gene has a profound effect on brain development and, most strikingly, on language. Failure of expression of other, maternally imprinted gene(s), gives rise to less severe learning disability but, instead, presents with a particular spectrum of behaviours that are increasingly seen as characteristic of the PWS – i.e. over-eating, obsessive–compulsive behaviours, temper control and insensitivity to pain. In the case of PWS the 'cognitive and behavioural phenotype' continues to be extensively studied. Our own population-based data indicates that IQ is normally distributed but with a mean approximately 40 points lower than the general population. This suggests that a single major genetic effect may be influencing brain development in a particular manner. In a population sample of people with PWS we have also found evidence of greater than expected phenotypic variation.

Both syndromes raise important issues that are directly relevant to the understanding of normal and abnormal human brain development and therefore, intellectual, social and emotional development, and particularly to our understanding of the 'behavioural phenotypes' of people with specific syndromes (see Brodsky & Lombroso, 1998, for discussion). Some of these are as follows.

What accounts for phenotypic differences in both PWS and AS? In the case of PWS it is likely that more than one gene gives rise to the phenotype, thus genotypic variation might account for phenotypic differences. In the case of AS, it is the failure of expression of a single gene that would appear to be important, but the loss of expression of one copy of other genes in those with the deletion form may also influence the phenotype (e.g. as with pigmentation).

What is the relative influence of genotype and environment on cognitive and behavioural outcomes? In the case of PWS there is some early evidence that critical periods of development and/or the occurrence of life events may result in the onset of serious psychiatric disorder. Little is known about the relationship between factors that can be modified (e.g. weight) and outcome.

Gender specific genomic imprinting is the particular genetic mechanism that gives rise to a failure of gene expression and to either AS or PWS. The implication of gender specific genomic imprinting is that maternal and paternal genomes are not equivalent. Animal studies indicate that paternal and maternal genomes have different roles in brain development and, furthermore, that gender specific genomic imprinting varies across tissues. If imprinting is not stable over time, or across development, and varies between tissues then this gives rise to another genetic mechanism that might account for differences in both normal and abnormal development in humans. This may be especially so for those genes concerned with brain development where imprinting may be of particular significance (see Keverne, 1997; Falls et al., 1999, for reviews).

Thus PWS and AS have illustrated the importance of a specific genetic mechanism on human development and how the expression or not of specific imprinted gene(s) has radically different effects on development and behaviour. As yet this understanding has not led to new treatments and there remains the task of identifying the mediating brain mechanisms that link gene expression to abnormal cognitive development and behavioural manifestations.

Table 9.1. Summary of clinical features of Prader–Willi and Angelman syndromes

Prader-Willi syndrome

This syndrome is associated with high rates of physical and psychiatric morbidity, associated with significant levels of mortality. These become particularly apparent in early adult life.

The most serious and potentially life-threatening behaviour associated with this syndrome is severe over-eating. With age, strategies to supervise and control the 'eating environment' become crucially important to prevent severe obesity.

Angelman syndrome

The main clinical features of people with this syndrome include antero-posterior flattening of the head, jerky movements of the limbs, bursts of uncontrollable laughter and very limited spoken language development. Severe sleep disturbance and epilepsy are common, and the person may have an apparent fascination with objects.

This syndrome is due to the loss of expression of one paternally imprinted gene (UBE3A), as opposed to Prader-Willi syndrome which is likely to be due to the loss of expression of more than one maternally imprinted gene.

See Table 9.1 for a summary of the clinical features of PWS and AS.

Acknowledgements

Our thanks to Robbie Patterson for administrative support. J.W. and JB are employed on a grant from the Wellcome Trust and we are grateful to the Trust for their support.

Glossary

Genomic imprinting a process whereby genes are switched on or off. Specific genes on chromosome 15 are normally imprinted (and therefore not expressing mRNA) depending on whether they are on the chromosome of maternal or paternal origin.

Uniparental disomy this is an abnormal state in which the two copies of a particular chromosome (chromosome 15 in the case of PWS or AS) are inherited from one parent, rather than one from each parent.

Gametogenesis the gametes are the spermatozoa (resulting from spermatogenesis) and ovum (resulting from oogenesis). These differ from other cells in that they contain only one copy of each chromosome and on fertilization give rise to cells with two copies of each of the 22 autosomes, and either two

X chromosomes for females, or an X and Y chromosome for males. Gamteogenesis involves a two-stage process referred to as meiosis.

Contiguous gene syndrome this is the term given to a syndrome whose genetic cause is usually a specific chromosomal deletion resulting in loss of expression of those genes that have been deleted. The loss of expression of more than one gene is considered necessary for the full phenotype of the syndrome to be present.

Epigenetic effects the indirect effects of gene expression. For example, the process leading to the differentiation of different organ systems.

REFERENCES

Akefeldt, A., Akefeldt, B. & Gillberg, C. (1997). Voice, speech and language characteristics of children with Prader–Willi syndrome. *Journal of Intellectual Disability Research*, **41**: 302–11.

Akefeldt, A. & Gillberg, C. (1999). Behaviour and personality characteristics of children and young adults with Prader–Willi syndrome: A controlled study. *Journal of American Academy of Adolescent Psychiatry*, **38**: 761–9.

Angelman, H. (1965). 'Puppet' children: a report on three case. *Developmental Medicine and Child Neurology*, **7**: 681–8.

Berntson, G.G., Zipf, W.B., Dorisio, O., Hoffman, J.A. & Chance, R.E. (1993). Pancreatic polypeptide infusions reduce food intake in Prader–Willi syndrome. *Peptides*, **14**: 497–503.

Boer, H., Clarke, D., Whittington, J., Butler, J. & Holland, A. (2001). Prader–Willi syndrome and psychosis. *11th World Congress of the International Association for the Scientific Study of Intellectual Disabilities (IASSID)*, Seattle, Washington, USA. Seattle: *Journal of Intellectual Disability Research*.

Brodsky, M. & Lombroso, P.L. (1998). Molecular mechanisms of developmental disorders. *Development and Psychopathology*, **10**: 1–20.

Butler, M.G., Moore, J., Morawiecki, A. & Nicolson, M. (1998). Comparison of leptin protein levels in Prader-Willi syndrome and control individuals. *American Journal of Medical Genetics*, **75**: 7–12.

Cassidy, S.B., Forsythe, M., Heeger, S., Nicholls, R.D., Schork, N., Benn, P. & Schwartz, S. (1997). Comparison of phenotype between patients with Prader–Willi syndrome due to deletion 15q and uniparental disomy 15. *American Journal of Medical Genetics*, **68**: 433–40.

Cassidy, S.B. & Schwartz, S. (1998). Prader–Willi and Angelman syndromes disorders of genomic imprinting. *Medicine*, **77**: 140–51.

Clarke, D. (1998). Prader-Willi syndrome and psychotic symptoms: 2. A preliminary study of prevalence using the Psychopathology Assessment Schedule for Adults with Developmental Disability checklist. *Journal of Intellectual Disability Research*, **42**: 451–4.

Clarke, D.J., Boer, H., Chung, M.C., Sturmey, P. & Webb, T. (1996). Maladaptive behaviour in Prader–Willi syndrome in adult life. *Journal of Intellectual Disability Research*, **40**: 159–65.

Clayton-Smith, J., Driscoll, D.J., Waters, M.F., Webb, T., Andrews, T., Malcolm, S., Pembrey, M.E. & Nicholls, R.D. (1993). Difference in methylation patterns within the D15S9 region of chromosome 15q11-13 in first cousins with Angelman syndrome and Prader–Willi syndrome. *American Journal of Medical Genetics*, **47**: 683–6.

Clift, S., Dahlitz, M. & Parkes, J.D. (1994). Sleep apnoea in the Prader–Willi syndrome. *Journal of Sleep Research*, **3**: 121–6.

Conroy, J.M., Grebe, T.A., Becker, L.A. et al. (1997). Balanced translocation 46, XY, t(2;15) (q37.2; q11.2) associated with atypical Prader-Willi syndrome. *American Journal of Human Genetics*, **61**: 388–94.

Curfs, L.M.G., Wiegers, A.M., Borghgraef, M. & Fryns, J.-P. (1991). Strengths and weaknesses in the cognitive profile of youngsters with Prader–Willi Syndrome. *Clinical Genetics*, **40**: 430–44.

Dan, B., Boyd, S.G., Christiaens, F., Cowtens, W., Van Maldergem, L. & Kahn, A. (2000). Atypical features in Angelman syndrome due to imprinting defect of uniparental disomy of chromsome 15. *Neuropediatrics*, **31**: 109–10.

Dunn, H.G. (1968). The Prader–Labhart–Willi syndrome review of the literature and report of nine cases. *Acta Paediatrica Scandinavica*, **186**(Suppl): 1–38.

Dykens, E.M. & Cassidy, S.B. (1995). Correlates of maladaptive behavior in children and adults with Prader–Willi syndrome. *American Journal of Medical Genetics*, **60**: 546–9.

Dykens, E.M., Cassidy, S.B. & King, B.H. (1999). Maladaptive behavior differences in Prader–Willi syndrome due to paternal deletion versus maternal uniparental disomy. *American Journal on Mental Retardation*, **104**: 67–77.

Dykens, E.M., Leckman, J.F. & Cassidy, S.B. (1996). Obsessions and compulsions in Prader–Willi syndrome. *Journal of Child Psychology and Psychiatry*, **37**: 995–1002.

Ehara, H., Ohno, K. & Takeshita, K. (1993). Growth and developmental patterns in Prader–Willi syndrome. *Journal of Intellectual Disability Research*, **37**: 479–85.

Falls, J.G., Pulford, D.J., Wylie, A.A. & Jirtle, R.L. (1999). Genomic imprinting: implications for human disease. *American Journal of Pathology*, **154**: 635–47.

Forssman, H. & Hagberg, B. (1964). Prader–Willi syndrome in a boy of ten with pre-diabetes. *Acta Paediatrica Scandinavica*, **53**: 70–8.

Gabreels, B.A., Swaab, D.F., de Kleijn, D.P.V., Seidah, N.G., Van de Loo, J.-W., Van de Ven, W.J.M., Martens, G.J.M. & van Leeuwen, F.W. (1998). Attenuation of the polypeptide 7B2, Prohormone convertase PC2 and vasopressin in the hypothamalmus of some Prader–Willi patients: indications for a processing defect. *Journal of Clinical Endocrinology and Metabolism*, **83**: 591–9.

Gillessen-Kaesbach, G., Robinson, W., Lohmann, D., Kaya-Westerloh, S., Passarge, E. & Horsthemke, B. (1995). Genotype–phenotype correlation in a series of 167 deletion and non-deletion patients with Prader–Willi syndrome. *Human Genetics*, **96**: 638–43.

Glenn, C.C., Saitoh, S., Jong, M.T.C., Filbrandt, M.M., Surti, U., Driscoll, D.J. & Nicholls, R.D. (1996). Gene structure, DNA methylation, and imprinted expression of the human SNRPN gene. *American Journal of Human Genetics*, **58**: 335–46.

Greenswag, L.R. (1987). Adults with Prader–Willi syndrome: a survey of 232 cases. *Developmental Medicine and Child Neurology*, **29**: 145–52.

Hersh, J.H., Zimmerman, A.W., Dinno, N.D., Greenstein, R.M., Weisskopf, B. & Reese, A.H. (1981). Behavioural correlates in the happy puppet syndrome: a characteristic profile? *Developmental Medicine and Child Neurology*, **23**: 792–800.

Holland, A.J. (1998). Understanding the eating disorder affecting people with Prader-Willi Syndrome. *Journal of Applied Research in Intellectual Disabilities*, **11**: 192–206.

Holland, A.J., Treasure, J., Coskeran, P., Dallow, J., Milton, N. & Hillhouse, E. (1993). Measurement of excessive appetite and metabolic changes in Prader-Willi syndrome. *International Journal of Obesity*, **17**: 527–32.

Holland, A.J. & Wong, J. (1999). Genetically determined obesity in Prader-Willis Syndrome: the ethics and legality of treatment. *Journal of Medical Ethics*, **25**: 230–6.

Holm, V.A., Cassidy, S.B., Butler, M.G., Hanchett, J.M., Greenburg, F., Whitman, B. & Greensway, L.R. (1992). Diagnostic criteria for Prader–Willi syndrome. In *Prader-Willi Syndrome and Other Chromosome 15q Deletion and Disorders*, ed. S.B. Cassidy. pp. 105–17. Berlin: Springer-Verlag.

Holm, V.A., Cassidy, S.B., Butler, M.G., Hanchett, J.M., Greenswag, L.R., Whitman, B.Y. & Greenberg, F. (1993). Prader–Willi syndrome: consensus diagnostic criteria. *Pediatrics*, **91**: 398–402.

Jong, M.T.C., Gray, T.A., Ji, Y., Glenn, C.G., Saitoh, S., Driscoll, D.J. & Nicholls, R.D. (1999). A novel imprinted gene encoding a RING zinc-finger protein and overlapping antisense transcript in the Prader–Willi syndrome critical region. *Human Molecular Genetics*, **8**: 783–93.

Keverne, E. (1997). Genomic imprinting in the brain. *Current opinion in Neurobiology*, **7**: 463–8.

Laurance, B.M. (1961). Hypotonia, obesity, hypogonadism and mental retardation in childhood. *Archives of Diseases in Childhood*, **36**: 690.

Laurance, B.M. (1967). Hypotonia, mental retardation, obesity, and cryptorchidism associated with dwarfism and diabetes in children. *Archives of Diseases in Childhood*, **42**: 126–39.

Ledbetter, D.H., Riccardi, V.M., Airhart, S.D., Strobel, R.J., Keenan, B.S. & Crawford, J.D. (1981). Deletions of chromosome 15 as a cause of the Prader–Willi syndrome. *New England Journal of Medicine*, **304**: 325–9.

Magenis, E., Toth-Fejel, S., Allen, L.J., Black, M., Brown, M.G., Budden, S., Cohen, R., Friedman, J.M., Kalousek., Zonana, J., Lacy, D., LaFranchi, S., Lahr, M., Macfarlane, J. & Williams, C.P.S. (1990). Comparison of the 15q deletions in Prader–Willi and Angelman syndromes: specific regions, extent of deletions, parental origin, and clinical consequences. *American Journal of Medical Genetics*, **35**: 33–49.

Magenis, R.E., Brown, M.G., Lacy, D.A., Budden, S. & LaFranchi, S. (1987). Is Angelman syndrome an alternate result of del(15)(q11q13)? *American Journal of Medical Genetics*, **28**: 829–38.

Matsuura, T., Sutcliffe, J., Fang, P., Galjaard, R.J., Jiang, Y.H., Benton, C.S., Rommens, J.M. & Beaudet, A.L. (1997). De novo truncating mutations in E6-AP ubiquitin-protein ligase gene (UBE3A) in Angelman syndrome. *Nature Genetics*, **15**: 74–7.

Miller, L., Angulo, M., Price, D. & Taneja, S. (1996). MR of the pituitary in patients with Prader–Willi syndrome: size determination and imaging findings. *Pediatric Radiology*, **26**: 43–7.

Nakada, Y., Taniura, H., Uetsuki, T., Inazawa, J. & Yoshikawa, K. (1998). The human chromosomal gene for necdin, a neuronal growth suppressor, in the Prader–Willi syndrome deletion region. *Genetics*, **213**: 65–72.

Nicholls, R.D. (1993). Genomic imprinting and uniparental disomy in Angelman and Prader–Willi syndromes: a review. *American Journal of Medical Genetics*, **46**: 16–25.

Nicholls, R.D., Knoll, J.H.M., Butler, M.G., Karam, S. & Lalande, M. (1989). Genetic imprinting suggested by maternal heterodisomy in non-deletion Prader–Willi syndrome. *Nature*, **342**: 281–7.

Nicholls, R.D., Saitoh, S. & Horsthemke, B. (1998). Imprinting in Prader–Willi and Angelman syndromes. *Trends in Genetics*, **14**: 194–200.

Ohta, T., Gray, T.A., Rogan, P.K., Buiting, K., Gabriel, J.M., Saitoh, S., Muralidhar, B., Bilienska, B., Krajewska-Walasek, M., Driscoll, D.J., Horsthemke, B., Butler, M.G. & Nicholls, R.D. (1999). Imprinting – mutation mechanisms in Prader–Willi syndrome. *American Journal of Human Genetics*, **64**: 397–413.

Pembury, M., Fennell, S.J., Berghe, J. et al. (1989). The association of Angelman's syndrome with deletions within 15q11-13. *Journal of Medical Genetics*, **26**: 73–7.

Prader, A., Labhart, A. & Willi, H. (1956). Ein syndrom von Adipositas, Kleinwicys, Kryptorchismus und Oligophrenie nach myatonieartigem Zustand im Neugeborenalter. *Schweizerische Medizinische Wochenschrift*, **86**: 1260–1.

Reed, M.L. & Leff, S.E. (1994). Maternal imprinting of human SNRPN, a gene deleted in Prader-Willi syndrome. *Nature Genetics*, **6**: 163–7.

Richards, A., Quaghebeur, G., Clift, S., Holland, A., Dahlitz, M. & Parkes, D. (1994). The upper airway and sleep apnoea in the Prader-Willi syndrome. *Clinical Otolaryngology*, **19**: 193–7.

Richdale, A.L., Cotton, S. & Hibbit, K. (1999). Sleep and behaviour disturbance in Prader-Willi syndrome: a questionnaire study. *Journal of Intellectual Disability Research*, **43**: 380–92.

Rinchik, E.M., Bultman, S.J., Horsthemke, B., Lee, S.T., Strunk, K.M., Spritz, R.A., Avidano, K.M., Jong, M.T. & Nicholls, R.D. (1993). A gene for the mouse pink-eyed dilution locus and for human type II oculocutaneous albinism. *Nature*, **361**(6407): 72–6.

Robb, S.A., Pohl, K.R.E., Baraitser, M., Wilson, J. & Brett, E.M. (1989). The 'happy puppet' syndrome of Angelman: review of the clinical features. *Archives of Diseases in Childhood*, **64**: 83–6.

Roof, E., Stone, W., MacLean, W., Feurer, I., Thompson, T. & Butler, M.G. (2000). Intellectual characteristics of Prader–Willi syndrome: comparison of genetic subtypes. *Journal of Intellectual Disability Research*, **44**: 25–30.

Schulze, A.C.H., Skakkebaek, N.E., Brondum-Nielson, K., Ledbetter, D.H. & Tommerup, N. (1996). Exclusion of SNRPN as a major determinant of Prader–Willi syndrome by a translocation breakpoint. *Nature Genetics*, **12**: 452–4.

Selikowitz, M., Sunman, J., Pendergast, A. & Wright, S. (1990). Fenfluramine in Prader–Willi syndrome: a double blind, placebo controlled trial. *Archives of Diseases in Childhood*, **65**: 112–14.

Smith, A., Buchholz, T. & Robson, L. (1997). Diagnostic testing for Prader–Willi and Angelman syndromes: response [letter]. *American Journal of Human Genetics*, **61**: 241–4.

Summers, J.A., Allison, D.B., Lynch, P.S. & Sadler, L. (1995). Behaviour problems in Angelman syndrome. *Journal of Intellectual Disability Research*, **39**: 97–106.

Summers, J.A. & Feldman, M.A. (1999). Distinctive pattern of behavioural functioning in Angelman Syndrome. *American Journal on Mental Retardation*, **104**: 376–84.

Swaab, D.F., Purba, J.S. & Hofman, M.A. (1995). Alterations in the hypothalamic paraventricular nucleus and its oxytocin neurons (putative satiety cells) in Prader–Willi syndrome: a study of five cases. *Journal of Clinical Endocrinology and Metabolism*, **80**: 573–9.

Symons, F.J., Butler, M.G., Sanders, M.D., Feurer, I.D. & Thompson, T. (1999). Self-injurious behavior and Prader–Willi syndrome: behavioral forms and body locations. *American Journal on Mental Retardation*, **104**: 260–9.

Verhoeven, W.M.A., Curfs, L.M.G. & Tuinier, S. (1998). Prader–Willi syndrome and cycloid psychosis. *Journal of Intellectual Disability Research*, **42**: 455–62.

Waters, J., Clarke, D.J. & Corbett, J.A. (1990). Educational and occupational outcome in Prader–Willi syndrome. *Child Care and Health Development*, **16**: 271–82.

Williams, C.A., Angelman, H., Clayton-Smith, J., Driscoll, D.J., Hendrickson, J.E., Knoll, J.H.M., Magenis, R.E., Schinzel, A., Wagstaff, J., Whidden, E.M. & Zori, R.T. (1995). Angelman syndrome: consensus for diagnostic criteria. *American Journal of Medical Genetics*, **56**: 237–8.

Zipf, W.B. & Bernston, G.G. (1987). Characteristics of abnormal food-intake patterns in children with Prader–Willi syndrome and study of effects of naloxone. *American Journal Clinical Nutrition*, **46**: 277–81.

Zipf, W.B., Dorisio, O., Cataland, S. & Dixon, K. (1983). Pancreatic polypeptide responses to protein meal challenges in obese but otherwise normal children and obese children with Prader-Willi syndrome. *Journal of Clinical Endocrinology and Metabolism*, **57**: 1074–80.

Zori, R.T., Hendrickson, J., Woolven, W., Whidden, E.M., Gray, B. & Williams, C.A. (1992). Angelman syndrome: clinical profile. *Journal of Child Neurology*, **7**: 270–80.

10

Rett Disorder

Alison Kerr

Introduction

Since it was described in 1966 by the Viennese neurologist Andreas Rett, the Rett syndrome has become familiar as a striking and consistent phenotype, affecting girls who look remarkably normal but display unusual behaviours associated with disturbed cognition, movement and autonomic control. In the final months of 1999 the underlying genetic problem was identified at Xq28, in the gene *MECP2* (Amir et al., 1999; Wan et al., 1999; Cheadle, Gill & Fleming, 2000) and a simple and reliable genetic test for the disorder will now certainly be developed. However clinical recognition must come before such a test can be correctly applied or interpreted and this recognition will depend on awareness by health professionals of the picture they should expect to meet in clinical practice. Over 950 families have contributed health information about their affected daughters to the British Isles Rett Survey (see Kerr, 1992a). Of these, 472 are aged over 18 years, the two eldest being 66 years. I have drawn extensively on my experience with all these people in writing this chapter.

The task has now begun of matching the longitudinal health information from this and other clinical studies with the known anatomical and biochemical abnormalities in the brain and relating these to the *MECP2* defects. Although parents are usually the first to identify problems, the early symptoms may not be recognized by clinicians. Thus, girls with Rett syndrome may appear, at any age, before puzzled nurses, teachers, general practitioners, paediatricians, neurologists, psychiatrists, psychologists, orthopaedic surgeons, anaesthetists, nutritionists and others, often without a previous diagnosis other than 'severe or profound intellectual disability'. The aim of this chapter is briefly to outline what is now known about the abnormalities underlying the syndrome; to describe how the disorder may present at various stages of life; and how the associated problems may be dealt with.

Implications of recent genetic discoveries

The *MECP2* gene, which is transcribed into the active MeCP2 protein (methyl CpG binding protein 2), is believed to suppress the transcription (activation) of many other genes in cells throughout the body (Nan, Campoy & Bird, 1997; Hendrich, 2000), silencing them as their task is completed and so orchestrating the activities of every cell. The gene is a long one with at least two active domains and at the time of going to press more than 100 mutations have been identified in Rett syndrome, although the search is still incomplete. In the United Kingdom (UK), 84% of the people with classic Rett syndrome who have been tested have a mutation (Amir et al., 1999; Wan et al., 1999; Cheadle et al., 2000; Vacca et al., 2001).

No case with a *MECP2* mutation has been found without Rett problems but it is clear that the range of severity is much wider than the narrowly defined classic syndrome. One reason to expect such a wide range of severity is that since one of the female's two X chromosomes is inactivated in each cell and this inactivation may favour one or other X chromosome (skewing of X inactivation), severity varies according to the proportion of cells and tissues using the faulty gene. A boy with Klinefelter syndrome has more than one X chromosome and so such a boy may also show the classic Rett syndrome and this has been reported (Salomao Schwartzman et al., 1999). A boy with XY and a Rett mutation would be expected to have very severe Rett disease if he survives to birth and this too has been documented (Schanen & Franke, 1998). Recurrence of Rett disorder in a family is very uncommon (estimated at less than 1 in 300) and so far the mutation found in a girl with Rett syndrome has rarely been found in any of her relatives, suggesting that the disorder in that girl has arisen as a fresh mutation in the germ cells of one of her parents. It is thought to be very uncommon for such a germ cell mutation to affect more than one offspring. An individual who acquires the disorder through such a mutation will however be expected to carry a 50% (dominant) risk to any of her own offspring and this too has been reported (Witt Engerstrom & Forslund, 1992). If a girl acquires a mutation but X inactivation is exceptionally skewed it is possible for her to show the disease in such a mild form as to miss detection, when she may pass on the disorder to her children (Schanen & Franke, 1998; Wan et al., 1999). In the uncommon situations when more than one member of a family has been affected the same mutation has been found in each case (Wan et al., 1999; Cheadle et al., 2000). Early reports also indicated the likelihod of male cases (Philippart, 1990).

The defects in the nervous system

There are indications that the whole body is disadvantaged by a Rett mutation but the brain is most vulnerable, probably because of its early and complex developmental programme. Brain growth is relatively poor, with brain weight reduced out of proportion to other organs (Armstrong, 1992, 1995). Migration of neurones and myelination of axons seems to be normal and there is no evidence of cell destruction, nor accumulation of abnormal metabolites. Although superficially the brain looks remarkably normal, dendritic territories are reduced early in life, particularly in the anterior, temporal and hippocampal cortex (Armstrong, 1992, 1995). Cortical speech areas have been found to be partially differentiated (Belichenko, 2001) and later changes have been reported in the substantia nigra and cerebellum (Kitt & Wilcox, 1995). Immaturities in cardiac connecting tissues have also been reported in several cases (Kearney, Armstrong & Glaze, 1997).

There are severe early disturbances of sleep rhythms in Rett syndrome suggesting early involvement of the monoamine system (Nomura, Segawa & Hasegawa, 1984; Segawa & Nomura, 1990; Nomura & Segawa, 1990, 1992). Very low (neonatal) levels of central cardiac parasympathetic (vagal) tone have been noted, which appear to leave the sympathetic system unopposed at times of stress (Julu et al., 1997, 1998; Julu, 2001). Visual, auditory and somatic evoked responses show slight or no delay (Badr, Witt Engerstrom & Hagberg, 1987; Pelson & Budden, 1987; Badr & Hagne, 1993; Saunders, McCulloch & Kerr, 1995). Electromagnetic stimulation of the motor cortex demonstrates shortened conduction time in the corticospinal tract, probably due to inadequate central processing (Eyre et al., 1990; Heinen & Korinthenberg, 1996). Uvebrant et al. (1992) found reduced blood flow in the frontal cortex, midbrain and brainstem using SPECT (single photon emission computed tomography) techniques.

Recent research has indicated increased receptor binding of serotonin in the brain stem nuclei comparable to the situation expected in infancy (Armstrong, 2001). Blue and her colleagues (1999a,b) demonstrated increased receptor density for NMDA, AMPA, GABA and glutamate in the superior frontal gyrus of young girls with Rett syndrome, with a reduction in older women as compared to controls, and altered development of glutamate and GABA receptors in the basal ganglia. Choline acetyl transferse activity has also been found to be reduced (Wenk & Hauss-Wegrzyniak, 1999). Immunoreactivity of microtubule associated protein 2 was reduced in the neocortex in cases reported by Kaufmann, Naidu & Budden, 1995; Kaufmann, 2001). This substance

Table 10.1. Abbreviated international criteria for classic Rett syndrome and how these compare with the characteristics of girls with Rett mutations but with a wider range of disabilities

1. Normal pregnancy and birth	A number has been premature
2. Early infancy development within the accepted range for some weeks or months	Girls and boys with Rett mutations may be clearly delayed from birth
3. OFC normal or near normal at birth, falling from original centile	In milder case there may be no fall off of OFC
4. No coexisting disorder which might itself cause the disability	This is still under investigation
5. Hand stereotypy (mouthing patting or squeezing)	In mild cases this may be seen only during agitation
6. Late infancy or early childhood regression in hand and speech skills	Regression may occur before 6 months or after 4 years and mild cases may stagnate without regression. Some speech and hand skills remain and may improve
7. Gait dyspraxia	Many never walk, mild cases may run and climb steps

is present in the base plate through which motor neurones travel to the cortex; its local expression is controlled by neurotransmitters and its function relates to dendritic and synaptic development and maintenance.

It is thus clear that the brain is immature in the Rett disorder and remains poorly equipped for the demands of maturation and ageing. The various defects so far identified correspond closely with the patterns of disability encountered but much work is still required to discover where the biochemical cascade begins and where intervention is likely to be effective.

Syndrome and disorder

The criteria for 'classic' Rett syndrome were agreed by international consensus in order to facilitate comparison between cases from different centres (Diagnostic Criteria Work Group et al., 1988). However it became clear from early studies of monozygotic twins (Kerr, 1992a) and other familial cases that the disorder encompassed a wider range of severity than the classic syndrome. Now that the genetic defect is known it is expected that previously unsuspected cases will come to light and previously unrecognized clinical signs of the disorder will also emerge. Although the strictly defined classic syndrome remains a useful description it is also important to be aware of variations. Table 10.1 lists the abbreviated 'classic' criteria with indications of how these relate to the characteristics of girls and women now known to have Rett mutations. This chapter focuses mainly on the well researched 'classic' picture but refers also to the wider range of the disorder.

Epidemiology

Prevalence of the classic syndrome in the UK is estimated at 1 in 10 000 females at 14 years (Kerr, 1992b) although higher and lower estimates have been published elsewhere (Asthana et al., 1990; Hagberg & Hagberg, 1997). This number is based on referrals to the British survey, not a systematic search, and the continuing referral rate indicates that it is still an underestimate. Nevertheless, this figure suggests that at least 1 in 10 females with profound intellectual and physical disability is affected by the Rett disorder.

In 1993, the estimated death rate for people with classic Rett syndrome in the British survey was 1.2% annually (Kerr et al., 1997). Of 31 classic cases, 15 (48%) were those with the most severe initial disease and these people usually died in adolescence or early adult life. Characteristically the body weight was low, a consequence of severe feeding difficulty, sometimes with aspiration. Epilepsy also contributed to early deaths. One-fifth (8) of the deaths recorded in the UK were unexpected and unexplained in healthy and active girls and women. These deaths occurred at any age, and it is now suspected that immature autonomic regulation may be involved (Sekul et al., 1994; Julu et al., 1997, 1998; Julu, 2001). Extrapolating from the British mortality figures, the risk of unexpected deaths is greater than 10% even for more able and healthy individuals, across a 50-year life span.

Developmental patterns in early childhood

Pregnancy and birth are usually unexceptional (Rett, 1966; Holm, 1986). The newborn infant is normal in appearance, weight, length and head circumference and for some weeks or months general development and growth continue (Percy, 1992; Budden, 1995). In the 'classic' syndrome, head circumference remains close to the third centile without crossing the centile lines, but more commonly there is some slowing of growth in early childhood, with resumption of growth later (Figure 10.1; Percy, 1992). Although the baby appears normal and passes routine screening tests, an almost invariable early sign is placidity (Kerr & Stephenson, 1985, 1986; Kerr, Montague & Stephenson, 1987; Witt Engerstrom, 1987, 1992; Witt Engerstrom & Forslund, 1992; Leonard & Bower, 1998). Typically, the infant is described as 'very good' and undemanding, but experienced parents may find her less responsive than expected (Naidu, 1997). Some babies have feeding difficulties but most suck well, thrive and pass the early milestones of sitting, reaching out and transferring objects from hand to hand. Mobility is usually poor, crawling uncommon and walking late (Nomura & Segawa, 1990). The latter problem is the commonest reason for seeking medical advice. Skills commonly plateau around the 9 to 12-month stage when concerns begin to be voiced, usually first by parents rather than health professionals. Words may develop but phrases are rare. Pointing and inventive play are poor or absent (Kerr & Stephenson, 1985, 1986; Kerr et al., 1987; Witt Engerstrom, 1987, 1992; Witt Engerstrom & Forslund, 1992).

The plateau in developmental progress is followed by a period of regression which is often quite dramatic, occurring over a few days or many months. This may begin as early as 4 months or as late as 4 years and its onset is more abrupt than its end. The child seems to forget the skills that have been gained, words usually disappear and hand skills diminish, being replaced by hand patting, clapping, squeezing or mouthing stereotypies. Irregular breathing appears towards the end of the regression period and at the same time a general coarse tremor is often noticed. Most distressing for the family is a transient withdrawal

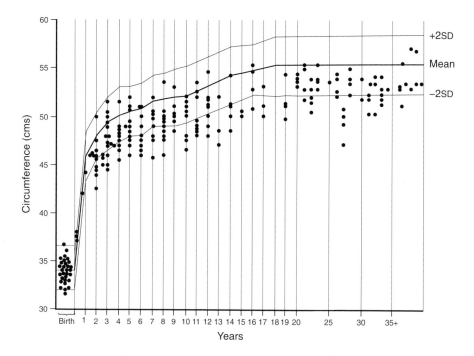

Figure 10.1. Occipito-frontal circumference measurements (OFC) for people with classic Rett syndrome at birth and after 18 months (from the British survey, Kerr, 1992a).

from contact by a child who has previously seemed sociable, and this may give rise to suspicions of autism. There is generally no external event that is associated with this regression although minor illnesses have been reported.

By the end of the regression period the main features of the disorder are obvious, with disturbance of voluntary movement, the presence of involuntary movement, abnormal posture, breathing irregularity, agitation, feeding difficulties, gaseous distension, constipation and severe to profound difficulties in cognitive skills, understanding and communication. After the regression period (usually by 5 years) there is improvement in contact, and skills recover to some extent. Head circumference usually continues to increase, the mean lying close to the second standard deviation (Figure 10.1). It is important to note on this graph that growth usually continues after the regression period. Abnormal muscle tone is an important constituent of the clinical problem, and is well discussed by Nomura & Segawa (1992).

The transition to adulthood

Although severe to profound intellectual impairment is characteristic of Rett syndrome, the clinical picture in adulthood is profoundly influenced by the initial severity of the disease, the age of the individual and the quality of care received. Neurological examination indicates abnormal muscle tone, reduced in the younger person and increasing with age, showing features of spasticity, rigidity and dystonic posturing. Following regression, deep tendon reflexes are brisk. Ankle clonus is usually present but the Babinski sign is absent. Table 10.2 relates the clinical range to the predominant abnormality of muscle tone (tone subtype) (Kerr & Stephenson, 1985, 1986). The most severely affected adults tend to be those who were most severely hypotonic from birth, with poorer head growth, earlier regression and more severe difficulties in feeding and posture than the other groups. In this subtype the breathing irregularity may be unremarkable to the casual observer and yet provide inadequate gas exchange. Severe hypotonia usually changes to severe hypertonia and dystonia, although some women remain hypotonic throughout life.

Babies with milder hypotonia also become increasingly hypertonic and dystonic after regression and remain so as adults. Individuals who are hypertonic and dystonic tend to be the most agitated, with very obvious and forceful breathing irregularity. The least severely affected women with Rett syndrome often have more normal muscle tone than the others, although the tendency for tone to increase is always present. These individuals often have better head growth, more normal posture and mobility, and a wider repertoire of communication and hand skills than the more severely affected groups. The relatively high proportion of older women seen in the mildest group to some extent reflects the better prognosis of mildly affected people.

There can be no rigid division of individuals into these subtypes as many people have features of more than one subtype and most move from one subtype to another. However, they do represent commonly encountered clinical presentations and to have them in mind may assist detection.

It should be appreciated that the prognosis depends on the standard of care given as well as the initial severity of the condition. Tables 10.3 and 10.4 indicate the changing pattern of skills and behaviour from childhood to adulthood in cohorts of girls and women involved in the British survey (Kerr, 1992a).

Table 10.2. The clinical subtypes in classic Rett syndrome, before and during regression and later in life

Tone subtype	Before regression	During regression	After regression
Hypotonic (subtype 1)	Floppy and placid	Slight decline in already poor skills; remains placid	May be obese if feeding difficulties permit. Shallow, sometimes inadequate breathing; passive; prone to contractures
	Few skills, lost early, no speech		
	Proportion of cases: 80%	Percentage falls during regression	About 5%, falls steadily
Hypertonic and dystonic (subtypes 2 and 3)	Odd postures and stereotyped movements, but skills gained	Abrupt skill loss; breathing irregularity is obvious	Walks if encouraged with dystonic posture, prone to scoliosis and contractures; extreme agitation; valsalva breathing
	Proportion of cases: 1%	Percentage rises during regression	Rises to about 70%
Mildly increased muscle tone (subtype 4)	'Good baby', placid, lacking initiative but gaining skill, often considered normal	Breathing may be less obvious; regression is less severe and later; less reduction in OFC growth	Prone to scoliosis but walks well; some hand use and speech; hyperactive with mood swings
	Proportion of cases: 19%	Percentage remains stable	Remains about 25%

OFC, occipito-frontal circumference.

Table 10.3. Changing skills with age in classic Rett syndrome. Figures are given for a cohort aged 15–40 years with additional early childhood data

Reported skill	Pre-regression n = 46–80 (%)	5–10 years n = 17–80 (%)	15–20 years n = 20–64 (%)	25–30 years n = 15–25 (%)	35–40 years n = 6–9 (%)
Take spoon or cup	61	21	18	21	14
Walk alone	56	60	48	67	14
Use words	75	22	20	4	0
Understand words	91	54	50	35	25
Major feeding difficulty	6	18	35	73	67
Moderate or severe scoliosis	0	9	52	59	56
Epilepsy	0	61	73	48	38

Table 10.4. Comparing behaviour in 10 adolescents and 10 adults (randomly selected from the British survey)

Reported by family / carer	Adolescent (n)	Adult (n)
Agitation	10	10
Injury to self	4	5
Injury to others	0	3
Night sleep disturbed	4	9
Day time sleep	7	7
Irregular breathing	10	9
Gaseous distension	5	9
Menstrual difficulty	1	5

Growth, feeding, nutrition and metabolism in adults with Rett disorder

With few exceptions, adults with Rett syndrome are shorter than the rest of their family. The dwarfing becomes evident within the first 2 years of life and average adult height is around 136 cm, i.e. 30 cm below the population mean (Holm, 1986; Percy, 1992). Feet and hands tend to be slim and there is shortening of the fourth digits, metacarpals and metatarsals, which becomes more obvious with age (Kerr, Robertson & Mitchell, 1993; Kerr, Mitchell &

Robertson, 1995; Glasson et al., 1998; Leonard et al., 1999a). Weight is also well below average (Percy, 1992) but difficulties in eating certainly contribute to this and women with least difficulty in eating may become obese. More agitated individuals with marked breathing irregularity are usually thin and although the resting metabolic rate has not been found to be elevated it is likely that agitation and forceful breathing consume excessive energy (Schultz et al., 1993; Motil et al., 1994; Rice & Haas, 1998). A 50% increase in calorie intake quickly results in their regaining the appropriate weight for height. When the calorie requirement cannot be taken orally, percutaneous tube feeding (PEG) can provide satisfactory nutrition without sacrificing the pleasure of oral feeding. Six per cent of those involved in the British survey used PEG feeding but to be successful it must be instituted and supervised by a team based in a gastro-enterological unit, with specialist help directly available to the carer. The difficulties experienced by carers in feeding people with Rett syndrome include problems due to posture, difficulties in chewing and swallowing, obstructive involuntary movements of the tongue and jaws, regurgitation or vomiting, excessive secretions, poor apetite and usually total dependence on others. Accepting fluids may be particularly difficult. All these difficulties tend to worsen in adult life as the tongue suffers the same increase in tone as other muscles (Morton et al., 1997).

Constipation was a problem amongst almost all adults in the British survey, perhaps due to the low parasympathetic tone as well as to poor fluid intake and lack of activity. Fortunately this is usually controlled without recourse to medication, through the combination of physical activity, plenty of fluid and fibre and regular toilet training. In my experience virtually every girl and woman can be habit trained for bowel motions, provided that her posture allows comfortable seating on a secure toilet.

Gastrointestinal reflux is another common problem in adults (Morton et al., 1997), causing pain and loss of appetite. Poor posture, difficulties with feeding technique and gaseous distension probably contribute, and low parasympathetic tone may be implicated. Careful clinical assessment and observation of the feeding technique is essential. If necessary, pH measurements may be used to detect acid entering the oesophagus, together with video fluoroscopy to observe mastication and swallowing. Conservative medical management is usually successful but if reflux persists and particularly if aspiration occurs, PEG feeding may become necessary. Although this can correct nutrition, allow healing of the oesophagus and allow removal of excess air from the stomach, the introduction of increased amounts of food into the stomach may actually increase reflux. The surgeon may wish to consider modifying the gastro-

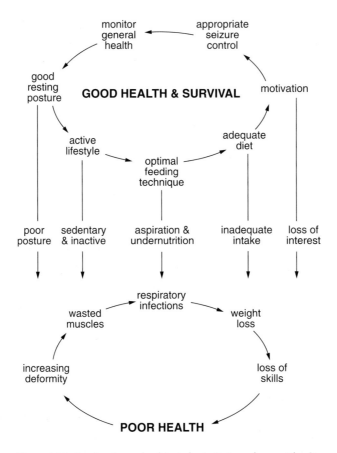

Figure 10.2. Good and poor health circles in Rett syndrome. The diagram indicates how attention or failure to attend to principles of care readily lead into good or adverse health cycles.

oesophageal junction at the same time as introducing a PEG (Gauderer, 1991).

In some older women, appetite fails periodically. This may be the consequence of discomfort including reflux, toothache, oral thrush or simply a change in the daily routine or meal time procedure. Loss of appetite is commonly reported when a woman has moved from her home into professionally supported accommodation. Frank depression should be also looked for although Sansom et al., (1993) failed to find signs of this. Low weight alone can lead to lethargy with anorexia and it may be helpful to break the 'vicious circle' of ill health by using PEG (Figure 10.2).

Osteoporosis

This is more common in adults with Rett syndrome than in others with severe learning disabilities and occurs even among actively walking adolescents

(Leonard et al., 1999b). A nutritious diet and daily exercise, with adequate protection from boisterous behaviour is the mainstay of management. It is a mistake to stop activities in an effort to avoid fractures since inactivity compounds the essential problem.

Muscle tone, posture and mobility in adults

In the adults who have been the most hypotonic babies – neither standing nor walking independently – posture is apt to be poor and contractures can develop rapidly at any age unless there is early and continuing support with passive and active exercise. Even in less severely affected adults posture is poor, perhaps due both to lack of position sense and to abnormal muscle tone. Women who can walk tend to stoop or hold themselves to one side, and foot posture is often abnormal with internal or external rotation. Tip-toe walking with a tight tendo-achilles is common in stronger individuals. In spite of these difficulties most women with Rett syndrome can walk and enjoy doing so, with or without support. However, this is a fragile skill, easily lost and not easily regained so it is a challenge to carers and providers of support services to ensure that the means are available to allow these women to continue to use their walking skills in a safe environment, without risk of injury to themselves or their attendants. Good supported seating should be provided at rest but when the individual is active a good posture is often best achieved by arranging positioning that encourages her to sit upright without additional back support. Horse riding seems to stimulate a good postural response in many people and so does movement to music. Pool physiotherapy is particularly effective and movement in warm water with good support is often better than on land, and some girls and women have learned to walk during pool activities. As with normal adults, active movement leads to improved posture and healthy joints and in Rett syndrome it appears that the motor pathways for spontaneous movement are less affected by the disorder than the voluntary pathways.

Joint deformities

These can occur due both to the nature of the disease and to a lack of expert advice and care. Light ankle–foot prostheses are often sufficient to limit ankle contractures but these need regular adjustment as the slim Rett foot is easily chafed by an ill-fitting prosthesis. If a prosthesis cannot hold the foot in a good posture for action, botulinus toxin (Botox) injections may be useful, both to relieve the muscle tightening in the short-term and also to allow the orthopaedic surgeon to plan how to correct severe tightening operatively. Few women require ankle surgery if there is good conservative care. Perhaps the greatest threat to walking is flexion contracture at the knees and with good positioning and physiotherapy this is entirely preventable, even in those with the most severe disorder. The head of the femur is liable to dislocate especially in women who are not standing or walking. Adductor tenotomy can be undertaken, cutting or weakening the strong muscles that pull the hip towards the midline. This requires careful follow-up with intensive physiotherapy and encouragement to full activity, otherwise scarring during the healing process may reverse the correction. Hand, wrist, elbow and shoulder joints are all at risk from contracture and since spontaneous movements are limited, passive exercises are required to maintain the full range of movement. When the corrective movements have been explained and demonstrated to carers they should become part of the daily routine throughout adult life.

Over 90% of adults with classic Rett syndrome have a degree of scoliosis and in over half this becomes moderate or severe (Table 10.3). This seems likely to be due to the uneven muscle tension and poor position sense combining to produce fixed rotation and flexion at the vertebral joints. It is certainly the most difficult of the contractures to control externally and worsens with the general increase in muscle tone. The ability of the person to respond actively to riding and swimming is a great advantage and these activities should be encouraged. At rest, however, there should be good, symmetric support for the back and hips. Splinting may restrain a mild scoliosis but needs very careful supervision to ensure that it is not unduly restrictive. Splinting cannot prevent progression of a severe deformity and if scoliosis is progressing rapidly, despite all the strategies described above, then surgical correction is advisable since extreme scoliosis compromises respiratory and gut function, causes discomfort and prevents activity.

The age of the individual and severity of Rett disorder are not a bar to successful scoliosis surgery (Roberts & Connor, 1988; Loder et al., 1989; Stokland, Lidstrom & Hagberg, 1993). Data from the British survey indicate that the chance of success is greatest if the woman is active and well nourished; the risks of surgery are increased if pre-operative nutrition and health are poor. The surgical team should meet the family and become familiar with the individual's personal needs and difficulties before she enters hospital. Unexpected breath holding, hyperventilation, vacant spells and epileptic seizures can lead to panic and unnecessary resuscitative efforts. It is wise to invite a parent or carer to stay in hospital to explain and assist.

The surgical correction must be thorough and robust. In the UK, a combined anterior and posterior, full spinal approach has been the most successful in preventing recurrence. The correction must be strong enough to withstand an epileptic seizure during recovery and allow mobilization within a few days to avoid loss of precarious skills and exacerbation of osteoporosis. In spite of these difficulties the woman with Rett syndrome is typically an ideal patient, uncomplaining and ready to be mobilized as soon as encouraged to be so. Healing appears to be normal and complications uncommon. Anaesthetics are generally well accepted and the women are remarkably tolerant of pain and restrictions. Correction of a rapidly progressing scoliosis protects skills, improves nutrition and quality of life and greatly eases the burden of care. The British survey indicates that it takes about one year for nutrition and activity to recover to pre-operative levels and for the full benefits to be enjoyed, so it is worthwhile to achieve the best possible health before surgery.

Manual dyspraxia

This is one of the chief problems associated with Rett disorder. It is present before regression (Kerr, 1995) but it is during the regression period that voluntary movement seems to disintegrate. A child who has previously fed herself may find this impossible or extraordinarily difficult. Thus, she may watch or circle the object of her interest with evident desire while her hands are engaged in continuous stereotypy, or she may be apparently unaware of her hands even when an object is placed between them. Dyspraxia is present even in the least affected adults although many people with the classic Rett syndrome do retain some voluntary control over their hand movements, can feed themselves to some extent and may acquire new hand skills (Table 10.3). When voluntary movements do occur they may be unpredictable, slow or fast, suggesting that the neural infrastructure is difficult to access and hard to control. The manipulative dyspraxia reflects the same essential problem as affects posture and locomotion, and receptive and perceptual difficulties seem to play as important a part as executive and motor ones. As with postural skills, useful and fluent spontaneous movements are occasionally seen. Unruly hair may be lifted from the face or an itchy place scratched without apparent difficulty. This capacity for useful spontaneous movement is a valuable asset and can be used therapeutically, although there is a danger of overestimating the voluntary abilities. The best results are achieved when a situation invites spontaneous action, and when direct commands seem to be counterproductive.

Involuntary movements

These account for much of the behaviour of the adult with Rett disorder. When carefully monitored, such movements can be seen to occur throughout the waking day. They follow a highly predictable pattern, with the same range, sequence, rate and rhythm established in early childhood changing little (apart from some reduction in amplitude) throughout life. The most hypotonic and placid people have the least noticeable movements and the most agitated have the most dramatic but the patterns are recognizable in all. Movements involve the jaws and tongue, neck and spine, lower and upper limbs and most notably the hands. In the young child these are usually in the mouth or hair; in the older child usually together at chest or waist level, and in adults often at the sides or held apart. There is no reason to interrupt or restrict these movements unless there is injury to the skin due to chafing or knocking against the teeth, or to other people. The level of activity is proportional to the individual's state of alertness. A light elbow splint may be employed to prevent injury but this should do no more than limit the damaging contact for as long as necessary to allow healing. Restraint of the hand movement may be justified if this is found to benefit other voluntary activities but individuals should normally be free of restraint. A coarse background tremor is typical. Dystonic spasms lasting for seconds or minutes are particularly common, especially in hypertonic and dystonic women, often affecting sterno-mastoid and the hip adductors and may remit and recur. Medication does not seem to reduce these involuntary movements although antispasmodics, muscle relaxants and Parkinsonian drugs have been tried (Zappella, 1990).

Defective autonomic regulation

This is an important facet of the Rett disorder, probably related to persisting immaturity of the brain stem nuclei (Sekul et al., 1994; Julu et al., 1997, 1998; Witt Engerstrom & Kerr, 1998; Guideri et al., 1999; Julu, 2001). This is responsible for most of the non-epileptic vacant spells which are an important feature of the condition and a problem in adult management (Kerr, 1992b, 1995). Central parasympathetic (vagal) tone is very low throughout life, comparable to that of a normal neonate, while sympathetic tone is normal. This leads to autonomic imbalance with unrestrained sympathetic activity, and is most marked when the woman is alerted (Julu et al., 1997). The unrestrained sympathetic activity is clearly reflected in the typical flushed face, dilated pupils, cold feet and agitation, and in stressful situations it may be dangerous (Julu et al., 1997, 2001; Julu, 2001).

The low central parasympathetic tone is associated with dysrhythmic breathing. Thirteen different rhythms have been described and the pattern changes with age (Julu et al., 1997; 1998; Witt Engerstrom & Kerr, 1998; Julu, 2001;). The breathing dysrhythmia is closely associated with the alert state (Southall et al., 1988; Kerr et al., 1990). Apneusis (delay in terminating an inspiration) is common. Serotonin produces the stimulus to end inspiration through serotonin 1A receptors and this has formed the basis for attempts to treat this particular dysrhythmia using a serotonin 1A agonist (Kerr et al., 1998). The apneustic pattern persists in many adults although it becomes less prominent with age. In older women valsalva breathing may become obvious. This occurs when the breath leaves the chest only after strong contractions of the expiratory muscles with the airway closed. The ineffective effort to expel air leads to a sudden drop in the return of venous blood to the heart and therefore to a sudden fall in blood pressure, which may lead to fainting. As the air is finally expelled from the chest there is a characteristic sound and air may enter the stomach leading to gaseous distension which is a feature of the disorder in most older people and some younger ones. Central apnoea, which is the failure to initiate a fresh inspiration, increases in middle childhood and is also commonly seen in adults with severe Rett disorder. This may give rise to severe hypoxia and fainting. Because this breathing rhythm is quiet it may not be recognized unless there are very marked colour changes.

At present there is no specific therapy for difficulties of this kind. It is helpful, however, to monitor the breathing abnormality to distinguish the vacant spells from epilepsy. This also allows carers to understand what is going on and to appreciate that these behaviours are not under the individual's control but are strongly physiologically driven events that interrupt other activities. Avoidance of excessive stimulation may be helpful since this worsens the problem, but careful planning may be needed to achieve a balance between quietness and the activity and interest needed for good health.

Measurements of the QT interval (the time for ventricular contraction and electrical recovery) from the ECG indicate that this is prolonged in some people with Rett disorder and QTc (corrected for age) should be routinely measured if vacant spells are troublesome. There is a known risk of cardiac arrhythmia developing in any person in the presence of a prolonged QTc and this might contribute to sudden and unexpected death (Sekul et al., 1994; Ellaway et al., 1999; Guideri et al., 1999).

Failure to restrain the sympathetic system results in the small cold feet that are characteristic of the Rett disorder. When scoliosis surgery involves sympathetic gangliectomy, both colour and growth of the foot improve and it has been suggested that planned sympathectomy should also be considered when such surgery is intended (Naidu et al., 1987). Among the girls in the British survey, a less invasive chemical sympathectomy has also been reported to be helpful (Kerr, 1992a).

Epileptic seizures

Around 75% of people with the Rett disorder have had an epileptic seizure at some time, usually soon after regression, and epilepsy continues in about 50% of adults (Glaze et al., 1987; Hagne, Witt-Engerstrom & Hagberg, 1989; Cooper, Kerr & Amos, 1998). These may be generalized motor, focal or atypical seizures and more rarely infantile spasms, but the true 'three per second spike and wave' petit mal pattern has not been reported. Usually epilepsy responds to the drugs appropriate to the type of seizure. In the UK cohort, carbamazepine, sodium valproate and lamotrigine are in frequent use as single agents, but seizures are intractable in a minority of girls and women and more than one drug is necessary. Although 'classic' Rett syndrome excludes cases in whom seizures are the first sign of regression, it is now clear that girls with the Rett disorder and a mutation may present with severe seizures at regression. The EEG is helpful but not diagnostic (Cooper et al., 1998). It is usually reported as normal before regression although on careful scrutiny immaturities may be detected (Bieber et al., 1990; Cooper et al., 1998). Gross abnormalities usually appear towards the end of the regression period (Cooper et al., 1998), with generalized bursts of slow wave with or without spikes, characteristically accentuated at rest and asleep. Theta rhythms predominate in later adult life (Ishizaki, 1992; Cooper et al., 1998). Since the abnormality and even epileptogenic spikes may be present without clinical seizures a routine EEG is of limited value in diagnosing epilepsy. However, when there is doubt about the nature of lapses in consciousness in adults an ambulatory EEG should be conducted. If vacant spells are not accompanied by epileptic spikes on ambulatory EEG then cardio-respiratory and autonomic monitoring is indicated. This can be achieved in a readily tolerated one hour non-invasive procedure, measuring ECG, EEG, respiratory rhythm, blood gases, blood pressure and central vagal tone (Julu, 1992, 2001; Julu et al., 1997, 2001).

Sleep disturbance

This is present early and remains prominent in adults with the Rett disorder (Table 10.4). Although the abnormality may result from fundamentally disrupted circadian rhythm it does seem to respond in adult life to the same simple measures recommended for toddler training: active days; night time baths; a quiet and secure sleeping area and minimal intervention at night without speech or additional lights; drinks of water; and silent change of clothes as necessary. It is not advisable for the person with Rett to sleep with a parent, sibling or carer as this reinforces the pattern of night waking. A sound alarm can be used to reassure the parent, and the sleeping area can be made safe with a low mattress or high cot sides. To help re-establish a normal sleep pattern melatonin or a night sedative may be used, but this should be short-term (McArthur & Budden, 1998). A family or carer suffering broken nights should have the option of night nursing relief at home and readily accessible overnight respite care.

Mood in adults with Rett disorder

The quiet and placid baby with Rett disorder becomes agitated at regression, with sudden attacks of screaming. This is the stage when glutamate levels in the brain become inappropriately high and it seems likely that the impact of external stimulation is enhanced (Blue et al., 1999a,b; Mitchell & Silver, 2000). It is during this period that the EEG becomes abnormal, breathing becomes irregular and there may be transient metabolic disturbances suggesting additional stress (Philippart & Brown, 1984). Following regression, although mood improves, the level of alertness remains heightened and moods can change rapidly and unaccountably from contented to agitated or distressed. As adolescence ends, general mood improves further and many parents comment that the young woman is happier and more quietly communicative than ever before. Periodic crying and distress continue to affect many women but depression does not seem to be common (Sansom et al., 1993). A minority of the most hypotonic women remain placid throughout life.

In trying to understand the mood changes of any individual it is important to exclude disorders that can affect all healthy people and may lead to distress or anger – e.g. unrecognized toothache, earache, headache, flatulence, gastro-oesphageal reflux, eczema, candida in the mouth, vagina or skin infestations, urinary infections, and so on. Both renal and biliary stones have occurred in people with Rett disorder. Although asthma, allergies and food intolerances do not appear to be more frequent in people with Rett disorder, these are common and easily overlooked so should be kept in mind. Change, particularly unexpected change may also be very difficult for someone with Rett syndrome to cope with, although problems can be minimized if she is well prepared in advance. The intense agitation and awareness of the adult with Rett may make her less tolerant than others and her inability to make her needs known may be frustrating. To establish an effective means of communication is therefore a priority.

Understanding and communication in adults with Rett disorder

After the transient withdrawal from contact which is seen at regression, the girl with Rett disorder becomes sociable, clearly preferring close contact with another person to inanimate objects. The human face seems to be peculiarly attractive, even when understanding is very poor (Kerr, Montague & Stephenson, 1987; Lindberg, 1991). If words are used they are directed to people. Even if speech is absent there is a clear desire to communicate (Burford & Trevarthen, 1997; Trevarthen & Burford, 2001). This can make a woman with Rett syndrome very popular provided that her restless activities can be accommodated.

Among those with classic Rett syndrome who have speech, the use of this facility is clearly enjoyed, but even in this minority, other means of communication often prove more useful. Some women learn to use gestures effectively and a few will learn to associate written words with objects. Learning to use a computer screen or to type may give pleasure but rarely seems to lead to independent communication, at least in the classic syndrome. Levels of understanding and communication may be better in the less severe cases. There should always be a comprehensive assessment of the potential for communication and a variety of alternatives should be offered, beginning with the simplest and allowing for development. The aim is to find means of communication that will be entirely under the control of the individual herself and which will extend her ability to control her environment. *Speech* should not necessarily be the principal goal. However, Zappella has reported on a group, the 'preserved speech variant' who appear to have the Rett disorder and later develop true speech (Zappella, 1997).

It can be difficult to determine comprehension levels in a disorder that so severely restricts movement and communication. It appears from what is now known of the genetic cause that most individuals who inherit a mutation on *MECP2* will use the normal and mutated gene equally while a small number will have skewed inactivation and use more or less of the abnormal gene in some or all tissues. Considerable variation is thus expected in the level of intellectual disability and the extent to which the specific Rett profile of disabilities is manifest (Schanen & Franke, 1998; Amir et al., 1999; Wan et al., 1999; Cheadle et al., 2000). For example, in the classic Rett syndrome, understanding, prediction and calculation appear to be at an early developmental level while spontaneous and emotional sensitivities appear less affected (Lindberg, 1991; Von Tetzchner, 1997), but there is a well documented case of a young woman carrying a *MECP2* mutation, which led to severe Rett disorder and early death in her son and the classic Rett syndrome in her daughter. She herself was only mildly affected and able to benefit from a normal education (Schanen & Franke, 1998; Kerr & Witt Engerstrom, 2001). Meticulous and individual assessment is clearly essential in every case.

Music

While the use and understanding of words is limited for most people with the classic Rett syndrome there is no doubting the appeal of music, which is listened to with great attention and some discrimination (Kerr et al., 1987; Lindberg, 1991; Merker & Wallin, 2001; Trevarthen & Burford, 2001). Music clearly gives pleasure, has the capacity to alter mood and encourages participation, and for these reasons it has a central role in enriching experience and encouraging interaction. Experience within the British Rett survey indicates that each person has favourite music. In the youngest girls this is often jaunty with a quick beat, clear melody and wide range of pitch, often including the human voice. Adolescents tend to favour popular groups. Some girls and women choose different music according to their mood, and families learn how to use this to soothe or alert. Individual music therapy can help to develop reciprocal communication and to improve interaction in a variety of situations. The music therapist should be an essential part of the communication team for adult assessment and therapy.

Behaviours in adults that may disturb others

These behaviours are generally involuntary and successful management is almost always through environmental modifications (Kerr, 2000).

Inadvertent ejection of saliva is uncommon but troublesome and seems to be the result of several factors – the seeking of personal contact, the habitually open mouth with pooling of secretions and the forceful effort required in expiration. Many active older women seem able to breathe out while awake only by means of a forceful valsalva manoeuvre.

Tooth grinding is troublesome to others and may wear down the teeth. A simple solution is to request the dentist to coat the teeth with a clear, light plastic. The temptation to drown the sound of grinding by loud music should be firmly resisted but intermittent use of a low volume personal stereo may help to produce relaxation and so reduce the amount of grinding, and this is often used by families to good effect.

Active and agitated girls and women may cause injury to their own hands and face or may pinch others with their stereotyped hand movements. It seems likely that this is due to a combination of the regular hand stereotypy, which is present whenever the girl is alert, even when she is alone and, in the case of pinching, her search for human contact and response. Adjustment to the daily routine to ensure that the individual has frequent and sufficient contact with the people around her, should reduce the problems without unduly restraining her spontaneous movements.

The strengths of people with Rett disorder

Vision and hearing are significantly better than in other disabled groups (Saunders et al., 1995). Eye defects are uncommon and when spectacles are needed they are usually well tolerated. It is of some interest that during regression, a squint is common but later improves spontaneously, suggesting that an effort is made to regain control of the eye movements. It is clear that much pleasure is derived from vision as girls and women often come repeatedly to scrutinize people and objects and show distinct preferences. It is therefore important to have sight tested regularly and offer spectacles when they may be of value. It is also helpful to mark on the spectacles whether they should be worn for close or distant vision.

Hearing is usually excellent but may be impaired by accumulation of wax and recurrent ear infections. The earliest signs are often difficult to detect, since the individual cannot indicate what is wrong, but disturbed behaviour may be an indication. The ears should be regularly examined and hearing tests should be arranged at intervals of 1 or 2 years.

The interest and curiosity of the person with Rett disorder is particularly endearing. Families with other children comment that their affected daughter is just 'one of the crowd' when something of interest is happening in the family, as she displays real enthusiasm and is keen to participate. People with Rett syndrome also often enjoy being the centre of attention and visiting new places. Visits to theme parks are frequently a success, and if there is a risk it is over excitement.

Although she may experience sad moods, happiness is yet another gift of the individual with Rett disorder and the ability to laugh without malice when other people in the family are gloomy is very endearing. Combined with her enjoyment of people and total lack of self-pity this gives the strong impression that she has empathy with the feelings of others. Not only is a woman with Rett disorder willing to try new experiences but she also retains the capacity to learn new skills. Some have learned to swim or to walk first as adults, and hand skills are capable of significant development over time.

Figure 10.3, provided with full permission by the family, shows just how attractive a woman with Rett syndrome may be.

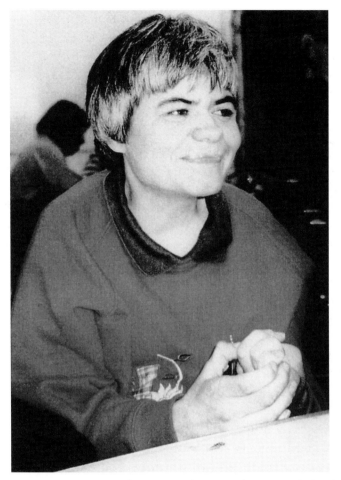

Figure 10.3. A woman of 36 years with Rett syndrome (supplied and published with the full agreement of her family).

Sexual preference, menstruation and fertility

People with Rett syndrome like to be with others, unless they are noisy or threatening, and many families confirm a preference for male company. It is important to appreciate that the Rett disorder does not appear to prevent conception and child birth, and young women will require protection from un-chosen pregnancy, in which the offspring carry a (dominant) 50% risk of inheriting the Rett disorder. Even with contraceptive measures in place the young woman is at risk from sexual abuse.

If a young woman is well nourished, menstrual periods usually begin normally and give no special problems. Early appearance of pubic hair has been reported but menstruation before 11 years is uncommon. Median onset of menstruation in the British survey was 13 years.

Periodic comprehensive clinical reassessment

A comprehensive assessment should be arranged at least once in every five years throughout adult life. This is true for everyone with significant disabilities and in Rett is particularly important since disabilities and skills are known to fluctuate and the consequences of neglect are severe and often irreversible. Such routine assessments should provide specialist advice on posture and mobility, nutrition, seizures, non-seizure vacant spells, communication, vision and hearing as well as general health. The individual and primary carer should participate and a clear explanation be provided for them of any new diagnoses or treatment. At each review a date should be set for the next assessment.

Management and medication in Rett disorder

At present symptomatic treatment is all that can be offered but this will change as it becomes understood exactly how the mutations on *MECP2* affect neuronal function. It is clear that the major neurotransmitters, serotonin, glutamate, GABA and acetylcholine are disturbed and since drugs are being developed to compensate for neurotransmitter defects there is hope of intervention at this level. Gene therapy may also become appropriate as techniques are refined.

Medication is justified for severe and persistent epilepsy and should be chosen according to the type of seizure. When there is doubt about the clinical diagnosis of epilepsy it is important to assess the breathing and autonomic abnormality which leads to non-epileptic vacant spells. Even in those with confirmed epilepsy, vacant spells are also common and it is important to avoid unnecessary medication on the assumption that they are epileptic.

For the breathing dysrhythmia no treatment is currently recommended except in the case of protracted inspiration, which in a few cases has been found to respond favourably to buspirone, a serotonin 1A receptor agonist (Kerr et al., 1998; Witt Engerstrom & Kerr, 1998). The rationale for this treatment depends on the fact that serotonin normally acts to end inspiration and has been found to be of value in treating protracted inspiration due to brain stem injury to the respiratory nuclei (Wilken et al., 1997). At present buspirone can be prescribed for children in the UK only on an individual basis. The recommended dose begins at 5 mg rising by 5 mg every 3 days to 25 mg daily. It should be stopped if it has not proved helpful in the first month, or if side-effects are troublesome. Experience in the British survey suggests that extreme agitation may be treated successfully in a few cases with the use of a serotonin reuptake inactivator.

Other medications have been suggested on the rationale that the brain may require more of the vitamins and other substances known to be involved in energy supply to neurones. These include the vitamins, serotonin, L-carnitine and gamma linolenic acid (evening primrose oil). However, there has been no convincing evidence that any of these makes a radical difference to the course of the disorder. The dangers of drug over-dosage and interactions should be borne in mind as well as the expense to the family and the discomfort to the individual herself of multiple medication.

There is a need for formal double blind trials to assess the effects and side-effects of potential therapies. A major difficulty remains the selection of appropriate outcome measures. As progress is made in understanding the whole sequence of events in the brain it seems likely that sufficiently sensitive, non-invasive methods will become available including functional brain imaging and EEG spectral analysis. Non-invasive autonomic monitoring is already of value when monitoring therapy directed to improve autonomic control and breathing rhythm.

Care provision for the adult with Rett disorder

Her natural home, or a small quiet house with consistent professional carers, seems to suit the woman with Rett disorder. The burden of physical care at home is such that additional professional support should be supplied and as parents grow older a small staffed house becomes the best arrangement. A successful transition can be well managed if respite care is provided from early in life on a regular basis, with parents and professional staff involved in both places to ensure that the needs, expectations and communications of the woman are understood and met. When a move takes place, continuing contact with the family should be encouraged. A suitable house for a person with Rett disorder will have a small number of residents (six or less) who are tempera-mentally compatible. If the woman is able to walk it must be made possible for her to do this safely. Staff require training in feeding techniques and non-verbal communication, and require the necessary aids to allow the individual to continue to be active – e.g. walking, exercising in water and enjoying such activities as supported riding. The move into new accommodation can be a crisis for the person with Rett disorder who appears to be very sensitive to change and to disturbance of close relationships. Crying spells and food refusal

Table 10.5. Essential components of interventions for adults with Rett disorder

- Clinical and genetic diagnosis
- Regular (active) exercise
- Encouragement of new skills
- Lifelong physiotherapy
- Nutritional supervision
- Protection from trauma
- Family genetic counselling
- Family respite provision
- Maintained contact with family
- Routine health surveillance and 5-yearly reassessment
  (including posture, movement, communication, nutrition, seizure, non-epileptic vacant spells, vision, hearing)

commonly follow such a move. This important life-event should therefore be carefully planned and phased if possible.

A summary of the essential components of interventions for adults with Rett disorder is given in Table 10.5.

Acknowledgements

I am pleased to acknowledge the professional support of my numerous colleagues, and the advice of Dr Robin Prescott, director of medical statistics at Edinburgh University. My post has been supported by the UK and National Rett Associations, Glasgow University, the Economic and Social Research Council and Quarriers Homes. I am indebted to the women and families who have faithfully shared information and so contributed to the advances in understanding of the Rett disorder.

REFERENCES

Amir, R.E., Van Den Veyver, I.B., Wan, M., Tran, C.Q., Franke, U. & Zoghbi, H. (1999). Rett syndrome is caused by mutations in X-linked MECP2, encoding methyl CpG binding protein 2. *Nature Genetics*, **23**: 185–8.

Armstrong, D.D. (1992). The neuropathology of the Rett syndrome. *Brain and Development*, **14**: 89–98.

Armstrong, D.D. (1995). The neuropathology of Rett syndrome – overview 1994. *Neuropediatrics*, **26**: 100–4.

Armstrong, D.D. (2001). The neuropathology of the Rett disorder. In *Rett Disorder and the*

Developing Brain, ed. A.M. Kerr & I. Witt Engerstrom, pp. 57–84. Oxford: Oxford University Press.

Asthana, J.C., Sinha, S., Haslam, J.S. & Kingston, H.M. (1990). Survey of adolescents with severe intellectual handicap. *Archives of Disease in Childhood,* **65**: 1133–6.

Badr, G.G., Witt Engerstrom, I. & Hagberg, B. (1987). Brain stem and spinal cord impairment in Rett syndrome: somatosensory and auditory evoked responses investigations. *Brain and Development,* **9**: 517–22.

Badr, G. & Hagne, I. (1993). Neurophysiological diagnosis. In *Rett Syndrome – Clinical and Biological Aspects,* ed. B. Hagberg, M. Anvret & J. Wahlstrom, pp. 72–9. London: MacKeith Press.

Belichenko, P. (2001). The morphological substrate for communication. In *Rett Disorder and the Developing Brain,* ed, A.M. Kerr & I. Witt Engerstrom, pp. 277–301. Oxford: Oxford University Press.

Bieber Nielsen, J., Friberg, L., Lou, H., Lassen, N.A. & Sam, I.L.K. (1990). Immature pattern of brain activity in Rett syndrome. *Archives of Neurology,* **47**: 982–6.

Blue, M.E., Naidu, S. & Johnson, M.V. (1999a). Development of amino acid receptors in the frontal cortex from girls with Rett syndrome. *Annals of Neurology,* **45**: 541–5.

Blue, M.E., Naidu, S. & Johnson, M.V. (1999b). Altered development of glutamate and GABA receptors in the basal ganglia of girls with Rett syndrome. *Experimental Neurology,* **156**: 345–52.

Budden, S.S. (1995). Management of Rett syndrome: a ten year experience. *Neuropediatrics,* **26**: 75–7.

Burford, B. & Trevarthen, C. (1997). Evoking communication in Rett syndrome: comparisons with conversations and games in mother–infant interaction. *European Child and Adolescent Psychiatry,* **S6**: 26–30.

Cheadle, J.P., Gill, H., Fleming, N. (2000). Long-read sequence analysis of the MECP2 gene in Rett syndrome patients: correlation of disease severity with mutation type and location. *Human Molecular Genetics,* **9**: 1119–29.

Cooper, R.A., Kerr, A.M. & Amos, P.M. (1998). Rett syndrome: critical examination of clinical features, serial e.e.g. and video-monitoring in understanding and management. *European Journal of Paediatric Neurology,* **2**: 127–35.

Diagnostic Criteria Working Group, Trevarthen, E., Moser, H.W. & Opitz, J.M. (1988). Diagnostic Criteria for Rett syndrome. *Annals of Neurology,* **23**: 425–8.

Ellaway, C.J., Sholler, G., Leonard, H. & Christodoulou, J. (1999). Prolonged QT interval in Rett syndrome. *Archives of Disease in Childhood,* **80**: 470–2.

Eyre, J.A., Kerr, A.M., Miller, S., O'Sullivan, M.C. & Ramesh, V. (1990). Neurophysiological observations on corticospinal projections to the upper limb in subjects with Rett syndrome. *Journal of Neurology, Neurosurery and Psychiatry,* **53**: 874–9.

Gauderer, M.W.L. (1991). Percutaneous endoscopic gastrosectomy: a 10 year experience with 220 children. *Journal of Paediatric Surgery,* **26**: 288–94.

Glasson, E.J., Thomson, M.R., Leonard, S., Rousham, E., Christodoulou, J., Ellaway, C. & Leonard, H. (1998). Diagnosis of Rett syndrome: can a radiograph help? *Developmental Medicine and Child Neurology,* **40**: 737–42.

Glaze, D.G., Frost, J.D., Miller, H.Y. & Percy, A.K. (1987). Rett's syndrome: correlation of electroencephalographic characteristics with clinical staging. *Archives of Neurology*, **44**: 1053–6.

Guideri, F., Acampa, M., Hayek, C., Zappella, N. & Di Perri, T. (1999). Reduced heart rate variability in patients affected with Rett syndrome. A possible explanation for sudden death. *Neuropediatrics*, **30**: 146–8.

Hagberg, B. & Hagberg, G. (1997). Rett syndrome: epidemiology and geographical variability. *European Child and Adolescent Psychiatry*, **6**: 5–7.

Hagne, I., Witt-Engerstrom, I. & Hagberg, B. (1989). EEG development in Rett syndrome. A study of 30 cases. *Electroencephalography and Clinical Neurophysiology*, **72**: 1–6.

Heinen, F. & Korinthenberg, R. (1996). Does transcranial magnetic stimulation allow early diagnosis of Rett syndrome? *Neuropediatrics*, **27**: 223–4.

Hendrich, B. (2000). Human genetics: Methylation moves into medicine. *Current Biology*, **10**: R60–R63.

Holm, V.A. (1986). Physical growth and development in patients with Rett syndrome. *American Journal of Medical Genetics*, **24**: 119–26.

Ishizaki, A. (1992). Electroencephalographical study of the Rett syndrome with special reference to the monorhythmic theta activities in adult patients. *Brain and Development*, **14**: S31–S36.

Julu, P.O.O. (1992). A linear scale for measuring vagal tone in man. *Journal of Autontomic Pharmacology*, **12**: 109–15.

Julu, P.O.O. (2001). The central autonomic disturbance in Rett. In *Rett Disorder and the Developing Brain*, ed A.M.Kerr & I. Witt Engerstrom, pp. 131–82. Oxford: Oxford University Press.

Julu, P.O.O., Kerr, A.M., Hansen, S., Apartopoulos, S.F. & Jamal, G.A. (1997). Functional evidence of brainstem immaturity in Rett syndrome. *European Child and Adolescent Psychiatry*, **6**: 47–54.

Julu, P.O.O., Kerr, A.M., Hansen, S., Apartopoulos, F. & Jamal, G. (1998). Cardio-respiratory instability in Rett Syndrome suggests medullary serotonergic dysfunction. Meeting report. Workshop on autonomic function in Rett syndrome Swedish Rett Centre, Froson, Sweden, May 1998, ed. I. Witt Engerstrom & A.M. Kerr, *Brain and Development*, **20**: 323–6.

Julu, P.O.O., Kerr, A.M., Apartopoulos, F., Al-Rawas, S., Witt Engerstrom, I., Engerstrom, L., Jamal, G.A. & Hansen, S. (2001). Characterisation of breathing and associated autonomic dysfunction, in the Rett disorder. *Archives of Disease in Childhood*, **85**: 29–37.

Kaufmann, W.E. (2001). Cortical development in Rett syndrome: molecular, neurochemical and anatomical aspects. In *Rett Disorder and the Developing Brain*, ed. A.M. Kerr & I. Witt Engerstrom, pp. 85–110. Oxford: Oxford University Press.

Kaufmann, W.E., Naidu, S. & Budden, S. (1995). Abnormal expression of microtubule protein 2 (MAP2) in neocortex in Rett Syndrome. *Neuropediatrics*, **26**: 109–13.

Kearney, D., Armstrong, D.L. & Glaze, D.G. (1997). The conduction system in Rett Syndrome. *European Child and Adolescent Psychiatry*, **6**(Suppl. 1): 78–9.

Kerr, A.M. (1992a). A review of the respiratory disorder in the Rett syndrome. *Brain and Development*, **14**(Suppl.): 43–5.

Kerr, A.M. (1992b). Rett syndrome British longitudinal study (1982–1990) and 1990 survey. *Mental Retardation and Medical Care, April 21–24 1991*, ed. J.J. Roosendaal, pp. 143–5. Den Haag: Uitgeverij Kerckbosch.

Kerr, A.M. (1995). Early clinical signs in the Rett disorder. *Neuropediatrics*, **26**: 67–71.

Kerr, A.M. (2000). Behaviour in the Rett disorder. In *Developmental Disability and Behaviour*, ed. C. Gillberg & G. O'Brien, pp. 43–55. Lavenham: McKeith Press.

Kerr, A.M., Armstrong, D.D., Prescott, R.J., Doyle, D. & Kearney, D.L. (1997). Analysis of deaths in the British Rett Survey. *European Child and Adolescent Psychiatry*, **6**: 71–4.

Kerr, A.M., Julu, P.O.O., Hansen, S. & Apartopoulos, F. (1998). Serotonin and breathing dysrhythmia in Rett syndrome. In *New Developments in Child Neurology*, ed. M.V. Perat, pp. 191–5. Bologna: Monduzzi Editore.

Kerr, A.M., Mitchell, J.M. & Robertson, P. (1995). Short fourth toes in Rett syndrome: a biological indicator. *Neuropediatics*, **26**: 72–4.

Kerr, A.M., Montague, J. & Stephenson, J.B.P. (1987). The hands, and the mind, pre- and post-regression in Rett syndrome. *Brain and Development*, **9**: 487–90.

Kerr, A.M., Robertson, P.E. & Mitchell, J. (1993). Rett syndrome and the 4th metatarsal. *Archives of Disease in Childhood*, **68**: 433.

Kerr, A.M., Southall, D., Amos, P., Cooper, R., Samuels, M., Mitchell, J. & Stephenson, J. (1990). Correlation of electroencephalogram, respiration and movement in the Rett syndrome. *Brain and Development*, **12**: 61–8.

Kerr, A.M. & Stephenson, J.P.B. (1985). Rett's syndrome in the west of Scotland. *British Medical Journal*, **291**: 579–82.

Kerr, A.M. & Stephenson, J.B.P. (1986). A study of the natural history of Rett syndrome in 23 girls. *American Journal of Medical Genetics*, **24**: 77–83.

Kerr, A.M. & Witt Engerstrom, I. (2001). The clinical background to the Rett disorder. In *Rett Disorder and the Developing Brain*, ed. A.M. Kerr & I. Witt Engerstrom, pp. 1–26. Oxford: Oxford University Press.

Kitt, C.A. & Wilcox, B.J. (1995). Preliminary evidence for neurodegenerative changes in the substantia nigra of Rett Syndrome. *Neuropediatrics*, **25**: 114–18.

Leonard, H. & Bower, C. (1998). Is the girl with Rett syndrome normal at birth? *Developmental Medicine and Child Neurology*, **40**: 115–21.

Leonard, H., Thomson, M.M., Lasson, E., Fyfe, S., Leonard, S., Ellaway, C., Christodoulou, J. & Bower, C. (1999a). Metacarpophaloangeal pattern profile and bone age in Rett syndrome: further radiological clues to the diagnosis. *American Journal of Medical Genetics*, **83**: 88–95.

Leonard, H., Thomson, M.R., Glasson, E.J., Fyfe, S., Leonard, S. & Bower, C. (1999b). A population-based approach to the investigation of osteopenia in Rett syndrome. *Developmental Medicine and Child Neurology*, **41**: 323–8.

Lindberg, B. (1991). *Dealing with Rett Syndrome – A Practical Guide for Parents, Teachers and Psychologists*. Toronto: Hogrefe & Huber.

Loder, R.T., Lee, C.L. & Stephens Richards, B. (1989). Orthopaedic aspects of Rett syndrome: a multicentre review. *Journal of Pediatric Orthopedics*, **9**: 557–62.

McArthur, A.J. & Budden, S.S. (1998). Sleep dysfunction in Rett syndrome: a trial of exogenous melatonin treatment. *Developmental Medicine and Child Neurology*, **40**: 186–92.

Merker, B. & Wallin, N.L. (2001). Musical responsiveness in the Rett disorder. In *Rett Disorder and the Developing Brain*, ed. A.M. Kerr & I. Witt Engerstrom, pp. 327–38. Oxford: Oxford University Press.

Mitchell, S.J. & Silver, R.A. (2000). Glutamate spillover suppresses inhibition by activating presynaptic mGluRs. *Nature*, **404**: 498–502.

Morton, R.E., Bonas, R., Minford, J., Kerr, A. & Ellis, R.E. (1997). Feeding ability in Rett syndrome *Developmental Medicine and Child Neurology*, **39**: 331–5.

Motil, K.J., Schultz, R., Brown, B., Glaze, D.G. & Percy, A.K. (1994). Altered energy balance may account for growth failure in Rett Syndrome. *Journal of Child Neurology*, **9**: 315–19.

Naidu, S. (1997). Rett syndrome: a disorder affecting early brain growth. *Annals of Neurology*, **42**: 3–10.

Naidu, S., Chattergee, S., Murphy, M., Uematsu, S., Philipart, M. & Moser H. (1987). Rett syndrome: new observations. *Brain and Development*, **9**: 525–8.

Nan, X., Campoy, F.J. & Bird, A. (1997). MeCP2 is a transcriptional repressor with abundant binding sites in genomic chromatin. *Cell*, **88**: 471–81.

Nomura, Y. & Segawa, M. (1990). Clinical features of the early stage of the Rett syndrome. *Brain and Development*, **12**: 16–19.

Nomura, Y. & Segawa, M. (1992). Motor symptoms of the Rett syndrome: abnormal muscle tone, posture, locomotion and stereotyped movement. *Brain and Development*, **14** (Suppl.): 21–8.

Nomura, Y., Segawa, M. & Hasegawa, M. (1984). Rett syndrome – clinical studies and pathophysiological considerations. *Brain and Development*, **6**: 475–86.

Pelson, R.O. & Budden, S. (1987). Auditory brain stem response findings in Rett syndrome. *Brain and Development*, **9**: 514–16.

Percy, A.K. (1992). Neurochemistry of the Rett syndrome. *Brain and Development*, **14**: S57–S62.

Philippart, M. (1990). The Rett syndrome in males. *Brain and Development*, **12**: 33–6.

Philippart, M. & Brown, W.J. (1984). Dystonia and lactic acidosis: new features of Rett's syndrome. *Annals of Neurology*, **16**: 387.

Rett, A. (1966). Uber ein eigenartiges hirnatrophisches Syndrome bei hyperammonamie im Kindsalter. *Wiener Medizinische Wochenschrift*, **116**: 723–6.

Rice, M.A. & Haas, R.H. (1998). The nutritional aspects of Rett syndrome. *Journal of Child Neurology*, **3** (Suppl.): S35–S42.

Roberts, A.P. & Connor, A.N. (1988). Orthopaedic Aspects of Rett's syndrome: short report. *Journal of Bone and Joint Surgery*, **70**: 2079–95.

Salomao Schwartzman, J., Zatz, M., Vasquez, L.dos R., Gomez, R. R., Koiffmann, C.P., Fridman, C. & Otto, P.G. (1999). Rett syndrome in a boy with 47, XXY karyotype. *American Journal of Human Genetics*, **64**: 1781–5.

Sansom, D., Krishnan, V.H.R., Corbett, J. & Kerr, A. (1993). Emotional and behavioural aspects of Rett syndrome. *Developmental Medicine and Child Neurology*, **35**: 340–5.

Saunders, K.J., McCulloch, D.L. & Kerr, A.M. (1995). Visual function in Rett syndrome. *Developmental Medicine and Child Neurology*, **37**: 496–504.

Schanen, C. & Franke, U. (1998). A severely affected male born into a Rett syndrome kindred supports X-linked inheritance and allows extension of the exclusion map. *American Journal of Human Genetics*, **63**: 267–9.

Schultz, R.J., Glaze, D.G., Motil, K.J., Armstrong, D.D., Del Junco, D.J. & Percy, A.K. (1993). The pattern of growth failure in Rett syndrome. *American Journal of Disease in Childhood*, **147**: 633–7.

Segawa, M. & Nomura, Y. (1990). The pathophysiology of the Rett syndrome from the standpoint of polysomnography. *Brain and Development*, **12**: 55–60.

Sekul, E.A., Moak, J.P., Schultz, R.J., Glaze, D.G., Dunn, J.K & Percy, A.K. (1994). Electrocardiographic findings in Rett syndrome: an explanation of sudden death. *Journal of Pediatrics*, **125**: 80–2.

Southall, D.P., Kerr, A.M., Tirosh, E., Amos, P., Lang, M.H. & Stephenson, J.B.P. (1988). Hyperventilation in the awake state: potentially treatable component of Rett syndrome. *Archives of Disease in Childhood*, **63**: 1039–48.

Stokland, E., Lidstrom, J. & Hagberg, B. (1993). Scoliosis in Rett syndrome. In *Rett Syndrome – Clinical and Biological Aspects*, ed. B. Hagberg, M. Anvret & J. Wahlstrom, pp. 72–9. London: MacKeith Press.

Trevarthen, C. & Burford, B. (2001). Early infant intelligence and Rett syndrome. In *Rett Disorder and the Developing Brain*, ed. A.M. Kerr & I. Witt Engerstrom, pp. 303–26. Oxford: Oxford University Press.

Uvebrant, P., Bjure, J., Sixt, R., Witt Engerstrom, I. & Hagberg, B. (1992). Regional cerebral blood flow: SPECT as a tool for localisation of brain dysfunction. In *Rett Syndrome – Clinical and Biological Aspects*, ed. B. Hagberg, pp. 80–5. London: MacKeith Press.

Vacca, M., Filippini, F., Budillon, A. et al. (2001). Mutation analysis of the MECP2 gene in British and Italian Rett syndrome females. *Human Molecular Genetics*, **11**: 648–55.

Von Tetzchner, S. (1997). Communication skills among females with Rett syndrome. *European Child and Adolescent Psychiatry*, **S6**: 33–7.

Wan, M., Lee, S.S.J.L., Zhang, X., Houwink-Manville, I., Song, H-R., Amir, R.E., Budden, S., Naidu, S., Pereira, J.L.P., Lo, I.F.M., Zoghbi, H.Y., Schanen, N.C. & Francke, U. (1999). Rett syndrome and beyond: recurrent spontaneous and familial MECP2 mutations at CpG hotspots. *American Journal of Human Genetics*, **65**: 1520–9.

Wenk, G.L. & Hauss-Wegrzyniak, B. (1999). Altered cholinergic function in the basal forebrain of girls with Rett syndrome. *Neuropediatrics*, **30**: 125–9.

Wilken, B., Lalley, P., Bischoff, A.M., Christen, H.J., Behnke, J., Hanefeld, F. & Richter, D.W. (1997). Treatment of apneustic respiratory disturbance with a serotonin-receptor agonist. *Journal of Pediatrics*, **130**: 89–94.

Witt Engerstrom, I. (1987). Rett syndrome: a retrospective pilot study of potential early predictive symptomatology. *Brain and Development*, **9**: 481–6.

Witt Engerstrom, I. (1992). Rett syndrome: the late infantile regression period – a retrospective analysis of 91 cases. *Acta Paediatrica Scandinavica*, **81**: 167–72.

Witt Engerstrom, I. & Forslund, M. (1992). Mother and daughter with Rett syndrome. *Developmental Medicine and Child Neurology*, **34**: 1022–3.

Witt Engerstrom, I. & Kerr, A.M. (1998). Workshop on autonomic function in Rett syndrome. Swedish Rett Centre, Froson, Sweden, May 1998. *Brain and Development*, **5**: 323–6.

Zappella, M. (1990). A double blind trial of bromocriptine in the Rett syndrome. *Brain and Development*, **12**: 148–50.

Zappella, M. (1997). The preserved speech variant of the Rett complex: a report of 8 cases. *European Child and Adolescent Psychiatry*, **6**: S23–S25.

11

Tuberous sclerosis

Petrus J. de Vries and Patrick F. Bolton

Introduction

Tuberous sclerosis is a complex genetic disorder, characterized by benign growths in many organs including the heart, kidney, skin and brain. It has a prevalence rate of around $1:10\,000$ (O'Callaghan, 1999). Brain abnormalities include cortical tubers (CT), subependymal nodules (SEN) and subependymal giant cell astrocytomas (SEGA). The two genes (TSC1 and TSC2) that cause tuberous sclerosis have been identified in recent years. The TSC1 gene is located on the long arm of chromosome 9 and the TSC2 gene on the short arm of chromosome 16 (The European Chromosome 16 Tuberous Sclerosis Consortium, 1993; van Slegtenhorst et al., 1997). About one-third of cases are familial and inherited in autosomal dominant fashion. The remaining two-thirds of cases are due to spontaneous mutations (Povey et al., 1994).

In addition to the spectrum of physical manifestations, tuberous sclerosis is associated with a wide range of behavioural, psychological and neuropsychiatric problems including epilepsy, learning disabilities, autism and multiple disruptive behaviours.

In a review of the genetics of learning disabilities, Simonoff and colleagues highlighted the need to expand knowledge of the effects of genetic abnormalities on the nervous system and on the biological mechanisms of learning disabilities (Simonoff, Bolton & Rutter, 1996). They emphasized the importance of considering not only the direct effects of genetic abnormalities on brain and behaviour, but also the indirect effects that stem from gene-environment correlations and interactions. This conceptual framework can be usefully applied to tuberous sclerosis when considering the ways in which associations with psychopathology arise. Firstly, the genotype of the disorder has now unequivocally been located to two genes, and knowledge of mutations, the molecular mechanisms and protein products is developing rapidly (Jones et al., 1997; Maheshwar et al., 1997; van Slegtenhorst et al., 1997; Soucek et al., 1998). Secondly, tuberous sclerosis presents with a number of brain manifestations

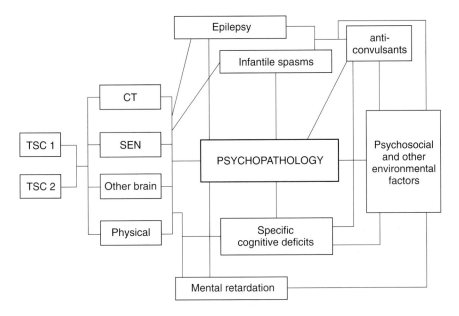

Figure 11.1. The diagram represents the spectrum of factors potentially involved in the psychopathologies of tuberous sclerosis (TSC). Outcome and development in TSC may be related to genotype–phenotype relations, brain or physical abnormalities, the epilepsies and epilepsy-control, general learning disabilities or specific cognitive deficits, as well as the important psychosocial and environmental domain. SEN, subependymal nodules; CT, cortical tubers.

that can be identified and accurately localized through neuro-imaging techniques (Griffiths & Martland, 1997). Thirdly, the disorder is associated with a spectrum of neuropsychiatric manifestations including epilepsy, learning disabilities, autism and disruptive behaviours (Harrison & Bolton, 1997; de Vries & Bolton, 1999; P. de Vries & P. Bolton, unpub. data).

Figure 11.1 is a diagrammatic representation of potential pathways to the behavioural, psychological and neuropsychiatric problems of tuberous sclerosis as broadly outlined above. Research in the field focuses on different aspects of these pathways in an attempt to elucidate important links and associations. Outcome and development in tuberous sclerosis will obviously be affected by some or even all of these factors. It is clear from the onset that tuberous sclerosis is a neurodevelopmental disorder with a wide range and complexity of manifestations. A particular challenge is posed by the variability of expression in the disorder. There is a huge range in the presence and severity of features between individuals, both in physical manifestations and in the psychopathologies. Even within the same family, one affected individual can be extremely mildly affected with only a few physical features, no epilepsy and normal intelligence, while a sibling may have severe learning disabilities, marked physical problems, autism and prominent disruptive behaviours. This variability of expression in the disorder can cause problems in diagnosis and in providing genetic counselling as to the nature and severity of the condition in future offspring.

For all the above reasons, predicting development and outcome and summarizing appropriate interventions is no mean feat. In this chapter we aim to delineate the most salient factors in the outcome of tuberous sclerosis. We begin with a brief historical overview of the tuberous sclerosis complex (TSC). We proceed to review current knowledge about the genotype, the physical phenotype and the behavioural phenotype. We then highlight the lifespan issues relating to outcome, before summarizing the key issues in assessment and intervention for children and adults with TSC.

Historical overview

A brief look at the historical 'development' of the disorder is extremely informative about changes in the understanding and conceptualization of the condition. Since the 1980s, historical changes have had a major impact on the prediction of outcome, and, as research provides further evidence of brain–behaviour associations in the disorder, our views of development and outcome will have to be revised.

Bourneville is the French physician historically associated with the term 'tuberous sclerosis' and with the first case report of the disorder. In his 1880 report, he described a 3-year-old girl admitted to la Salpetriere Hospital in Paris with seizures and learning disabilities (Bourneville, 1880). Her seizures reportedly started in infancy. At age 15 she had facial skin lesions, which Bourneville called 'acne rosacee' and attributed to the bromide that had been used to treat her epilepsy. He described frequent tonic–clonic seizures until her death as a consequence of the epilepsy. Post-mortem examination of the brain revealed multiple cortical tubers ('hypertrophic sclerosis of portions of the cerebral convolutions' resembling the cut surfaces of potatoes – hence the French term *sclerose tubereuse*) and multiple small nodules in the walls of the lateral ventricles in the region of the striatum (a glossary of this and other terms can be found at the end of the chapter).

One year later Bourneville and Brissaud reported pathological findings on a 4-year-old boy with a history of unilateral seizures starting at 4 months of age, delayed motor milestones (walked at age 2 years) and language delay (could only say one syllable at age 4 years). Again post-mortem revealed 'sclerotic hypertrophic convolutions' (Bourneville & Brissaud, 1881). The ventricles of the child's brain were normal in size but were covered with many small sclerotic tumours in the lateral walls. The heart was enlarged and hypertrophic. The kidneys showed yellow-white tumours.

TSC remained a pathological diagnosis made at post-mortem examination until 1908 when Henrich Vogt discovered the association between brain lesions and the facial angiofibromas (Vogt, 1908). Thus the triad of deficits classically associated with tuberous sclerosis (adenoma sebaceum, epilepsy and learning disabilities) was established and TSC became a clinical diagnosis.

Gradually other lesions associated with TSC were described. Van der Hoeve (1920) suggested that the eye and skin tumours of TSC were similar to those seen in neurofibromatosis and von Hippel-Lindau disease and hence developed the concept of the phakomatoses. He was also the first to introduce the idea that not all patients with TSC died at an early age, nor were they 'epileptic idiots', and recognized the variability of expression in TSC. Moreover, he suggested that hereditary (genetic) factors may cause the condition (van der Hoeve, 1932).

The term epiloia, a conjunction of *epi*lepsy and an*oia* (or mindlessness) was introduced by Sherlock (1911). Current terminology favours the use of tuberous sclerosis complex to reflect the multi-system nature of the disorder.

Critchley & Earl (1932) gave the first detailed description of the spectrum of abnormal behaviours associated with TSC, but clear evidence of behavioural, psychological and psychiatric problems over and above the presence of learning disabilities only began to emerge in the 1980s (Hunt, 1983). Gomez (1979) was the first to report the presence of a large group (37%) of TSC patients with normal intelligence. Both these findings represented major conceptual shifts from the earlier impressions that learning disabilities were inevitable in TSC and that behavioural problems were purely secondary to the learning disabilities. Interestingly, recent work suggests that even in individuals with TSC who have normal intelligence and no obvious behavioural problems, specific cognitive deficits may exist (de Vries & Bolton, 1999; Harrison et al., 1999; P. de Vries & P. Bolton, unpub. data; P. de Vries et al., unpub. data). Clearly, such findings may well influence our expectations of outcome.

The work of Gomez and colleagues at the Mayo Clinic led to the first set of diagnostic criteria, revised by Osborne (1988) to separate primary and secondary features. The current diagnostic criteria were adopted at a Consensus Conference on TSC held in Annapolis, Maryland (USA) in July 1998 (Roach, Gomez & Northrup, 1998). These criteria are set out in Table 11.1.

Table 11.1. Revised diagnostic criteria for tuberous sclerosis complex (TSC) (Roach et al., 1998)

Major features

1. Facial angiofibromata or forehead plaque
2. Non-traumatic ungual or peri-ungual fibroma
3. Hypomelanotic macules (more than three)
4. Shagreen patch (connective tissue nexus)
5. Multiple renal nodular hamartomas
6. Cortical tuber (a)
7. Subependymal nodule
8. Subependymal giant cell astrocytoma
9. Cardiac rhabdomyoma, single or multiple
10. Lymphangiomyomatosis (b)
11. Renal Angiomyolipoma (b)

Minor features

1. Multiple randomly distributed pits in dental enamel
2. Hamartomatous rectal polyps (c)
3. Bone cysts (d)
4. Cerebral white matter radial migration lines (ade)
5. Gingival fibromas
6. Non-retinal hamartoma (c)
7. Retinal achromic patch
8. 'Confetti' skin lesions
9. Multiple renal cysts (c)

Definite TSC: 2 major features *or* 1 major feature + 2 minor features

Probable TSC: 1 major + 1 minor feature

Possible TSC: 1 major feature *or* 2 + minor features

(a) When cerebral cortical dysplasia and cerebral white matter migration tracts occur together, they should be counted as one rather than two features of tuberous sclerosis

(b) When both lymphangiomyomatosis and renal angiomyolipomas are present, other features of tuberous sclerosis should be present before a definite diagnosis is made

(c) Histological confirmation is suggested

(d) Radiological confirmation is sufficient

(e) One panel member felt strongly that three or more radial migration lines should constitute a major sign

See Glossary for explanation of terms used.

The genotype

Tuberous sclerosis is caused by mutations in either the TSC1 or TSC2 gene (Povey et al., 1994). The TSC1 gene is located at 9q34 (van Slegtenhorst et al., 1997) and the TSC2 gene on 16p13.3 (The European Chromosome 16 Tuberous Sclerosis Consortium, 1993). TSC2 is a large and complex gene with 41 exons. It produces a 200 kDa protein product, termed tuberin (Maheshwar et al., 1997). TSC1 is a smaller gene with 21 coding exons and a protein product, hamartin, which has no known homology to other vertebrate proteins. Both genes have been shown to act as tumour suppressors (Soucek et al., 1997, 1998). Hamartin and tuberin have been shown to co-immunoprecipitate, interact in yeast two-hybrid system and co-localize on immunofluorescence, suggesting that the proteins participate in at least some common pathways (Jones et al., 1999). Even though tuberin has been suggested to act as a cytosolic 'chaperone' for hamartin (Nellist et al., 1999), more recent findings suggest that tuberin and hamartin may well contribute differentially to the central nervous system (CNS) pathology in TSC (Gutmann et al., 2000).

The mechanism proposed to account for the variability of expression in tuberous sclerosis is based on Knudson's 'two hit model' of tumour pathogenesis (Knudson, 1971). According to the model, affected individuals with TSC either inherit one abnormal copy of the TSC gene from a parent (in autosomal dominant fashion) or develop an abnormal copy as a spontaneous mutation. Phenotypic manifestations then occur only after a so-called 'second hit' event knocks out the remaining normal copy allele. This occurs during cell division and results in inactivation of the TSC gene and its protein product. In the normal embryological brain, for instance, progenitor cells in the ventricular zone proliferate and migrate towards the cortical plate to form the cortex. In tuberous sclerosis one of the TSC genes is already mutated, so when a second hit occurs randomly during cell division, there is gene knock-out and loss of expression of tuberin or hamartin. This causes dysregulation of the cell cycle and increases cell proliferation. The abnormally proliferating progeny migrates towards the cortex in a disorganized manner to form cortical tubers. Subependymal nodules are formed when abnormally differentiated and proliferated cells do not migrate from the periventricular zone.

No clear qualitative differences have been shown between the phenotypes of TSC1 and TSC2, with the exception of a contiguous gene deletion syndrome involving TSC2 and the polycystic kidney disease (PKD) gene on chromosome 16 (Jones et al., 1997). However, recent reports have suggested that TSC1 and TSC2 may differ in the severity of manifestation, with TSC1 being less likely to

Table 11.2. Physical manifestations of tuberous sclerosis complex (TSC)

1. Dermatological manifestations

Facial angiofibromata

Hypomelanotic macules

Shagreen patches (connective tissue nexus)

Ungual fibromas

Cafe-au-lait spots

Soft fibromas

2. Renal abnormalities

Angiomyolipomas

Renal cysts

3. Cardiac manifestations

Rhabdomyomata

4. Opthalmological manifestations

Retinal abnormalities: hamartomas, pigmentary and vascular changes

Non-retinal abnormalities: cataracts, field defects, nystagmus, vitreous haemorrhage and

papilloedema

5. Other visceral manifestations of TSC include:

Lungs: lymphangiomyomatosis

Spleen: hamartomas

Liver: hamartomas

Digestive tract: mouth, teeth, pancreas, rectum

Endocrine organs: thyroid, adrenal, pancreatic islets, gonads, hypothalamus, pituitary

Skeleton: bone cysts and other sclerotic lesions

give rise to learning disabilities (Jones et al., 1997; de Vries & Bolton, 2000). The findings can only be considered preliminary and there are various methodological issues concerned with the ascertainment of cases and the evaluation of intelligence and psychopathology that still need to be ironed out. However, if TSC1 and TSC2 are found to differ in severity, then genotype–phenotype research will have brought us one step closer to predicting outcome.

The physical phenotype

Tuberous sclerosis can give rise to lesions in virtually any part of the body. A glance at the diagnostic criteria (see Table 11.1) highlights the spectrum of features in the skin, eyes, heart, lungs and the CNS. Physical features are listed in Table 11.2. The third edition of *Tuberous Sclerosis Complex* contains detailed

Table 11.3. Central nervous system features of tuberous sclerosis

---

1. Radiologically/Histologically confirmed

Cortical tubers

Subependymal nodules

Subependymal Giant Cell Astrocytomas

Other white matter and migrational changes

2. Clinical manifestations

Learning disabilities

Epilepsies

Psychopathologies

---

sections on the spectrum of physical manifestations and interested readers may find this a useful reference (Gomez, 1999).

Central nervous system manifestations

Involvement of the CNS in tuberous sclerosis is the most consistent finding and is associated with the greatest number of clinical problems. Table 11.3 summarizes the CNS features of TSC.

Radiologically/histologically confirmed features

Brain size is normal in most cases of tuberous sclerosis although both microcephaly and megalencephaly are well recognized (Griffiths & Martland, 1997). The most typical findings in the cerebrum are cortical tubers – firm, hard cortical nodules within abnormally broad gyri. Magnetic resonance imaging (MRI) has been shown to be the best way to detect cortical tubers (Martin, et al., 1987; McMurdo et al., 1987; Nixon, et al., 1989; Iwasaki, et al., 1990). More recently, Maeda and colleagues (1995) found that fluid attenuated inversion recovery (FLAIR) MRI sequences were even better than the more traditionally-used T2 weighted MRI images. Cortical tubers may calcify, usually following degeneration of the central portion of the tuber. Once calcified, they can be identified using a computed tomography (CT) scan. Tubers are most frequently identified in the frontal, temporal, parietal and occipital lobes of the brain. Cerebellar tubers have been found in 8–15% of subjects with TSC (Griffiths & Martland, 1997). Histologically, tubers are composed of abnormal glial and neuronal cells and exhibit prominent demyelination.

Subependymal nodules (SEN) represent the other pathological hallmark of tuberous sclerosis (Griffiths & Martland, 1997), and tend to be found in the walls of the lateral and third ventricles of the brain and less frequently in the fourth ventricle or aqueduct. SENs are firm and, when calcified, stone hard. They occur most frequently in the striato-thalamic groove between the caudate nucleus and thalamus in the region of the foramen of Monro (a special opening in the ventricular system of the brain, that allows the fluid surrounding the brain to circulate freely). In spite of their close proximity to the foramen of Monro, they do not usually lead to obstruction of the flow of cerebrospinal fluid (CSF). CT scanning is the traditional technique to detect calcified SENs. Nodules consist of swollen glial cells, mostly giant and multinucleated astrocytes with a peripheral ependymal cover.

In 5–10% of cases SENs develop into subependymal giant cell astrocytomas (SEGAs) (Harrison & Bolton, 1997). Histological distinction between SEN and SEGA can be very difficult (Harding, 1992) and radiological diagnosis can also be complicated (Griffiths & Martland, 1997). When a SEGA does grow, it can obstruct the foramen of Monro and lead to raised intracranial pressure. This produces nausea, vomiting, sensitivity to bright light and, if severe and untreated, coma and death. SEGAs may present more subtly with onset of epilepsy, change in seizure-control or with changes in behaviour or deterioration of scholastic performance.

Clinical CNS manifestations
Learning disabilities
In the earliest reports of tuberous sclerosis, learning disabilities were considered to be almost invariably present (Critchley & Earl, 1932). However, population-based studies have shown that the true frequency of learning disabilities lies somewhere between 38% and 80% (Webb, Fryer & Osborne, 1991; Shepherd & Stephenson, 1992; Gillberg, Gillberg & Ahlsen, 1994). Harrison & Bolton (1997) point out that studies did not undertake standardized assessment of IQ and adopted different ascertainment strategies. The much reduced rate (38%) of learning disabilities in the secondarily ascertained sample (i.e. families where one member had been diagnosed, a subsequent child born, screened and then diagnosed with TSC), suggested that ascertainment in the population was truncated. However, there is still uncertainty about the true rate of learning disabilities and well-replicated figures are needed to aid in genetic counselling and planning of services. Uncertainty also remains about the nature of the IQ distribution in TSC, despite the fact that clarification of this issue would help to narrow down the focus on the mechanisms giving rise to learning disabilities. Harrison & Bolton (1997) pointed out that the limited available evidence suggested a bimodal distribution of IQ with individuals either normal or severely handicapped. Preliminary findings from more recent epidemiological

surveys seem to support this suggestion (Bolton et al., 2000; Needham et al., 2000). The early suggestion that males are at greater risk of learning disabilities (Clarke, Cook & Osborne, 1996; Webb, Fryer & Osborne, 1996) has not been substantiated by more recent research (Needham et al., 2000). In our survey of 510 UK families, a bimodal IQ distribution was reported but no sex difference was found (P. de Vries & P. Bolton, unpub. data).

There is a paucity of information about the overall neuropsychological profile of people with tuberous sclerosis and little knowledge about the rate of specific cognitive impairments in TSC individuals of normal intelligence. Initial findings suggested that adults with IQs above 70 may be prone to having specific cognitive impairments (Harrison et al., 1999). These early suggestions were confirmed in a neuropsychological case-control study (P. de Vries et al., unpub. data). Computerized tasks selected for differential sensitivity to fronto-striatal functioning revealed significant impairment in spatial working memory and attentional set-shifting tasks. Taken together, the findings suggested that adults with TSC may have significant difficulty with learning generalization and attentional control, in spite of the fact that they have no general intellectual impairment. In an epidemiologically-derived sample of 20 TSC children with normal or near-normal intelligence, de Vries & Bolton (1999) reported significant deficits in selective attention, sustained attention and attentional control independent of age, IQ and sex. Children had relative strengths in visual selective attention tasks, but performed particularly poorly on auditory sustained attention and dual tasks. Further work is needed to explore specific cognitive strengths and deficits in children and adults with TSC, and the link with behaviour and performance in daily life.

Epilepsy

Reported rates of epilepsy vary from 90% in a postal survey of members of the Tuberous Sclerosis Association (Hunt, 1993) to 62% in a sample of secondarily ascertained children with TSC (Webb et al., 1991). The full range of epilepsies is found, often in complex combinations, and seizures are often difficult to treat. Gomez (1999) suggests that approximately 84% of all individuals with TSC will have epileptic seizures at some point in their lives, with the majority developing seizures by 5 years of age.

Behavioural, psychological and psychiatric problems

It is now generally accepted that TSC is associated with a spectrum of behavioural, psychological and psychiatric problems. Critchley & Earl (1932) made some clear observations of autism-like and other abnormal behaviours in their early review of TSC. Moolten (1942) reported the renal abnormalities and adenoma sebaceum in a 15-year-old girl who 'had always been nervous, shy and sensitive'. In the first edition of *Tuberous Sclerosis*, Gomez (1979) reported cases of childhood schizophrenia, autism and adult dementia in association with TSC. However, it was not until the 1980s that systematic collection of behavioural data on individuals with TSC started to confirm the presence of a wide range of psychopathologies over and above the rates expected due to epilepsy or learning disabilities (Hunt, 1983). Of all the complexities of the disorder, parents were most often concerned about their child's behaviour and communication. In her report of 58 children, Hunt listed hyperactivity (in 38%), screaming (24%), destructiveness (16%), temper tantrums (16%), aggressiveness (16%), sleeplessness (12%), self-mutilation (12%), masturbation (3%) and expulsion from school (5%). Only 41% of the children were reported not to have any behavioural problems.

Hunt & Dennis (1987) followed with a more detailed assessment of 90 individuals, also gathered through the UK Tuberous Sclerosis Association. The study reported a markedly higher prevalence rate of autism and hyperkinetic disorder in the TSC children with infantile spasms compared with the rates reported in a Finnish study of children with infantile spasms without TSC (Riikonen & Amnell, 1981). The rate of psychiatric diagnoses in the TSC group was also very high in comparison to other children with similar levels of learning disabilities (Wing & Gould, 1979).

Two population-based studies reported high rates of autism (24–61%) and more broadly defined autism spectrum disorders (43–86%) (Hunt & Shepherd, 1993; Gillberg et al., 1994). Indirectly this suggested TSC as a medical 'cause' in 5–9% of children diagnosed with infantile autism. These studies highlighted the importance of considering a diagnosis of tuberous sclerosis in a child who presents with the triad of learning disabilities, epilepsy and autism.

Neither of the population-based studies used specialized instruments for the diagnosis of developmental disorders, attention deficit disorders or for the measurement of general intelligence. This might explain the difference between the reported rates of disorder in the two studies. Preliminary results from ongoing work in a population-based TSC sample undertaken by our research group using standardized assessment procedures have broadly confirmed a prevalence of 50% autism spectrum disorders with 25% core autism. There appears to be substantial overlap between attention deficit symptoms/disruptive behaviours and pervasive developmental disorder (Hunt & Shepherd, 1993; Gillberg et al., 1994; P. de Vries & P. Bolton, unpub. data).

A number of case reports has described other psychiatric problems in association with TSC, including mania (Khanna & Borde, 1989), recurrent depressed mood and command auditory hallucinations (Harvey, Mahr & Balon, 1995), hebephrenic schizophrenia (Herkert, Wald & Romero, 1972), Capgras syndrome (Holschneider & Szuba, 1992) and specific phobias (Smalley, McCracken & Tanguay, 1995). In the study of an extended kindred, Smalley, Burger & Smith (1994) reported very high rates of anxiety disorders (59%) and mood disorders (35%) in the family members affected with TSC in comparison to the unaffected members ($P = 0.016$ for anxiety and $P = 0.009$ for any psychiatric disorder). She suggested that a specific behavioural phenotype may be found in TSC gene carriers (TSC2 in her study) without learning disabilities, which could include anxiety disorders and perhaps autism/pervasive developmental disorders (PDD). She argued that, in the absence of a 'second hit' of a TSC2 gene, abnormal cell migration and differentiation may occur, not to form tubers and SENs, but sufficient to lead to changes in brain architecture that could underlie the behavioural, cognitive and psychiatric sequelae of the condition.

Smalley (1998) also reviewed the association between tuberous sclerosis and autism and suggested that there may be three main hypotheses to explain the observed link. Firstly, disruption of the TSC gene function in early stages of neurogenesis may lead to abnormal brain development in regions involved in autism or PDD; secondly, that a susceptibility gene for autism is in linkage disequilibrium with a TSC gene; and thirdly, that secondary effects of the TSC gene, such as seizures, learning disabilities or cortical tubers, result in brain abnormalities leading to autism or PDD. Bolton & Griffiths (1997) found evidence for a link between temporal lobe tubers and PDD. Learning disabilities and epilepsy do seem to be strongly associated with autism spectrum disorders in TSC, but neither are necessary nor sufficient for the development of the autism spectrum behaviours (P. de Vries & P. Bolton, unpub. data). Progress in the molecular genetics of TSC may shed light on these competing hypotheses.

Because of the relative dearth of information about behavioural, psychological and psychiatric problems in tuberous sclerosis, we recently conducted a survey of 510 UK families to enquire about the lifetime prevalence of such problems (P. de Vries & P. Bolton, unpub. data). Table 11.4 summarizes the spectrum of problems reported by parents and carers in children and adults with TSC in this study. Results should be regarded as a 'birds-eye view' of the range of difficulties associated with TSC. Further research will provide more detailed information about outcome and add to the understanding of genetic and neural underpinnings of behavioural, psychological and neuropsychiatric problems.

Table 11.4. Psychopathologies associated with the tuberous sclerosis complex

The rates of behavioural, psychological and psychiatric problems in 510 children and adults with tuberous sclerosis. The table represents the overall frequency of features and is adapted from R. de Vries & P. Bolton, unpub. data

Psychopathologies	Overall frequency (%)
Learning disabilities	63
Severe/profound	36
Moderate	16
Mild	11
None	37
Pervasive developmental disorders	
Autism spectrum disorders	46
Poor eye contact	44
Repetitive and ritualized behaviour	54
Disruptive behaviours and attention deficit symptoms	
Overactivity	50
Restlessness	52
Impulsive behaviour	48
Aggressive outbursts	56
Temper tantrums	49
Self injury	36
Mood and emotional symptoms	
Anxiety	45
Depressed mood	29
Extreme shyness	18
Specific phobias	26
Sleep problems	54
Language (in subjects over 5 years)	
No communicative language	39
Normal language with no delay	28

TSC across the lifespan

Information about the natural history of the physical and behavioural manifestations of tuberous sclerosis is limited. Although Lishman (1998) suggests that the course is virtually inevitably progressive when the disease is declared in childhood, this view has not been confirmed. Because of the enormous variability of expression and variety of neurological manifestations, there is no typical developmental course in TSC. However, it does appear that course and outcome are in part related to the severity of the disease, as judged by the number of benign growths (especially in the brain), the age of presentation, additional physical problems and the presence and type of seizure disorder.

Infancy and the pre-school period

Cardiac abnormalities usually present in the antenatal or postnatal period with rhabdomyomas identified on antenatal ultrasound or as neonatal arrhythmias (O'Callaghan et al., 1998). These may remit completely in the first years of life. Most children with TSC first present with seizures in the early years (Gomez, 1999). The most frequent types are partial seizures (sometimes with secondary generalization) and infantile spasms, which occur in up to two-thirds of children (Hunt, 1993). Infantile spasms commonly start 2 months after birth, with a peak onset between 4 and 6 months. Spasms may be associated with arrest of psychomotor development and a hypsarrhythmic EEG pattern, to produce the typical picture of West syndrome (Gastaut et al., 1965). Infantile spasms can however also be quite atypical in form (Gomez, 1999). It is common for infants with TSC to present with a mix of infantile spasms and partial seizures.

In the second year of life, the seizures may evolve into a Lennox–Gastaut syndrome, associated with difficult to control mixed seizures and progressive intellectual deterioration. This is, however, not a frequent occurrence in tuberous sclerosis. During the childhood years complex partial seizures (with or without secondary generalization) are the most common seizure type. The treatment of seizures in TSC can be very challenging. At the onset, seizures may be difficult to recognize and classify, so the choice of treatment is not always straightforward. In addition, there are often several types of seizures present and the clinical presentation can change over time. Furthermore, it is common for the seizures to be partially resistant or refractory to anti-epileptic drugs. As a result, children may often require several different types of medication in order to gain some control of the fits, with the possibility of adverse side-effects.

The other physical feature usually evident in the early years is the presence of ash-leaf macules (white patches on the skin). The combination of these depigmented skin patches and epilepsy often leads clinicians to suspect TSC and the diagnosis may then be confirmed by identifying TSC abnormalities on brain scan. The rate of learning disabilities in children presenting very early in development with severe epilepsy is very high. This has led to the view that the epilepsy may be the cause of the intellectual impairment and, therefore, that prompt effective treatment may really make a difference to long-term outcome. This, however, is not a universal view and others have argued that the strong link between epilepsy and learning disabilities seen in TSC results from the underlying brain abnormalities. At present there is no clear answer as to which of these views is correct. There is evidence to suggest, for example, that children who present with infantile spasms due to an unknown cause can develop normally (Gaily et al., 1999; Rantala & Putkonen, 1999). These findings would suggest that the spasms themselves are not necessarily damaging, although there is some, albeit very limited, evidence to suggest that outcome may be improved by effective treatment of uncontrolled epilepsy (Holmes et al., 1999; Jambaque et al., 2000). Of course, these two views are not mutually exclusive and it may turn out that cognitive and intellectual development are influenced by both the underlying structural abnormalities as well as the ensuing epilepsy.

Other developmental and psychiatric problems may be apparent as early as 2 or 3 years of age. Parents and health visitors often become concerned about absent or delayed language and about overactive and restless behaviours, which can occur whether or not seizures are well controlled. The first signs of autism spectrum disorders may also emerge during this period, with difficulties in social interaction and communication becoming more pronounced as the child is increasingly exposed to more complex social situations. The mechanisms that give rise to communication problems, autism and hyperactivity are poorly understood and similar considerations concerning the possible role of the brain abnormalities and epilepsy apply. Current evidence suggests that the likelihood of developing an autism spectrum disorder is increased if cortical tubers are located in the temporal lobes, or if the child presents with infantile spasms. As yet, the detail concerning the way in which these factors create an increased risk for autism spectrum disorders is not known (Bolton & Griffiths, 1997; Gutierrez, Smalley & Tanguay, 1998). Although the majority of the children who develop an autism spectrum disorder also has learning disabilities, this is not an inevitable finding (Gillberg et al., 1994; P. de Vries & P. Bolton, unpub. data).

The school years

Special schooling may be required for the more severely disabled children and various levels of learning support may be necessary for others. About a third of children with TSC have normal intelligence and are able to attend mainstream schools and lead independent lives. However, even in this group, behavioural problems and specific learning problems may occur. Autism spectrum disorders, disruptive behaviours and attention deficit problems, language delay and sleep problems have been reported both in clinic and research settings (P. de Vries & P. Bolton, unpub. data). It is therefore essential to be aware of the risks of developmental disorders even in children with normal intellectual levels. The current evidence indicates that attention deficits and hyperactivity may be one of the main problems in this more able group (de Vries & Bolton, 1999). As yet, the extent to which these difficulties are associated with tuber location (e.g. in the frontal lobes) or derive from the epilepsy is undetermined.

During the school years multiple problems may manifest. Specific scholastic difficulties may be identified, and educational progress may be hampered by more general factors such as epilepsy, hospitalization, attentional problems and global or pervasive developmental problems not yet diagnosed at the time. No systematic study has investigated the spectrum of scholastic difficulties in children with TSC, but clinical reports cover a wide range from reading, writing, arithmetic difficulties and marked receptive and/or expressive language problems.

There have been reports of specific phobias in children, but the incidence is not necessarily greater than in the general population (Smalley et al., 1995). Emotional problems such as depressed mood and anxiety have also been reported, but very limited information is available in children (Smalley, Burger & Smith, 1994).

In addition to the neurodevelopmental sequelae, children with TSC have associated physical stigmata. The facial rash and epilepsy can lead to problems with self-perception and confidence. Skin and other physical manifestations may progress with time. White patches are usually visible from birth, while shagreen patches tend to develop in early childhood. Facial angiofibromas may not be very pronounced in childhood or be avascular and only identified on very close inspection. Ungual fibromas may not develop until adulthood (Gomez, 1999). SEGAs are most likely to present in childhood and adolescence, at a median age of 9 years (Griffiths & Martland, 1997). Children typically present with signs of raised intracranial pressure including vomiting, photophobia, headaches and papilloedema. A sudden change in seizure-control or deterioration in scholastic skills or behaviour should also raise the suspicion of a SEGA.

Adolescence

The transition from childhood to adulthood is associated with enormous change in the psychological, sexual and social self of all adolescents. The child with tuberous sclerosis enters this phase with a wide range of physical and behavioural strengths and weaknesses. It is not difficult to imagine how, during the psychological phase of working towards an integrated image of the self, physical and neuropsychiatric problems can lead to difficulties. For children with severe and profound learning difficulties, progress through adolescence may not be at the same level of psychological sophistication as for the mildly affected teenagers, but sexual maturation, emotional development and the hormonal changes of puberty affect all. For these reasons, adolescence can be a particularly challenging stage for individuals with tuberous sclerosis and their families.

Facial angiofibromas may not be visible until middle childhood but often become more prominent during adolescence. In the adolescent patient they may be mistaken for acne vulgaris, a frequent feature of normal adolescence. Understandably, adolescents may become uncomfortable with their facial rash and seek cosmetic treatment such as laser therapy or other dermatological procedures (Gomez, 1999).

Renal abnormalities have a peak incidence around puberty (Roach et al., 1999). Presenting symptoms include haematuria, flank pain, hypertension and renal failure. These may require hospitalization, surgery, and/or dialysis, all of which can affect behaviour, school attendance and attainment, and peer relationships.

There are at least 11 case reports of precocious puberty in tuberous sclerosis (Zimmerman, 1999). This may be due to gonadal activation by the pituitary gland or to gonadal activation of gonadotropin-independent mechanisms. Other endocrinological abnormalities include growth hormone excess or deficiency. Age of maturation can affect adolescents' satisfaction with their appearance and body image. Early maturing boys tend to feel secure about their appearance during early to middle adolescence, but the later maturing boys often end up as the healthiest group in later adolescence (Petersen, 1989). In contrast, early maturing girls experience more depressed mood, anxiety and have lower self-esteem (Atkinson et al., 1996). For adolescents with learning disabilities and their families, the emergence of sexual maturity leads to new challenges in dealing with sexual urges, masturbation and decision-making about sexual activity. More able individuals become increasingly aware of the impact of the condition on their lives and future. The realization that they have a potentially life threatening condition and an increased risk of having affected children of their own, may prove extremely demoralizing. Not surprisingly, depression or emotional disturbances and reckless behaviour may develop as a reaction.

During adolescence, those with autism spectrum problems may become more marginalized from peers, and parents/carers sometimes report increased ritualistic behaviours at this time. Disruptive behaviours such as aggressive outbursts may become more unacceptable as a child grows older and can lead to further difficulties at home, in school and with peers.

Studies also report changes in seizure control, tic disorder and pica, but there are currently no systematic research data to indicate specific patterns of change among adolescents with tuberous sclerosis.

Adulthood

The normal adult goals of finding employment, living independently and making close and long-term relationships may represent real hurdles for many individuals with tuberous sclerosis. Adults with moderate to profound learning difficulties will obviously not be able to achieve many of these and instead will require support in daily living and work. Those with milder learning problems may have social communication difficulties or other specific difficulties necessitating support or supervision of various degrees.

Research data about the lifespan progress and outcome in TSC are very limited. In a follow-up of 23 people from age 5 years to adulthood, Hunt (1998) reported that there was little change in the abilities of those with severe learning disabilities. Epilepsy control did not change much, with overall control not markedly affected by the introduction of the newer generation of anti-epilepsy drugs. Symptoms of autism and hyperactivity decreased, but rates of aggression and self-harm remained unchanged. Importantly Hunt found no evidence of an 'inevitable decline' in functioning, as suggested in earlier reports (Bourneville, 1880; Critchley & Earl, 1932; Lishman, 1998).

With regards to physical problems, ungual fibromas are more prevalent in adults, and lung complications (lymphangiomiomatosis, pneumothorax, respiratory failure) tend to present in middle adulthood in a small proportion of cases. Renal angiomyolipomas can cause microscopic or macroscopic haematuria, requiring medical intervention. Late-onset seizures starting in adulthood have also been reported (Gomez, 1999).

Mood and emotional disorders become more prominent in adults and Smalley et al. (1994) suggested rates of 35% for depression and 59% for anxiety disorders in adults with TSC. Future research needs to address the role of the brain abnormalities, seizures, neurochemical factors and the obvious psychosocial components when trying to elucidate the underlying mechanisms.

Tuberous sclerosis has a major impact on the lives of all family members. The diagnosis of TSC can be made at any point in an individual's life. It may take a long time for the diagnosis of this rare disorder to be made or confidently confirmed. After diagnosis it may be difficult to predict what to expect in terms of outcome, due to the extreme variability and the large number of factors at play in the disorder. Understandably parents, siblings and other carers experience anger, guilt, frustration and severe anxiety at the diagnosis of the disorder (Whittemore, 1999). Parents may have to decide whether to attempt further pregnancies and risk having another child with TSC. An affected adult will have a 50% chance of having a child with tuberous sclerosis, as it is autosomal dominantly inherited. A family with a child where tuberous sclerosis is shown to have occurred due to a spontaneous mutation will have a 1–2% risk of having further children with TSC. Fortunately, prenatal diagnosis is now becoming available and will increasingly become helpful at this stage of decision-making. Caring for a child or adult with a chronic disorder or disability can lead to major changes in the lives of families. A parent may have to stop working, siblings may feel (or be) left out in the effort to take care of a child with major developmental problems, and lives may be severely disrupted by the child's pronounced routines, rituals, sleep problems or recurrent seizures.

Interventions for children and adults with TSC

Tuberous sclerosis is undoubtedly a disorder with a major potential impact on individuals and families alike, and the complex interplay of physical, behavioural and environmental factors affects outcome. It is important for health care professionals to understand the huge challenge that families and affected individuals face and to provide accurate information in a timely and supportive way.

As yet there are no specific interventions for tuberous sclerosis. The wide range of problems and large variation between people with TSC mean that an individualized treatment plan is mandatory for every person with the disorder. Research and clinical reports suggest a number of areas where health and social care workers should be alert to potential problems. These include learning difficulties, pervasive developmental disorders, hyperactivity, attention deficits, language, mood and emotional problems. Origins of these problems have to be considered in the context of the spectrum of potential pathways to the psychopathologies, as set out in Figure 11.1.

It is prudent to adopt a hierarchical approach to evaluating the relevance of each potential factor in causing psychiatric and behavioural disturbances. Physical factors are considered first: seizure-control, the risk of a giant cell astrocytoma, the effect of anti-epileptic medication (too much or too little) and renal complications. Next, consider the possible role of an associated developmental disorder or specific cognitive deficits. Finally, assess the responses of the individual, family, school and community and its consequences. Families and individuals are likely to require support in the process of seeking advice, diagnosis and decision-making about appropriate educational, residential or psychological/psychiatric treatment.

In the UK, US and a number of other countries worldwide, parent/carer associations are extremely active in supporting families in negotiating with health, social and educational services. Organizations such as the Tuberous Sclerosis Association (UK) or the Tuberous Sclerosis Alliance (US) support research in TSC and organize regular educational events for parents, carers, professionals and affected individuals. In the UK, a number of specialist TSC clinics have been set up with the financial support of the Tuberous Sclerosis Association. In addition, these organizations have a strong network of family care and support, aiming for an individual care approach for their members. In the UK, special groups for mildly affected adults with TSC and a sibling support group were recently launched. Tuberous Sclerosis International (TSI) was founded in 1986 as a world organization of national tuberous sclerosis organizations. The TSI website may be a useful initial source of contact for interested professionals, parents or carers (http://www.stsn.nl/tsi/tsi.htm). This extremely positive and pro-active approach to TSC does mean that professionals will often encounter tuberous sclerosis families with knowledge far superior to their own about the disorder. Health and social care professionals may need to join the family and individual with TSC in learning about tuberous sclerosis and its management.

The use of medication

The majority of children and adults with TSC will be prescribed anti-epilepsy medication at some stage during their lives. As previously noted, seizure control can be very difficult and many patients benefit from referral to a specialist epilepsy clinic. Vigabatrin was reported to be particularly effective for the treatment of infantile spasms in TSC, but recent reports of visual field defects have led to concerns and changes in prescription guidelines (Wilton, Stephens & Mann, 1999). Vigabatrin should now only be prescribed by epilepsy specialists and only used as a monotherapy for infantile spasms. For other epilepsies, monotherapy with an anti-epilepsy drug is preferable to combination therapy, particularly in view of increased adverse cognitive effects, such as memory impairment and reduced attentional abilities. However, it is often necessary to use several different drugs to control seizures. Changes in seizure-control, especially in middle childhood, should always alert the clinician to consider the likelihood of a SEGA.

In children with autism spectrum disorders there are reports of benefits from selective serotonin reuptake inhibitors (SSRIs) to reduce ritualistic, routinized and obsessive–compulsive types of behaviour, but the potential helpfulness needs to be considered against likely effects on seizure control and renal function. Stimulant medication (e.g. methylphenidate) has been used in children with disruptive behaviours and attention deficits with clear behavioural improvement. However, methylphenidate may have a risk of reducing seizure threshold and clinicians may prefer dexamphetamine in special cases. There are no studies to support either the benefits or adverse effects of psychotropic medication in TSC.

Mood disorders may benefit from treatment by appropriate antidepressant drugs in conjunction with psychological and physical support for those with and without learning disabilities.

Special investigations

Consensus guidelines for diagnostic assessment were published in 1999 (Roach et al., 1999). The guidelines distinguish between initial diagnosis and further evaluation of known patients. At the time of diagnosis, special investigations are performed to confirm the clinical diagnosis, to evaluate presenting symptoms such as epilepsy and to establish a baseline assessment of areas in which problems may develop. Special investigations recommended at diagnosis include a brain scan (preferably using MRI), EEG for those with seizures, renal ultrasound, echocardiography, eye examination and neurodevelopmental assessment. The consensus panel recommended detailed age-appropriate screening for behavioural and neurodevelopmental function at the time of diagnosis. Newly diagnosed adolescents and adults with no overt indication of social or cognitive difficulties may not require formal assessment, but if the presence of subtle cognitive deficits is robustly confirmed in the literature, this consensus recommendation may have to be reconsidered.

DNA testing for the TSC1 or TSC2 gene is not currently routinely available and further genotype–phenotype studies are needed to investigate the possible link between specific mutations and particular complications or deficits. At present unaffected family members can be tested to establish whether they carry a TSC mutation if the mutation in their affected family member has been identified. This will predict the likelihood of having a child with TSC (50% if mutation is present; 2% if mutation is not present). Genetic testing is currently of no value in predicting the likely outcome in terms of the severity of physical features, learning difficulties or other neurodevelopmental problems. If genotype–phenotype research does find robust correlations, DNA testing may

Table 11.5. Principal recommendations for clinicians working with tuberous sclerosis complex (TSC)

- Maintain a broad approach where physical, medication and behavioural factors are hierarchically considered for management and assessing outcome. Remember that TSC has no typical pattern of development and outcome
- Carefully examine for learning difficulties, subtle forms of epilepsy, autism spectrum disorders, disruptive behaviours and language disorders, especially in children
- In adults look out for mood and emotional disorders
- Remember that individuals with normal intelligence have a high risk of specific cognitive and behavioural problems
- Be aware that TSC is a severe and potentially life-threatening condition that can place a great demand on all family members

---

acquire a predictive role, associated with a new set of ethical dilemmas and decision-making.

Conclusions

Although in some senses tuberous sclerosis is a relatively simple genetic condition, it is nevertheless associated with an extraordinarily complex mix of physical, psychological and behavioural manifestations. Substantial advances have been made in mapping out the main features of the condition, but much remains to be done to determine the origins of many of the problems. Future research will have to focus in particular on the interplay between the brain abnormalities, epilepsy and correlated environmental influences in shaping intellectual, cognitive and behavioural development. Perhaps the most obvious gap in knowledge and the one most likely to help clarify some of the crucial issues is our understanding of the natural history of the condition. Current information of development and outcome in TSC is based entirely on cross-sectional data, and the gap will only really be filled by careful prospective longitudinal studies of representative populations.

See Table 11.5 for a summary of the principal recommendations for clinicians working with tuberous sclerosis.

Glossary

Ashleaf macules (hypomelanotic macules) White patches, typically leaf-shaped, occur most commonly over the trunk and buttocks. May be better visible under a Woods light, which accentuates the white patch.

Café-au-lait Oval or round areas of skin the colour of coffee with milk. They may be seen in tuberous sclerosis, neurofibromatosis and normal individuals.

Facial angiofibroma (Adenoma Sebaceum) Red to pink bilateral symmetrical rash over the cheeks in a butterfly pattern, sparing the upper lip. Very typical skin sign in over 80% of people with tuberous sclerosis complex.

Foramen of Monro The interventricular foramina of Monro are the openings through which cerebrospinal fluid flow from the lateral ventricles of the brain to the third ventricle.

Hamartomas Benign growths due to cells that have multiplied excessively in a particular organ in the body.

Hypertrophic The enlargement of tissue or an organ due to increase in the size of the cells that constitute the tissue or organ.

Infantile spasms (IS) Typical spasms consist of brief repeated flexor spasms of the trunk and limbs. So-called 'salaam spasms' are typical examples, but spasms may be more variable.

Lennox-Gastaut Syndrome A seizure–related syndrome with typical onset between the age of 1 and 8. Characterized by seizure-onset and associated intellectual decline.

Phakomatoses A term coined by Van der Hoeve (1920) to describe a group of autosomal dominant inherited disorders with similar well-circumscribed benign growths in various organs including the eyes. The phakomatoses currently include tuberous sclerosis, neuro-fibromatosis, von Hippel-Lindau and Sturge Weber disease.

Phenotype The observable characteristics of an organism, person or group associated with a specific genotype (genetic pattern). This could be a physical phenotype (observable physical features) or a behavioural phenotype (observable behavioural, psychological and neuro-psychiatric features).

Proband Genetic epidemiological term to describe the member of a family who was the first to bring attention to the presence of a disorder.

Renal angiomyolipomas Localized non-malignant proliferations of blood vessels, smooth muscles and fat in the kidneys.

Rhabdomyoma Benign growths of muscle fibres in the heart.

Sclerosis Derived from the Greek word *skleros*, meaning 'hard'.

Secondarily ascertained A family member born and diagnosed after someone else in the family had already been confirmed to have the disorder.

Shagreen patch 'Skin with the appearance of untanned leather'. Yellow-brown or pink uneven or course skin, usually in the lumbosacral region.

Soft fibromas Soft, baglike growths on the neck, trunk or extremities, sometimes referred to as 'skin tags'. These are not diagnostic of tuberous sclerosis complex.

Striatum The corpus striatum refers to an embryological aggregation of neurons which gives rise to two of the three nuclei of the basal ganglia of the cerebral cortex. The corpus striatum forms the caudate nucleus and the lentiform nucleus. The lentiform nucleus consists of the putamen and the globus pallidus.

Ungual fibroma Nodules arising from the nailbed. More common on toes than fingers.

West Syndrome Consists of the triad of infantile spasms, arrest of psychomotor development and a characteristic hypsarrthythmia pattern on EEG.

REFERENCES

Atkinson, R., Atkinson, R., Smith, E., Bem, D. & Nolen-Hoeksema, S. (1996). *Hilgard's Introduction to Psychology*, 12th edn. Fort Worth: Harcourt Brace College Publishers.

Bolton, P.F. & Griffiths, P.D. (1997). Association of tuberous sclerosis of temporal lobes with autism and atypical autism. *Lancet*, **349**: 392–5.

Bolton, P.F., Park, R., Crawley, R., Griffiths, P.D., Higgins, N. & de Vries, P.J. (2000). Brain factors underlying the intellectual impairments in tuberous sclerosis. Presented at the *TSC Millennium Research Symposium 2000, September 2000, Edinburgh, Scotland*.

Bourneville, D. (1880). Sclerose tubereuse des circonvolutions cerebrales: idiotie et epilepsie hemiplegique. *Archives of Neurology (Paris)*, **1**: 81–91.

Bourneville, D. & Brissaud, E. (1881). Encephalite ou sclerose tubereuse de circonvolutions cerebrales. *Archives of Neurology (Paris)*, **1**: 390–412.

Clarke, A., Cook, P. & Osborne, J.P. (1996). Cranial computed tomographic findings in tuberous sclerosis are not affected by sex. *Developmental Medicine and Child Neurology*, **38**: 139–45.

Critchley, M. & Earl, C.J.C. (1932). Tuberous sclerosis and allied conditions. *Brain*, **55**: 311–46.

de Vries, P.J. & Bolton, P.F. (1999). Neuropsychological attention deficits in children with tuberous sclerosis. *Molecular Psychiatry*, **4**: S51.

de Vries, P.J. & Bolton, P.F. (2000). Genotype-phenotype correlations in tuberous sclerosis. *Journal of Medical Genetics*, **37**: 3.

Gaily, E., Appelqvist, K., Kantola-Sorsa, E. et al. (1999). Cognitive deficits after cryptogenic infantile spasms with benign seizure evolution. *Developmental Medicine and Child Neurology*, **41**: 660–4.

Gastaut, H., Roger, J., Solayrol, R., Regis, H. & Loeb, H. (1965). Encephalopathie myoclonique infantile avec hypsarythmie (syndrome de West) et sclerose tubereuse de Bourneville. *Journal of Neurological Science*, **2**: 140–60.

Gillberg, I.C., Gillberg, C. & Ahlsen, G. (1994). Autistic behaviour and attention deficits in tuberous sclerosis: a population-based study. *Developmental Medicine and Child Neurology*, **36**: 50–6.

Gomez, M. (1999). Tuberous sclerosis complex. In *Developmental Perspectives in Psychiatry*, 3rd edn. ed. J. Harris, p. 31. New York: Oxford University Press.

Gomez, M.R. (1979). *Tuberous Sclerosis*. New York: Raven Press.

Griffiths, P.D. & Martland, T.R. (1997). Tuberous sclerosis complex: the role of neuroradiology. *Neuropediatrics*, **28**: 244–52.

Gutierrez, G.C., Smalley, S.L. & Tanguay, P.E. (1998). Autism in tuberous sclerosis complex. *Journal of Autism and Developmental Disorders*, **28**: 97–103.

Gutmann, D.H., Zhang, Y.J., Hasbani, M.J., Goldberg, M.P., Plank, T.L. & Henske, E.P. (2000). Expression of the tuberous sclerosis complex gene products, hamartin and tuberin, in central nervous system tissues. *Acta Neuropathologica*, **99**(3): 223–30.

Harding, B.N. (1992). Malformations of the nervous system. In *Greenfield's Neuropathology*, ed. L. Hume Adams & L.W. Duchen, pp. 521–638. London: Edward Arnold.

Harrison, J., O'Callaghan, F., Hancock, E., Osborne, J. & Bolton, P. (1999). Cognitive deficits in normally intelligent patients with tuberous sclerosis. *American Journal of Medical Genetics (Neuropsychiatric Genetics)*, **88**(6): 642–6.

Harrison, J.E. & Bolton, P.F. (1997). Annotation: tuberous sclerosis. *Journal of Child Psychology and Psychiatry*, **38**: 603–14.

Harvey, K.V., Mahr, G. & Balon, R. (1995). Psychiatric manifestations of tuberous sclerosis. *Psychosomatics*, **36**: 314–15.

Herkert, E.E., Wald, A. & Romero, O. (1972). Tuberous sclerosis and schizophrenia. *Diseases of the Nervous System*, **33**: 439–45.

Holmes, G., Sarkisian, M., Ben-Ari, Y. & Chevassus-Au-Louis, N. (1999). Effects of recurrent seizures in the developing brain. In *Childhood Epilepsies and Brain Development*, ed. A. Nehlig, J. Motte, S. Moshe & P. Plouin, pp. 263–78. London: John Libbey & Company Ltd.

Holschneider, D.P. & Szuba, M.P. (1992). Capgras' syndrome and psychosis in a patient with tuberous sclerosis. *Journal of Neuropsychiatry and Clinical Neurosciences*, **4**: 352–3.

Hunt, A. (1983). Tuberous sclerosis: a survey of 97 cases. III: Family aspects. *Developmental Medicine and Child Neurology*, **25**: 353–7.

Hunt, A. (1993). Development, behaviour and seizures in 300 cases of tuberous sclerosis. *Journal of Intellectual Disabilities Research*, **37**: 41–51.

Hunt, A. (1998). A comparison of the abilities, health and behaviour of 23 people with tuberous sclerosis at age 5 and as adults. *Journal of Applied Research in Intellectual Disabilities*, **11**: 227–38.

Hunt, A. & Dennis, J. (1987). Psychiatric disorder among children with tuberous sclerosis. *Developmental Medicine and Child Neurology*, **29**: 190–8.

Hunt, A. & Shepherd, C. (1993). A prevalence study of autism in tuberous sclerosis. *Journal of Autism and Developmental Disorders*, **23**: 323–39.

Iwasaki, S., Nakagawa, H., Kichikawa, K., et al. (1990). MR and CT of tuberous sclerosis: linear abnormalities in the cerebral white matter. *American Journal of Neuroradiology*, **11**: 1029–34.

Jambaque, I., Chiron, C., Dumas, C., Mumford, J. & Dulac, O. (2000). Mental and behavioural outcome of infantile epilepsy treated by vigabatrin in tuberous sclerosis patients. *Epilepsy Research*, **38**: 151–60.

Jones, A., Shyamsundar, M., Thomas, M. et al. (1999). Comprehensive mutation analysis of TSC1 and TSC2 and phenotypic correlations in 150 families with tuberous sclerosis. *American Journal of Human Genetics*, **64**: 1305–15.

Jones, A.C., Daniells, C.E., Snell, R.G. et al. (1997). Molecular genetic and phenotypic analysis reveals differences between TSC1 and TSC2 associated familial and sporadic tuberous sclerosis. *Human Molecular Genetics*, **6**: 2155–61.

Khanna, R. & Borde, M. (1989). Mania in a five-year-old child with tuberous sclerosis. *British Journal of Psychiatry*, **155**: 117–19.

Knudson, A.G. (1971). Mutation and cancer: statistical study of retinoblastoma. *Proceedings of the National Academy of Science USA*, **68**: 820–3.

Lishman, W.A. (1998). *Organic Psychiatry*, 3rd edn. Oxford: Blackwell Science.

Maeda, M., Tartaro, A., Matsuda, T. & Ishii, Y. (1995). Cortical and subcortical tubers in tuberous sclerosis and FLAIR sequence. *Journal of Computer Assisted Tomography*, **19**: 660–1.

Maheshwar, M.M., Cheadle, J.P., Jones, A.C. et al. (1997). The GAP-related domain of tuberin, the product of the TSC2 gene, is a target for missense mutations in tuberous sclerosis. *Human Molecular Genetics*, **6**: 1991–6.

Martin, N., de Broucker, T., Cambier, J., Marsault, C. & Nahum, H. (1987). MRI evaluation of tuberous sclerosis. *Neuroradiology*, **29**: 437–43.

McMurdo, S.K., Jr., Moore, S.G., Brant-Zawadzki, M. et al. (1987). MR imaging of intracranial tuberous sclerosis. *American Journal of Roentgenology*, **148**: 791–6.

Moolten, S.E. (1942). Hamartial nature of the tuberous sclerosis complex and its bearing on the tumour problem. Report of a case with tumour anomaly of the kidney and adenoma sebaceum. *Archives of Internal Medicine*, **69**: 589–623.

Needham, C.J., Harris, T.J.R., O'Callaghan, F.J.K., Osborne, J.P. & Bolton, P.F. (2000). Prevalence of cognitive deficits in an epidemiological sample of tuberous sclerosis. Presented at the *TSC Millennium Research Symposium 2000, September 2000, Edinburgh, Scotland.*

Nellist, M., van Slegtenhorst, M.A., Goedbloed, M., van den Ouweland, A.M., Halley, D.J. & van der Sluijs, P. (1999). Characterisation of the cytosolic tuberin-hamartin complex. Tuberin is a cytosolic chaperone for hamartin. *Journal of Biological Chemistry*, **274**(50): 35647–52.

Nixon, J.R., Houser, O.W., Gomez, M.R. & Okazaki, H. (1989). Cerebral tuberous sclerosis: MR imaging. *Radiology*, **170**: 869–73.

O'Callaghan, F. (1999). Tuberous sclerosis. *British Medical Journal*, **318**: 1019–20.

O'Callaghan, F.J., Clarke, A.C., Joffe, H. et al. (1998). Tuberous sclerosis complex and Wolff–Parkinson–White syndrome. *Archives of Disease of Childhood*, **78**: 159–62.

Osborne, J.P. (1988). Diagnosis of tuberous sclerosis. *Archives of Disease of Childhood*, **63**: 1423–5.

Petersen, A. (1989). Adolescent development. In *Annual Review of Psychology*, vol 39. ed. M. Rosenzweig & L. Porter, pp. 104–6. Palo Alto, CA.

Povey, S., Burley, M.W., Attwood, J. et al. (1994). Two loci for tuberous sclerosis: one on 9q34 and one on 16p13. *Annals of Human Genetics*, **58**: 107–27.

Rantala, H. & Putkonen, T. (1999). Occurrence, outcome, and prognostic factors of infantile spasms and Lennox-Gastaut syndrome. *Epilepsia*, **40**: 286–9.

Riikonen, R. & Amnell, G. (1981). Psychiatric disorders in children with earlier infantile spasms. *Developmental Medicine and Child Neurology*, **23**: 747–60.

Roach, E., DiMario, F., Kandt, R. & Northrup, H. (1999). Tuberous sclerosis consensus conference: recommendations for diagnostic evaluation. *Journal of Child Neurology*, **14**: 401–7.

Roach, E., Gomez, M. & Northrup, H. (1998). Tuberous sclerosis consensus conference: revised diagnostic criteria. *Journal of Child Neurology*, **13**: 624–8.

Shepherd, C.W. & Stephenson, J.B.P. (1992). Seizures and intellectual disability associated with tuberous sclerosis complex in the west of Scotland. *Developmental Medicine and Child Neurology*, **34**: 766–74.

Sherlock, F.B. (1911). *The Feeble-Minded*. London: McMillan and Co.

Simonoff, E., Bolton, P. & Rutter, M. (1996). Mental retardation: genetic findings, clinical implications and research agenda. *Journal of Child Psychology and Psychiatry*, **37**: 259–80.

Smalley, S. (1998). Autism and tuberous sclerosis. *Journal of Developmental Disorders*, **28**: 407–14.

Smalley, S.L., Burger, F. & Smith, M. (1994). Phenotypic variation of tuberous sclerosis in a single extended kindred. *Journal of Medical Genetics*, **31**: 761–5.

Smalley, S.L., McCracken, J.& Tanguay, P. (1995). Autism, affective disorders, and social phobia. *American Journal of Medical Genetics*, **60**: 19–26.

Soucek, T., Holzl, G., Bernaschek, G. & Hengstschlager, M. (1998). A role of the tuberous sclerosis gene-2 product during neuronal differentiation. *Oncogene*, **16**: 197–204.

Soucek, T., Pusch, O., Wienecke, R., DeClue, J.E. & Hengstschlager, M. (1997). Role of the tuberous sclerosis gene-2 product in cell cycle control. Loss of the tuberous sclerosis gene-2 induces quiescent cells to enter S phase. *Journal of Biology and Chemistry*, **272**: 29301–8.

The European Chromosome 16 Tuberous Sclerosis Consortium (1993). Identification and characterization of the tuberous sclerosis gene on chromosome 16. *Cell*, **75**: 1305–15.

van der Hoeve, J. (1932). Eye symptoms in phacomatoses. *Transactions of the Opthalmological Society UK*, **52**: 380–401.

van der Hoeve, J. (1920). Eye symptoms in tuberous sclerosis of the brain. *Transactions of the Opthalmological Society UK*, **40**: 329–34.

van Slegtenhorst, M., de Hoogt, R., Hermans, C. et al. (1997). Identification of the tuberous sclerosis gene TSC1 on chromosome 9q34. *Science*, **277**: 805–8.

Vogt, H. (1908). Zur Diagnostik der tuberosen Sklerose. *Erforsch Behandl jugendl Schwachsinns*, **2**: 1–12.

Webb, D.W., Fryer, A.E. & Osborne, J.P. (1991). On the incidence of fits and mental retardation in tuberous sclerosis. *Journal of Medical Genetics*, **28**: 395–7.

Webb, D.W., Fryer, A.E. & Osborne, J.P. (1996). Morbidity associated with tuberous sclerosis: a population study. *Developmental Medicine and Child Neurology*, **38**: 146–55.

Whittemore, V. (1999). The diagnosis of tuberous sclerosis complex: the impact on the individual and family. In *Tuberous Sclerosis Complex*, 3rd edn., ed. M. Gomez, pp. 324–30. New York: Oxford University Press.

Wilton, L., Stephens, M. & Mann, R. (1999). Visual field defect associated with vigabatrin: observational cohort study. *Lancet*, **319**: 1165–6.

Wing, L. & Gould, J. (1979). Systematic recording of behaviours and skills of retarded and psychotic children. *Journal of Autism and Childhood Schizophrenia*, **8**: 79–97.

Zimmerman, D. (1999). The endocrine system in tuberous sclerosis complex. In *Tuberous Sclerosis Complex*, 3rd edn., ed. M. Gomez, pp. 218–27. New York: Oxford University Press.

12

Williams and Smith-Magenis syndromes

Orlee Udwin

Introduction

Williams syndrome and Smith-Magenis syndrome are both rare, genetically determined conditions with an assumed prevalence of 1 in 25 000 live births, an equal sex ratio and an association with learning disabilities, mostly in the mild to severe range. Both syndromes are associated with distinctive patterns of cognitive and behavioural characteristics, although in each case the pattern of characteristics is different and carries very different implications for adjustment in adulthood and for educational and behavioural interventions.

While rare, these syndromes are becoming better known among health professionals, and more and more affected individuals are being identified. These individuals are also quite likely to be referred to health and mental health specialists because the particular behavioural and psychological characteristics associated with the conditions place them at increased risk for difficulties in adjustment and psychopathology in both childhood and adult life. In recent years there has been a growth in research on the psychological characteristics, difficulties and needs of children with Williams syndrome, and to a lesser extent Smith-Magenis syndrome. Research findings are also beginning to accrue on the long-term course of these conditions and adjustment in adulthood. This is vital for parents and professionals in order to facilitate the sharing of information about appropriate educational and behavioural approaches, to inform intervention efforts and to help plan for adulthood. Moreover, as Turk & Sales (1996) point out, the knowledge that particular behaviours are caused by, or at least associated with, underlying genetic abnormalities rather than parental handling or other environmental factors, can assist parents and other carers to generate a sense of control, rather than guilt, anger or helplessness in relation to their children's difficulties.

This chapter will briefly discuss the genetic underpinnings, physical features and natural history of Williams syndrome and Smith-Magenis syndrome, and the cognitive and behavioural characteristics associated with these conditions in childhood, and then go on to explore their long-term course, their effects on adjustment in adulthood and implications for support and intervention for affected individuals across the life span.

Williams syndrome

Aetiology, epidemiology and physical presentation

Williams syndrome is a developmental disorder involving the vascular, connective tissue and central nervous systems. Recent research indicates that it is a contiguous gene deletion syndrome, involving a microdeletion on chromosome 7 (at locus 7q 11.23) that includes the elastin gene (Ewart et al., 1993). Elastin is an important constituent of connective tissue, especially in arterial walls, and reduced or abnormal elastin could explain the vascular and connective tissue pathology found in the syndrome, as well as the atypical facial appearance. Other phenotypic features might be accounted for through the involvement of contiguous genes. Most cases of Williams syndrome are the result of a new mutation, although the condition can be inherited as an autosomal dominant disorder.

The mean birth weight of affected individuals is reduced, and cardiac murmurs and an unusual facial appearance are often noted at birth (Martin, Snodgrass & Cohen, 1984). Difficulties with feeding are a major problem in infancy, and with vomiting, constipation and irritability, lead to failure to thrive. A proportion of children are found to have raised levels of blood calcium. This subgroup is generally treated with a low-calcium and vitamin D-restricted diet, and serum calcium levels return to normal and the feeding difficulties improve with dietary treatment, or simply with the passage of time. However, other features of the condition persist. Physical features of the children include a distinctive face with full prominent cheeks, a wide mouth, long philtrum, a retroussé nose with a flat nasal bridge, heavy orbital ridges, medial eyebrow flare and stellate iris pattern (Joseph & Parrott, 1958); dental anomalies, including microdontia, missing teeth and enamel hypoplasia; and renal and cardiovascular abnormalities (most commonly supravalvular aortic stenosis and peripheral pulmonary artery stenosis) (Morris et al., 1988; Pober et al., 1993). The cardiovascular symptoms vary in severity and may change over time. Commonly found skeletal abnormalities include radio-ulnar synostosis, joint contractures and laxity. Gait abnormalities are common and include immature gait and abnormal stress gait, with early hypotonia giving way to hypertonia in older individuals (Chapman, du Plessis & Pober, 1996). Growth retardation, short stature and a hoarse voice are further frequent findings, and an early starting and fast progressing puberty has been reported in many cases.

Many adults with Williams syndrome appear to age prematurely, and greying hair and a coarse facial appearance are common even in the early to mid-twenties. Progressive multi-system medical problems have been identified in at least some adults, and can lead to premature death. These include cardiovascular complications, hypertension, gastrointestinal problems, urinary tract abnormalities and progressive joint limitations (Morris et al., 1988). However, it is not clear how common these problems are.

Cognitive and behavioural characteristics in childhood

Studies have highlighted a distinctive psychological profile, and unusual personality and behavioural characteristics that are associated with Williams syndrome that differentiate affected children from other groups with learning disabilities (Udwin, Yule & Martin, 1987; Udwin & Yule, 1991).

Approximately 95% of the children have mild to severe learning disabilities and the mean Full Scale IQ is around the mid-50s (Bennett, La Veck & Sells, 1978; Kataria, Goldstein & Kushnick, 1984; Udwin et al., 1987). Most of the school-aged sample investigated by Udwin and her colleagues required special schooling, and only about half were able to attain some score in reading and spelling. Language may be slow to develop in the pre-school years but by school-age verbal abilities are in most cases markedly superior to visuo-spatial abilities and to gross and fine motor skills. Most children with Williams syndrome have an unusual command of language: their comprehension is usually far more limited than their expressive language, which tends to be grammatically correct, complex and fluent at a superficial level, but verbose and pseudo-mature. The children tend to be very chatty, and their auditory memory, verbal processing and the social use of language are particularly well developed. They typically have a well-developed and precocious vocabulary, with excessive and frequently inappropriate use of clichés and stereotyped phrases, but accompanied by various syntactic, semantic and pragmatic deficits and problems with turn taking and topic maintenance (Udwin & Yule, 1990; Bellugi, Wang & Jernigan, 1994; Karmiloff-Smith et al., 1996, 1998). They also show significant deficits in the integration of visual–perceptual information, in sequencing, performance speed, and fine motor skills, when compared with their verbal abilities and with groups of children matched for verbal IQ (Crisco, Dobbs & Mulhern, 1988; Udwin & Yule, 1991). However, even in non-verbal areas there is an uneven profile, with consistent relative strengths on tasks of face recognition (Udwin & Yule, 1991; Bellugi et al., 1994).

Most children with Williams syndrome have poor relationships with peers but are outgoing, socially disinhibited and excessively affectionate towards adults, including strangers; they also appear acutely attentive to the feelings of others (Udwin et al., 1987; Dilts, Morris & Leonard, 1990; Gosch & Pankau, 1994; Dykens & Rosner, 1999). Their relatively good verbal abilities, engaging personalities and excessive sociability can be deceptive and result in an overestimation of their general cognitive abilities, as well as being a major worry for parents, particularly as the children approach adolescence.

Affected children show higher rates of emotional and behavioural disturbance when compared with the rates that have been reported for other children with learning disabilities, particularly in terms of overactivity, poor concentration and distractibility, attention seeking behaviours and generalized anxiety (Einfeld, Tonge & Florio, 1997; Udwin et al., 1987). Parents describe the children as worrying excessively about unfamiliar situations, anticipated events and all kinds of imagined disasters. They tend to be over-eager to please and constantly seek reassurance from adults. They show high rates of preoccupations and obsessions with particular activities, objects or topics such as electrical gadgets, cars, disasters and illness, and also particular people, for example a neighbour or a teacher at school. Over 90% of the children are hypersensitive to particular sounds, which may include electrical noises like vacuum cleaners, drills, music and thunder. The basis for this hyperacusis is not clear but it tends to diminish in frequency and severity in adulthood (Udwin et al., 1987; Klein et al., 1990).

It is important to note that although the characteristics described above are typical of Williams syndrome, they show some variability across children, and are not necessarily all present in every case.

Abilities, behaviour and adjustment in adult life

Recent studies of adults with Williams syndrome indicate that the characteristic cognitive and personality profile and typical behavioural difficulties that have been identified in affected children persist into adulthood with the same or even greater frequency. These characteristics can cause major difficulties for the individuals in terms of independent living, employment and in developing social and emotional relationships (Udwin, 1990; Davies, Howlin & Udwin, 1997; Davies, Udwin & Howlin, 1998; Udwin et al., 1998).

On assessment, most adults with Williams syndrome have mild learning disabilities (IQ between 50 and 70); only 4% of the group assessed by Howlin, Davies & Udwin (1998) had moderate to severe learning disabilities (IQ below 50), while 10% had borderline cognitive abilities. On the basis of a longitudinal study, Udwin, Davies & Howlin (1996) concluded that adults with Williams syndrome, at least within the 20–40 year age group, do not appear to show the decline in cognitive abilities over time that is found in certain other conditions, for example Down syndrome (Carr, 1994) and fragile X syndrome (Hagerman et al., 1989). Instead, as in the general population, there was a slight increase in IQ scores from WISC-R to WAIS-R re-testing. The pattern of cognitive functioning reported in the adults was very similar to that described in affected children; they tended to do relatively well on tests of vocabulary and abstract reasoning but performed poorly on tasks involving general knowledge, memory, numeracy and visual sequencing. Assessment of receptive and expressive language indicated persisting deficits in both areas, while attainments in reading, spelling and mathematical abilities, and functioning in the areas of communication, independence and socialization (as assessed on the Vineland Behaviour Scales) were poorer still. The average levels reached in all these areas were equivalent to the 6–8 year level. Thus, although general cognitive abilities appear to be well maintained in adults with Williams syndrome, they make little progress in literacy and numeracy beyond the early teenage years, and their ability to use these skills within a general social context appears to be extremely limited.

In line with this conclusion, Davies et al. (1997) reported that most of the adults in their study lived at home with their families (69%) or in sheltered accommodation (24%), and most required substantial amounts of supervision and support in the areas of self-care and daily living skills. According to their carers, about half of the sample required at least some assistance with washing and dressing and between 80% and 94% were wholly dependent on others for the preparation of food and domestic chores such as cleaning, shopping and laundry. Only one of the sample of 70 could use money appropriately and controlled her own finances. In all the remaining cases, the caregivers took responsibility for budgeting and shopping. Although 40% of the group were able to use public transport unaccompanied on familiar journeys, only two (3%) of the group were able to use public transport for unfamiliar journeys. Moreover, many carers reported being wary of letting the adults go out alone because their friendly and over-trusting nature made them vulnerable to exploitation, while their visuo-spatial difficulties and poor appreciation of speed and distance made crossing roads dangerous. Three adults (4%) were living independently but were receiving considerable supervision and support from family members and community workers to help them cope with the demands of daily life, particularly domestic chores and dealing with money.

Only one adult in the sample of 70 described by Davies et al. (1997) had an independent job and four worked in sheltered employment, as shop or kitchen assistants. A further five people had part-time voluntary jobs, while 11 were undertaking part-time work placements organized by their adult training centres or further education colleges, for example as packers, shop assistants or nursery helpers. Supervisors reported 'considerable difficulties' for about half of these adults, and 'at least some difficulties' for a further third. Thus, despite their relatively good cognitive abilities, most of the adults had very limited self-care and independence skills and required considerable supervision and support in their occupational and daily living environments.

Problems reported by carers, supervisors and employers, which necessitated supervision and prompting for most, even when performing routine tasks, included the adults' distractibility and poor persistence, anxiety, inappropriate social behaviours and motor difficulties, all characteristics that are typically associated with Williams syndrome. These characteristics appear to limit the levels of independence, self-care and occupational status attained by adults with Williams syndrome, when compared with other groups of adults with mild or moderate cognitive impairment (e.g. Dykens et al., 1992; Carr, 1994).

The characteristic behavioural and emotional difficulties described in children with Williams syndrome have been found to persist into adulthood with the same or greater frequency (Davies et al., 1998). Almost all of Davies et al.'s sample of 70 adults were reported to have difficulties making or maintaining friendships, and nearly three-quarters were said to be socially isolated. At the same time the majority continued to be socially disinhibited, over-friendly and too trusting of others. Over half were reported to be physically over-demonstrative, often seeking attention and affection in inappropriate ways such as touching, hugging and kissing others. While these characteristics are often regarded as endearing and appealing in children, they become increasingly problematic in adolescence and adulthood and can make individuals vulnerable to sexual exploitation and abuse. At least 20% of the sample had reportedly been victims of sexual abuse and in half of these cases police intervention had been sought. A particular problem, seen in over 50% of the adults, was the tendency to focus their attention and affection on television or film personalities or familiar people such as neighbours. In some cases these attachments developed into all encompassing infatuations, causing significant difficulties for those involved.

Preoccupations and circumscribed interests were highly characteristic of the adult sample and, as with affected children, typically centred on fascinations and obsessive interests in cars, electrical appliances, machinery, disasters and violence in the news, and future events such as birthdays and holidays. In many cases these preoccupations significantly disrupted daily life and restricted activities; for example some adults were reported to spend hours dismantling electrical appliances. Most adults with Williams syndrome exhibit high levels of anxiety, which tends to be triggered by excessive worries about perceived threat, inappropriate demands, uncertainty or changes in routine. Even relatively minor changes in the environment can prove very upsetting, while major life events, such as the death of a parent or a move to new accommodation, can result in prolonged periods of anxiety or depression (Davies et al., 1998). Ten per cent of the sample investigated by Davies et al., were said to have had a period of low mood or depression in their adult lives and a further 10% were said to have had marked mood swings. Phobias and hypochondria were reported in around half of the group and were often sufficiently intense to restrict activities. Excessive worries about their health often resulted in frequent visits to doctors and necessitated considerable reassurance about health-related matters. Hyperactivity, which is prominent in children with Williams syndrome, is reported to diminish considerably in adulthood, but concentration problems and distractibility continue to cause difficulties in 90% of cases. Stereotyped motor movements such as rocking, hand rubbing and skin picking, are also common, particularly when individuals become angry or anxious.

The characteristic cognitive and behavioural profiles of children and adults with Williams syndrome carry important implications for psychological and educational interventions. These will be examined in the following section.

Implications for interventions and educational and training approaches

As illustrated above, a diagnosis of Williams syndrome can help families and professionals to gain a better understanding of the strengths and difficulties of affected children and adults, and to plan to better meet present and future needs. Moreover, the finding that most psychological difficulties identified in childhood persist into adulthood highlights the need for early interventions to address these difficulties. Although research evidence on the effectiveness of interventions with this population is sparse, clinical experience suggests that the fact that particular behavioural and emotional difficulties are linked with this genetic condition does not mean that they are not amenable to modification. On the contrary, there are many reports that behaviourally-based interventions for characteristic difficulties such as overactivity, anxiety and social disinhibition can be as effective with individuals with Williams syndrome as they are with other groups. Moreover, the similarities identified in the patterns of learning and behaviour of these children and adults have helped to refine appropriate educational strategies and behavioural management approaches through the sharing of information and experiences between parents and professionals.

Given that feeding difficulties and delayed language development are characteristic in the early years, programmes to encourage pre-linguistic and feeding skills should be introduced early, with an emphasis on sucking, swallowing and chewing. Early speech and language therapy should focus on helping children to attend to and comprehend auditory stimuli, and on building up vocabulary, syntax and turn taking skills (Meyerson & Frank, 1987). The introduction of signing and other communication systems to augment speech expression and comprehension in the early years can also be beneficial. In addition, physiotherapy and occupational therapy input will be needed in areas of particular difficulty, including co-ordination, balance, gross and fine motor activities and visuo-spatial skills. These therapists can also advise on developing an array of self-help skills, including dressing, washing, eating with a knife and fork, and writing.

Udwin & Yule (1998a,b) have produced guidelines for parents and teachers of children with Williams syndrome, in which they describe the main features of the condition and advise on the management of behavioural difficulties using standard behavioural techniques, and on appropriate educational approaches. For example, given their characteristic social disinhibition and overfriendliness, parents and teachers are advised on the need to teach appropriate social skills and to set clear boundaries from the start, teaching appropriate greeting behaviours and discouraging the child from approaching strangers and from excessive and inappropriate verbalizations. Obsessions and preoccupations should, where possible, be nipped in the bud by diverting the child's attention and introducing new activities and interests. Where preoccupations are well established, carers should try to keep them within acceptable bounds, for example by allocating specific amounts of time to activities related to the preoccupations, and then gradually reducing the amount of time spent in this way. Alternatively, time spent engaged in the preoccupation could be used as a reward for desired behaviour in other areas. The obsessional interest could also be channelled into useful activity, for example practising pencil control by drawing or writing about a favourite topic.

Clinical experience suggests that temper outbursts and aggressive behaviours displayed by children with Williams syndrome can be effectively addressed with standard behaviour management approaches, including identifying triggers for such behaviours, anticipating these and diverting the child's attention elsewhere; teaching the child more appropriate ways of communicating needs, wants or frustrations, and removing adult attention when the child displays unacceptable behaviours. In general, children with Williams syndrome do best with a predictable schedule and a set routine, and they benefit from preparation before changes in activities or routines. Stress and anticipatory anxiety can often be reduced by talking the child through a change or difficult task ahead of time. Where children appear to be more nervous or anxious than usual, the home and school environments should be examined to ensure that excessive demands or pressures are not being placed on them.

Treatments for hyperacusis have not been systematically evaluated. Filtered ear-protectors are sometimes recommended, but since these may well filter out certain speech frequencies as well, their use should be limited. Reassurance and an explanation about the source of the noise often helps the child, and a warning just before predictable noises (e.g. before switching on a food processor) means that children can prepare themselves for the noise and leave the room if necessary. Parents report that the reactions will often diminish if the child is able to exercise some control over the sounds that cause discomfort, for example practising switching a vacuum cleaner on and off. Repeated, gentle exposure to the sounds may also help to desensitize the child, for example by tape recording distressing sounds and then encouraging the child to play these back, quietly at first, then gradually increasing the volume.

Since the children's good spoken language and outgoing personalities can give a false expectation of their functioning in other areas, careful assessment of their cognitive abilities and profile of strengths and weaknesses is essential. Most require special schooling, though some attend mainstream schools with additional support. Because of their unusual pattern of abilities they have special educational needs that are different from those of other children with learning disabilities, and it can be difficult to find a school that is exactly suited to their particular needs. Finding the most appropriate school will depend on the individual child's level of abilities and profile of strengths and weaknesses, and also on the provisions in the particular schools that are available locally. Because poor concentration, distractibility and hypersensitivity to sounds are among the most common problems of children with Williams syndrome, they are likely to concentrate best in one-to-one or small group settings that are as quiet and free from distractions as possible. Activities should be varied, of short duration and with frequent breaks, and regular prompting and reminders will help the child to stay on task. Programmes of positive reinforcement for remaining seated and on task for increasing lengths of time are also recommended, while self instructional training may be particularly effective with older children and adolescents. In a series of placebo-controlled case studies Bawden, MacDonald & Shea (1987) showed that treatment with methylphenidate benefited two children with Williams syndrome in terms of improved attention, and reduced activity, impulsivity and irritability, with no signs of serious side effects. No effects were discernible in the other two children included in the study. The trial used only a single dosage of medication, was of short duration and included just four children. Further trials are needed but it is likely that methylphenidate is a useful adjunct in the treatment of some children with Williams syndrome.

Advice to teachers might include suggestions for harnessing the children's superior spoken language abilities in training perceptual and motor skills to help them to focus their attention on the tasks, and on ways of providing verbal reinforcement and support for the activities, for example encouraging children to talk themselves through each step of an exercise while they are doing it. The use of topics and objects in which children have a particular interest can help to motivate them to work on activities that are not intrinsically interesting, for example practising eye–hand co-ordination and pencil control skills by copying and tracing over pictures of cars, washing machines, etc. (Udwin & Yule, 1998b). Thought should also be given to the way work is presented to the child with Williams syndrome; books and programmes with many pictures and colours may lead to visual overstimulation, and materials or worksheets with relatively little information on each may be preferable. In teaching reading, strategies that use the child's superior verbal skills (i.e. phonetic approaches) are likely to have the greatest success. Teaching through music and songs, which many children with Williams syndrome enjoy, can further speed up the learning process and make it more enjoyable. Finally, many of the children enjoy working on computers and may become very proficient in computer use. Such skills should be encouraged and can support school-based learning.

The needs of siblings of children with Williams syndrome should not be forgotten. Many siblings are poorly informed about the syndrome and may harbour unnecessary worries about the possibility that they may be at risk of having a child with the condition, or of developing the condition themselves. It is important for parents to give siblings information about the condition, its cause and long-term course since accurate information will serve to allay unnecessary fears and worries, and increase understanding among siblings of the Williams syndrome child's difficulties and needs.

Adults with Williams syndrome are probably easier to live with and to manage than individuals with certain other conditions, for example Prader-Willi syndrome (Greenswag, 1987). Parents frequently point out how helpful their adult Williams syndrome children are with both practical matters and in terms of providing emotional and social support (Udwin, 1990). However, given the significant medical, psychological and psychiatric difficulties identified in many adults, and their continued need for supervision and support, routine health screening and assessment of their cognitive profile, mood and behaviour are essential to ensure that their living and occupational environments are appropriate to their ability levels and needs, and to facilitate access to health and social services as necessary.

Moreover, given that many adults continue to live with their families into their 30s and 40s (Udwin et al., 1998), attention must be paid to the families' needs for support, advice on management issues and also occasional breaks from caring for their children. In reality, Udwin et al. (1998) found that most families caring for adults with Williams syndrome had minimal if any contact with medical or mental health professionals or with social services.

As already noted, most adults with Williams syndrome experience substantial difficulties in the work place and have severely limited self-care and independence skills, mostly due to the cognitive and personality characteristics known to be associated with the condition, notably anxiety, social disinhibition, poor social functioning, visuo-motor difficulties and distractibility. As a result, they require substantial supervision and support in everyday activities. Yet their comparatively good spoken language and outgoing personalities often give a false expectation of their abilities in other areas. This can lead to their being placed in residential, training and employment settings which place excessive demands on them, with a concomitant deterioration in behaviour and mood. Careful thought needs to be given to finding daytime occupations and living arrangements that are appropriate to their ability levels and take account of their particular personality traits and interests, and their characteristic profile of cognitive strengths and deficits. For example, routine manual tasks such as stacking shelves, packing or assembly-line work, which are typically considered suitable for people with learning disabilities, may not be appropriate for people with Williams syndrome because of their visuo-motor difficulties, lack of stamina and tendency to tire easily. Their distractibility means that they may get bored with repetitive tasks, though at the same time they tend to dislike change and are reported to perform better when given structured routine tasks to carry out. Many people with Williams syndrome get particular pleasure from meeting and helping others, and working in a helping capacity (e.g. as an assistant in a nursery or hospital) with adequate supervision may be appropriate in some cases. Noisy and busy work and living environments tend to be distressing because of the hypersensitivity of individuals to sounds and visuo-perceptual difficulties; quiet environments that are structured and ordered are to be preferred.

Psychiatric and psychological difficulties in adults with learning disabilities often go undiagnosed and untreated. The high levels of anxiety exhibited by many adults with Williams syndrome may be triggered by excessive worries

Table 12.1. Adults with Williams syndrome: implications of the cognitive and behavioural phenotype for carers and supervisors

- Considerable support and supervision are needed:
  - in self-care and daily living tasks
  - when out of the house, because over-friendliness and disinhibited behaviours place individuals at risk of exploitation and abuse
  - in the workplace, due to distractibility, poor persistence, anxiety, inappropriate social behaviours and motor difficulties
- Training in social skills and appropriate social behaviours will be required to address social isolation, inappropriate overfriendliness and disinhibition
- Working and living environments must be tailored to the individual's abilities. Placements that are too demanding may result in a deterioration in behaviour and mood
- A predictable environment and set routines are preferred. Where possible changes should be prepared for well ahead of time

Table 12.2. Implications of the Williams syndrome phenotype for health and mental health professionals

- Regular health checks to monitor cardiac and kidney function and blood pressure
- Assessment of the cognitive profile will help clarify areas of strengths and weaknesses, since individuals' superior expressive language and outgoing personalities may be misleading, resulting in an overestimation of underlying abilities.
- Psychological interventions, with or without medication, may be required for:
  - anxiety
  - depression
  - obsessions and preoccupations
  - phobias, hypochondria
- Carers will require support and advice on management issues

about perceived threat, inappropriate demands, uncertainty, or when faced with changes in routine. Major life events such as the death of a parent or a move to new residential accommodation can, in some cases, result in prolonged periods of anxiety or depression (Davies et al., 1998). Additional psychological support at such times to prepare individuals for change or to help them cope with unforeseen events may prevent long-term psychological difficulties. In addition, training in social skills, appropriate social behaviours and wariness of others is a priority for individuals with Williams syndrome, given their social disinhibition. Teaching independence in self-care, including dressing, washing, shopping and cooking is also important.

The above recommendations are based on clinical experience and reports from parents and professionals on approaches that have been found to be helpful with this population (Udwin, Howlin & Davies 1996a,b). Studies are urgently needed to examine their effectiveness under controlled conditions and in comparison with other intervention approaches.

For a summary of the implications of the cognitive and behavioural phenotype for carers and supervisors see Table 12.1 and for health and mental health professionals see Table 12.2.

Smith-Magenis syndrome

Aetiology, epidemiology and physical presentation

Like Williams syndrome, Smith-Magenis syndrome is a chromosomal disorder associated with learning difficulties and a specific pattern of physical, behavioural and cognitive characteristics. The syndrome was first described by Smith, McGavran and Waldstein in 1982 and is believed to have an incidence of at least 1 in 25 000 births, with an equal sex ratio (Greenberg et al., 1991). It is caused by an interstitial deletion of chromosome 17p11.2, and most cases are sporadic, suggesting a low recurrence risk for parents, although at least one case of vertical transmission of the deletion from mother to daughter has been reported (Zori et al., 1993). Several candidate genes have been identified in the deletion region (Chevillard et al., 1993; Zhao et al., 1995; Chen, Potocki & Lupski, 1996b; Elsea et al., 1996), but further investigations are required to clarify their significance to the clinical and behavioural phenotype.

Associated dysmorphic features reported in over two-thirds of affected individuals include a flat, broad head (brachycephaly) and prominent forehead, epicanthal folds, a broad nasal bridge, flat mid-face, abnormal ear shape and position, down-turned mouth with cupid's bow, broad hands with inbent fingers, small toes, short stature and a hoarse deep voice (Greenberg et al., 1991, 1996). The latter may be related to features such as polyps, nodules, paralysis of the vocal chords and structural vocal-fold abnormalities which have been reported in individuals with Smith-Magenis syndrome. With age there is a general coarsening of the facial features. Infantile hypotonia, early feeding difficulties, failure to thrive, and frequent ear infections leading to progressive hearing loss are common. Clinical signs of peripheral neuropathy have been found in approximately 75% of cases, which include decreased deep tendon reflexes, decreased sensitivity to pain and temperature, reduced leg muscle mass, gait disturbances and muscle weakness (Greenberg et al., 1996; Webber, 1999). Eye abnormalities are also common, and include iris anomalies, microcornea, strabismus, cataracts and myopia (Finucane et al., 1993; Chen et al., 1996a). Affected individuals are particularly prone to retinal detachment, possibly as a result of the combination of high myopia, self-injurious head banging, aggression and hyperactivity.

Less consistent features include cardiac defects (in 37% of cases), renal and thyroid abnormalities (in 35% and 29% of cases), scoliosis (in at least 24%), seizures (in 11–30%), and also genital abnormalities, and abnormal palmar creases. Several individuals in their 60s and 70s have been described in the literature (e.g. Greenberg et al., 1991), suggesting that life expectancy may be normal.

Cognitive and behavioural characteristics in childhood

There are relatively few published reports on the cognitive and behavioural characteristics of children with Smith-Magenis syndrome and these are mainly clinical descriptions of small samples. There is an urgent need for systematic investigations of representative samples using standardized instruments and appropriate comparison groups. Nevertheless, on the basis of the information available to date some general conclusions can be drawn regarding the cognitive and behavioural phenotype of Smith-Magenis syndrome.

It is suggested in the literature that all affected individuals have mild to severe learning disabilities, with the majority in the moderate range (IQ 40–50; Moncla et al., 1991; de Rijk-van Andel et al., 1991; Greenberg et al., 1996; Udwin, Webber & Horn, 2001). Of Udwin et al.'s sample of 29 school children, 26 attended special schools or units, mostly for children with mild, moderate or severe learning difficulties; only two of the younger children attended mainstream schools, and one attended a remedial class in a mainstream school. On the other hand, Crumley (1998) recently reported on a child cytogenetically diagnosed with Smith-Magenis syndrome who on assessment did not have associated learning difficulties in non-verbal areas of functioning. Clearly more able individuals with the syndrome are less likely to come to the attention of paediatricians and geneticists, and hence are less likely to be represented in the studies undertaken to date.

In contrast to the Williams syndrome phenotype, in Smith-Magenis syndrome speech delay tends to be more pronounced than motor delay, and expressive language abilities are more impaired than receptive language skills (Chen et al., 1996a; Moncla et al., 1991). Dykens, Finucane & Gayley (1997) examined the cognitive profiles in 10 children and adults, and identified relative weaknesses in sequential processing and in short-term memory, and relative strengths in long-term memory, alertness to the environment, attention to meaningful visual detail and reading. However, Udwin et al. (2001) failed to confirm a strength in reading ability in her sample of affected children.

Behaviourally, children with Smith-Magenis syndrome tend to pose severe management problems for their carers due to hyperactivity, aggressive outbursts, self-injurious behaviours and sleep disturbance (Smith et al., 1986; Stratton et al., 1986; Greenberg et al., 1991; de Rijk-van Andel et al., 1991; Dykens et al., 1997; Dykens & Smith, 1998; Webber, 1999). Between 50% and 100% of individuals investigated have been described as hyperactive, restless, impulsive and distractible, and 70% to 100% are reported to show attention-seeking behaviours, hostility, temper outbursts and aggression towards people and property. These rates are much higher than the rates reported for other groups of children with learning disabilities. The behaviours are often very severe and, according to parent and teacher reports, may be triggered by tiredness, frustration, changes in routine, inability to get one's own way, attempts to avoid situations, or they may have no identifiable triggers (Webber, 1999). Self-injurious behaviours have been observed in children as young as 18 months and are reported in between 67% and 100% of the samples investigated (Greenberg et al., 1991; de Rijk-van Andel et al., 1991; Dykens & Smith, 1998; Webber, 1999). These rates, too, are higher than the rates reported in children with learning disabilities of unknown aetiology but equivalent to rates of self-injury reported in some genetic syndromes, for example Lesch-Nyhan disease (Anderson & Ernst, 1994). The self-injury is often a response to frustration or anger and can be extreme, possibly due to the decreased sensation in the extremities and relative insensitivity to pain that is characteristic of affected individuals. Boredom or habit may be other reasons for self-injurious behaviours. The self-injurious behaviours typically include hand-biting, self-pinching/scratching and picking at sores, hitting the head or body, picking skin around the fingernails and tearing or pulling at the nails. Greenberg et al. (1991) reported two additional types of self-injurious behaviours as striking features of the syndrome – pulling out fingernails and toenails, and inserting foreign objects into bodily orifices. However, a systematic investigation by Webber (1999) found few examples of the latter two behaviours, and she concludes that these may not be characteristic of the syndrome. There have been anecdotal accounts of affected individuals who have strangled pets, possibly as a result of violent hugging which may be linked to reduced sensation in the hands (Smith, Dykens & Greenberg, 1998a; Webber, 1999).

Single cases have been described of children with Smith-Magenis syndrome who fulfil the diagnostic criteria for autism (Smith et al., 1986; Stratton et al., 1986; Vostanis et al., 1994), and autistic-type behaviours including resistance to change, repetitive questioning, and preoccupations with particular themes have been described in many cases. In the first systematic investigation of the association between autism and Smith-Magenis syndrome, Webber (1999) found that 93% of a sample of 29 children aged 6 to 16 years qualified for a diagnosis of autism using Wing's (1980) Schedule of Handicaps, Behaviour and Skills. While this instrument is considered by some to over-diagnose autism, Webber's findings highlight the high rates of autistic-type behaviours associated with the syndrome. At the same time children with Smith-Magenis syndrome are less impaired in their communicative abilities and sociability than one might expect from autistic children.

Severe sleep disturbance is a further hallmark of the syndrome and has been reported in up to 100% of children (Greenberg et al., 1996; Smith, Dykens and Greenberg, 1998b; Webber, 1999). The problems described include difficulties falling asleep, shortened sleep cycles, frequent and prolonged night awakings, early morning waking, excessive daytime sleepiness and daytime napping. Eighty per cent of Webber's sample of 29 children aged 6–16 exhibited two or more of these difficulties. Of the 25 (86%) who exhibited early waking (5.00 a.m. or earlier), 59% did this on a daily basis and about half of the total sample regularly slept during the day. Nocturnal enuresis is a common problem even in older children, possibly due to (or aggravated by) a hypotonic bladder. Abnormalities of REM sleep have been reported in over half of those studied with polysomnography (Greenberg et al., 1991). These abnormalities, abnormal melatonin levels and sleep cycle disturbances are suggestive of an underlying biological clock problem in the syndrome (Potocki et al., 1997).

On the positive side, children with Smith-Magenis syndrome are frequently described as loving and caring, eager to please and with a good sense of humour. They like adult attention and enjoy interacting with adults, though the desire for individual attention from adults may be intense. Many also love music, which can be used as a reinforcer as well as helping to calm children down. They react well to consistency, structure and routine. An unusual spasmodic upper body squeeze has been reported in 90–100% of affected individuals, comprising hand clasping and squeezing at chest or chin level, or crossing both arms tightly across the chest and spasmodically tensing the upper body. Excitement and pleasure can trigger this behaviour, which appears to be quite involuntary and may be an important diagnostic marker for the syndrome (Finucane et al., 1994; Webber, 1999).

The sizes of samples investigated to date, and the fact that the investigations are largely descriptive, limit the conclusions that can be drawn thus far about a cognitive and behavioural phenotype in Smith-Magenis syndrome. Moreover, it is likely that as case recognition improves an increasing number of less severely affected children will be identified and the figures on the rates of severe behavioural problems may fall. Nevertheless, the above findings are strongly suggestive of a set of behaviours and cognitive features that are characteristic of the syndrome and differentiate it from other disorders associated with learning disabilities.

Abilities, adjustment and behaviour in adult life

Little is known about the natural history of Smith-Magenis syndrome and the persistence of characteristic behavioural features into adulthood. Information currently available comes from a handful of descriptive studies of small, mixed samples of affected children and adults, and from one more systematic study of a sample of 21 adults aged 16–51 years undertaken by Udwin et al. (2001). Udwin et al. completed psychometric assessments on 19 affected adults; one adult scored at the floor of the test, a quarter had Full Scale IQs below 50, while just under three quarters had IQs within the mild learning disability range (IQ 50–69). IQs were on average somewhat higher than those reported for affected children. While this may be a result of the different cognitive tests that were used (WAIS versus WISC), it does suggest that adults with Smith-Magenis syndrome, at least those aged up to 50 years, do not show a decline in cognitive abilities over time. As is the case for children with the syndrome, long-term memory (for past events and routes), computing and perceptual skills were found to be areas of strength, while visuo-motor co-ordination, sequencing and response speed were highlighted as areas of weakness.

Despite their intellectual abilities falling largely in the mild learning disabilities range, the attainments of the adults in Udwin et al.'s sample in reading and spelling were on average only at a six to seven year level. Moreover, they showed little independence in daily living skills and were more dependent on carers than might be expected from their level of intellectual functioning. About 70% were unable to dress independently, while 85–90% could not cook a meal or undertake other household chores without supervision. No adults were able to travel any considerable distance on their own; 86% of the sample could only be left on their own for short periods of time, while 57% could only be left alone for a matter of minutes. No adult lived independently; around half lived with their families, while the remainder lived in residential communities or group homes. Only one adult worked in sheltered employment, as a kitchen assistant. The remainder attended day centres, adult training centres or college courses for people with learning disabilities. A few had work placements on day release programmes; in almost all cases these adults were reported by carers to require either substantial or continuous supervision.

A study by Horn (1999) confirmed previous reports of the persistence into adulthood of the severe behaviour difficulties associated with the syndrome. Most of the adults continued to show marked impulsivity and distractibility, although the rate of overactivity appears to decline in adolescence and adulthood. Over 80% were reported to exhibit high rates of verbal and physical aggression, and self-injurious behaviours were reported in 100% of cases. The behaviours had very similar triggers and were similar in type to those described in children. The pattern of persistence from childhood to adulthood was variable, with some showing improvement in adulthood, but others showing a worsening of the aggression and self-injury or no change. These findings are consistent with previous reports based on smaller samples of children and adults (Greenberg et al., 1991; Dykens et al., 1997), although the finding of 100% prevalence of self-injury is higher than rates previously reported. The rates of aggression and self-injury are unquestionably higher than those reported in general learning disability populations as well as in samples co-morbid for psychiatric disorders (Eyman & Call, 1977; Jacobson, 1982). They are, however, similar to those observed in certain other genetic syndromes, notably Lesch-Nyhan syndrome and Prader-Willi syndrome (Greenswag, 1987; Anderson & Ernst, 1994).

Horn (1999) highlighted the violent and alarming nature of the aggressive outbursts exhibited by some affected adults. In some cases, the outbursts were of such severity that the police had to be called; three adults had been admitted to hospital under a section of the Mental Health Act, and two were placed in regional secure units for people with learning disabilities. Five carers reported that adults had attempted to 'strangle' them on occasions when they were angry. Strangulation of pets was reported in two cases. As noted earlier, strangulation may be related to the self-hug that is characteristic of the syndrome, which in turn may be related to the peripheral neuropathy reported by Greenberg et al. (1996). If so, it is possible that this behaviour is not intentional, but rather that individuals with Smith-Magenis syndrome have difficulties gauging their own strength due to reduced sensation in their hands and arms.

Horn's (1999) study is the first to use a standardized instrument – the Diagnostic Interview for Social and Communication Disorders (Wing & Gould, 1994) – to examine autistic features in adults with Smith-Magenis syndrome. She found that 70% of her sample fulfilled diagnostic criteria for autism according to ICD-10 and DSM-IV criteria. This rate, and the rate reported by Webber (1999) for children with Smith-Magenis syndrome, are considerably higher than the rates reported in the general population (Fombonne, 1999), in populations of adults with moderate learning disabilities (Callacott et al., 1992) and in other genetic syndromes, including fragile X syndrome (Bailey et al., 1993). However, as Horn points out, while the behavioural characteristics associated with the syndrome might qualify for a diagnosis of autism on a standard diagnostic measure, they are quite distinct in a number of ways. Over 50% of adults with Smith-Magenis syndrome show marked stereotypic and repetitive behaviours, including a limited pattern of self-chosen activities, an insistence on sameness, repetitive questioning, a tendency to communicate around repetitive themes, and routine and stereotypical hand movements. Few show appropriate emotional responses, non-verbal communication or body postures, and social approaches are described as one-sided and on their own terms. Yet most affected individuals show some social awareness, are able to maintain eye-contact, greet people appropriately and seek social and physical comfort from others. Their communicative abilities, too, appear less impaired than might be expected for autistic individuals.

Sleep disturbance into adulthood continues to be a prominent feature of Smith-Magenis syndrome (Greenberg et al., 1996; Smith et al., 1998b; Horn, 1999). Seventy-five per cent to 100% of samples of adults are reported to have significant sleep problems which tend to be of a long-standing nature and are characterized primarily by night-time waking, early morning waking and difficulties falling asleep. These rates are significantly higher than rates for adults with general learning disabilities (Espie & Tweedie, 1991). The adults investigated by Horn (1999) woke an average of once or twice a night and took a mean time of 46 minutes to return to sleep. Their mean morning wake-up time was 6.00 a.m., though the majority woke at 5.00 a.m., and they slept for an average of 6 hours 40 minutes. Smith et al. (1998b) reported very similar findings, and also found that increased age was related to earlier wake-up times, shorter duration of sleep and an increased number of wakings in the night. Interestingly, carers reported that in most cases adults' sleep problems had shown some improvement over time (Horn, 1999). Horn concluded that this was not because adults slept for longer or woke less in the night, but because with age individuals became less disruptive during periods of wakefulness and were able to occupy themselves. Behaviours reported to have occurred during these periods in childhood, such as climbing out of windows, cooking breakfast and rearranging bedroom furniture, were replaced by more adaptive behaviours such as listening to tapes and watching television.

Horn (1999) and Webber (1999) found significant associations between severity of aggressive behaviours, severity of sleep disturbance and the presence of autistic features in their studies of children and adults. This combination of difficulties means that many affected individuals are extremely hard to manage. Given that many continue to live at home with their parents, the stress on families is likely to be considerable, and their need for support and input from health and social services is evident.

Implications for interventions

Given the physical and medical problems associated with Smith-Magenis syndrome, there is a need for regular medical checks, including eye examinations, hearing checks, ear, nose and throat examinations, heart and kidney investigations, and evaluations for thyroid function and scoliosis. Behaviourally, affected children and adults pose severe management problems for their carers, indicating a need for considerable support for families, as well as information about effective intervention approaches. Controlled treatment trials are lacking and urgently needed; however, anecdotal information gathered from parents, teachers and other carers has been useful in indicating that many of the behavioural difficulties described above may be modifiable, and in identifying helpful interventions and educational strategies for this population (Haas-Givler & Finucane, 1996; Smith et al., 1998a,b; Horn, 1999; Webber, 1999).

In childhood, oral motor and feeding training are important. Speech and language therapy using a total communication approach (including the use of sign and symbol systems) is likely to be helpful in promoting speech development and comprehension, and in alleviating frustration associated with poor expressive language skills (Smith et al., 1998a). Occupational therapy for difficulties with visuo-spatial skills, sequencing and co-ordination is also recommended. Since children with Smith-Magenis syndrome are typically distractible and overactive, they are likely to work best in classroom settings that are small, free from distractions and highly structured (Haas-Givler & Finucane, 1996). They are described as preferring consistency, structure and routine. Dykens et al. (1997) stress the need for teaching strategies that recognize their weaknesses in sequential processing and take advantage of their strengths in visual reasoning and other non-verbal areas. The use of visual cues in the form of pictures and symbols can aid recall of more complex sequential tasks and generally help with comprehension. Their particular interest in computers can also be used in teaching pre-reading and reading skills and promoting visuo-spatial skills. Individuals with Smith-Magenis syndrome tend to be eager to please and very responsive to adult attention; hence praise and attention from teachers and other adults, if used judiciously, can serve as useful reinforcers.

Parents and teachers describe a range of situations and characteristics that are likely to trigger aggressive outbursts and self-injurious behaviours (Haas-Givler & Finucane, 1996; Horn, 1999; Webber, 1999). These include an insatiable need for attention from adults and competition for their attention, transitioning from one activity or setting to another, unexpected changes in routine, tiredness, frustration, being reprimanded and not getting their own way. Attempts to anticipate and avoid such situations, for example by preparing the child for any change of routine well ahead of time, using clear instructions, rewards and distraction techniques (music, for example) are often effective in diffusing the situation. If not, ignoring aggressive behaviours or removing the child to another room and letting outbursts run their course may be the only remaining course of action. The range of triggers for aggressive behaviours and self-injury highlights the importance of carrying out a thorough functional analysis in each case so that appropriate interventions can be introduced. Moreover, in view of the prevalence of autistic-type behaviours in individuals with Smith-Magenis syndrome, it is recommended that multidisciplinary assessment for autistic spectrum disorders is undertaken. This would allow for a greater understanding of their communication difficulties and needs by parents and professionals, and could facilitate access to appropriate educational and mental health services.

A range of medications has been tried in an attempt to reduce the characteristic aggressive outbursts (Horn, 1999; Webber, 1999), but there have been no controlled trials of their effectiveness. Anecdotally, some medications have proven to be ineffective; others have been beneficial in some cases, but resulted in a worsening of behaviour for others. Clearly, if medication is going to be introduced for any one individual, it will need to be carefully monitored.

As regards the sleep difficulties of individuals with Smith-Magenis syndrome, parents' interventions have focused on keeping their children safe at night and attempting to minimize the disruption caused by night-waking. Implementing a firm and consistent approach, removing all small objects and breakables from the bedroom, locking the bedroom door or other doors in the house, use of blackout curtains to minimize light, firm and consistent instructions to return to bed, and providing soft toys, magazines, a tape recorder or television (in the case of older individuals), have all been reported to be helpful in minimizing night-time disruption in at least some cases, although not necessarily in increasing the amount of sleep (Smith et al., 1998b; Horn, 1999; Webber, 1999). Reducing daytime sleep is also effective for some individuals, though it can result in a worsening in behaviour in other cases. There have been anecdotal

Table 12.3. Smith-Magenis syndrome: implications of the phenotype for carers and professionals

---

- Regular medical checks should include:
  - eye examinations
  - hearing checks
  - ear, nose and throat checks
  - heart and kidney investigations
  - thyroid function
  - scoliosis
- Despite intellectual abilities mostly in the mild learning disabilities range, most individuals require substantial assistance with daily living skills and show little independence
- Severe behavioural difficulties requiring psychological interventions, and possibly also medication, include:
  - aggressive outbursts
  - self-injurious behaviours
  - sleep disturbance
  - hyperactivity and impulsivity
- Support and advice for carers is critical in view of severely challenging behaviours
- Assessment for autistic spectrum disorders is advisable in view of the high prevalence of autistic type behaviours in the syndrome

---

reports from the United States of improvements in sleep patterns with the administration of melatonin, but formal treatment trials are required before any recommendations can be made in this regard. Other medications for sleep have anecdotally shown mixed responses, with many individuals finding them ineffective (Horn, 1999; Webber, 1999).

The high prevalence rates of aggressive and self-injurious behaviours and the severe sleep disturbance found in both children and adults with Smith-Magenis syndrome underline the urgent need for research into effective management techniques and medications, and for appropriate and accessible mental health and social services provision for this population. There have been a number of cases in the UK and United States where concerns were raised about possible physical abuse by adults towards their children with Smith-Magenis syndrome, before the correct attribution of self-inflicted injuries by the children was made. In other cases parents have been blamed by teachers, social workers and others for the aggressive outbursts and excessive daytime sleepiness of their children. It is imperative that professionals have a good understanding of the implications of syndrome diagnosis for cognitive and behavioural characteristics, and that they are able to consider the often severe and disturbing behaviours exhibited by individuals with Smith-Magenis syndrome in the context of the underlying genetic syndrome.

For a summary of the implications of the phenotype for carers and professionals see Table 12.3.

REFERENCES

Anderson, L.T. & Ernst, M. (1994). Self-injury in Lesch-Nyhan Disease. *Journal of Autism and Developmental Disorders*, **24**: 67–81.

Bailey, A., Bolton, P., Butler, L. et al. (1993). Prevalence of the Fragile X anomaly among autistic twins and singletons. *Journal of Child Psychology and Psychiatry*, **34**: 673–88.

Bawden, H.N., MacDonald, G.W. & Shea, S. (1987). Treatment of children with Williams syndrome with methylphenidate. *Journal of Child Neurology*, **12**: 248–52.

Bellugi, U., Wang, P.P. & Jernigan, T.L. (1994). Williams syndrome: an unusual neuropsychological profile. In *Atypical Cognitive Deficits in Developmental Disorders*, ed. S.H. Broman & J. Grafman, pp. 22–56. New Jersey: L. Erlbaum.

Bennett, F.C., La Veck, B. & Sells, C.J. (1978). The Williams elphin faces syndrome; the psychological profile as an aid in syndrome identification. *Pediatrics*, **61**: 303–6.

Callacott, R., Cooper, S.A., Branford, D. & McGrother, C. (1992). Behaviour phenotypes for Down's syndrome. *British Journal of Psychiatry*, **172**: 85–9.

Carr, J. (1994). Long-term outcome for people with Down's syndrome. *Journal of Child Psychology and Psychiatry*, **35**: 425–39.

Chapman, C.A., du Plessis, A. & Pober, B.R. (1996). Neurologic findings in adults and children with Williams syndrome. *Journal of Child Neurology*, **11**: 63–5.

Chen, K.S., Lupski, J.R., Greenberg, F. & Lewis, R.A. (1996a). Ophthalmic manifestations of Smith-Magenis syndrome. *Ophthalmology*, **103**: 1084–91.

Chen, K.S., Potocki, L. & Lupski, J.R. (1996b). The Smith-Magenis syndrome [del(17)p11.2]: clinical review and molecular advances. *Mental Retardation and Developmental Disability Research Review*, **2**: 122–9.

Chevillard, C., Le Paslier, D., Passage, E. et al. (1993). Relationship between Charcot-Marie-Tooth 1A and Smith-Magenis regions: SnU3 may be a candidate gene for the Smith-Magenis syndrome. *Human Molecular Genetics*, **2**: 1235–43.

Crisco, J.J., Dobbs, J.M. & Mulhern, R.K. (1998). Cognitive processing of children with Williams syndrome. *Developmental Medicine and Child Neurology*, **30**: 650–6.

Crumley, F.E. (1998). Smith-Magenis syndrome. *Journal of the American Academy of Child and Adolescent Psychiatry*, **37**: 1131–2.

Davies, M., Howlin, P. & Udwin, O. (1997). Independence and adaptive behaviour in adults with Williams syndrome. *American Journal of Medical Genetics*, **70**: 188–95.

Davies, M., Udwin, O. & Howlin, P. (1998). Adults with Williams syndrome: preliminary study of social, emotional and behavioural difficulties. *British Journal of Psychiatry*, **172**: 273–6.

de Rijk-van Andel, J.F., Catsman-Berrevoets, van Hemel, J.O. & Hamers, A.J.H. (1991). Clinical and chromosome studies of three patients with Smith-Magenis syndrome. *Developmental Medicine and Child Neurology*, **33**: 343–55.

Dilts, C.V., Morris, C.A. & Leonard, C.O. (1990). Hypothesis for development of a behavioural phenotype in Williams syndrome. *American Journal of Medical Genetics*, **6**: 126–31.

Dykens, E.M., Finucane, B.M. & Gayley, C. (1997). Cognitive and behavioural profiles in persons with Smith-Magenis syndrome. *Journal of Autism and Developmental Disorders*, **27**: 203–11.

Dykens, M.D., Hodapp, R.M., Walsh, K. & Nash, L.J. (1992). Adaptive and maladaptive behaviour in Prader-Willi syndrome. *Journal of the American Academy of Child and Adolescent Psychiatry*, **31**: 131–6.

Dykens, M.D. & Rosner, B.A. (1999). Refining behavioural phenotypes: personality-motivation in Williams and Prader-Willi syndromes. *American Journal on Mental Retardation*, **104**: 158–69.

Dykens, E.M. & Smith, A.C.M. (1998). Distinctiveness and correlates of maladaptive behaviour in children and adolescents with Smith-Magenis syndrome. *Journal of Intellectual Disability Research*, **42**: 481–9.

Einfeld, S.L., Tonge, B.J. & Florio, T. (1997). Behavioural and emotional disturbance in individuals with Williams syndrome. *American Journal on Mental Retardation*, **102**: 45–53.

Elsea, S.A., Finucane, B., Juyal, R.C. et al. (1996). Smith-Magenis syndrome due to a submicroscopic deletion in 17p11.2 allows further definition of the critical interval. *American Journal of Human Genetics*, **59**(4): A257.

Espie, C.A. & Tweedie, F.M. (1991). Sleep patterns and sleep problems amongst people with mental handicap. *Journal of Mental Deficiency Research*, **35**: 25–36.

Ewart, A.K., Morris, C.A., Atkinson, D., Jin, W., Sternes, K., Spallone, P., Stock, A.D., Leppert, M. & Keating, M.T. (1993). Hemizygosity at the elastin locus in a developmental disorder, Williams syndrome. *Nature Genetics*, **5**: 11–16.

Eyman, R.K. & Call, T. (1977). Maladaptive behaviour and community placement. *American Journal of Mental Deficiency*, **82**: 137–44.

Finucane, B.M., Jaeger, E.R., Kurtz, M.B., Weinstein, M. & Scott, C.I. (1993). Eye abnormalities in the Smith-Magenis contiguous gene deletion syndrome. *American Journal of Medical Genetics*, **45**: 443–6.

Finucane, B.M., Konar, D., Haas-Givler, B., Kurtz, M.B. & Scott, C.I. (1994). The spasmodic upper-body squeeze: a characteristic behaviour in Smith-Magenis syndrome. *Developmental Medicine and Child Neurology*, **36**: 70–83.

Fombonne, E. (1999). The epidemiology of autism: a review. *Journal of Psychological Medicine*, **29**: 769–86.

Gosch, A. & Pankau, R. (1994). Social-emotional and behavioural adjustment in children with Williams syndrome. *American Journal of Medical Genetics*, **53**: 335–9.

Greenberg, F., Guzzetta, V., de Oca-Luna, R.M. et al. (1991). Molecular analysis of the Smith-Magenis syndrome: a possible contiguous-gene syndrome associated with del(17)(p11.2). *American Journal of Human Genetics*, **49**: 1207–18.

Greenberg, F., Lewis, R.A., Potocki, L. et al. (1996). Multi-disciplinary clinical study of Smith-Magenis syndrome (deletion 17p11.2). *American Journal of Medical Genetics*, **62**: 247–54.

Greenswag, L.R. (1987). Adults with Prader-Willi syndrome: a survey of 232 cases. *Developmental Medicine and Child Neurology*, **29**: 145–52.

Haas-Givler, B. & Finucane, B. (1996). "What's a teacher to do?": classroom strategies that enhance learning for children with Smith-Magenis syndrome. *Spectrum* (Newsletter of PRISMS), **2**(1): 6–8.

Hagerman, R.J., Schreiner, R.A., Kemper, M.B., Willenberger, M.D., Zahn, B. & Habicht, K. (1989). Longitudinal IQ changes in fragile X males. *American Journal of Medical Genetics*, **33**: 513–18.

Horn, I. (1999). *The Cognitive and Behavioural Phenotype of Smith-Magenis Syndrome.* Unpublished Doctoral Thesis, University of London.

Howlin, P., Davies, M. & Udwin, O. (1998). Cognitive functioning in adults with Williams syndrome. *Journal of Clinical Psychology and Psychiatry*, **39**: 183–9.

Jacobson, J.W. (1982). Problem behaviour and psychiatric impairment within a developmentally disabled population. I. Behaviour frequency. *Applied Research in Mental Retardation*, **3**: 121–39.

Joseph, M.C. & Parrott, D. (1958). Severe infantile hypercalcaemia, with special reference to the facies. *Archives of Disease in Childhood*, **33**: 385–95.

Karmiloff-Smith, A., Grant, J., Berthoud, I., Davies, M., Howlin, P. & Udwin, O. (1996). Language and Williams syndrome: how intact is "intact"? *Child Development*, **68**: 274–90.

Karmiloff-Smith, A., Tyler, L.K., Voice, K., Sims, K., Udwin, O., Howlin, P. & Davies, M. (1998). Linguistic dissociations in Williams syndrome: evaluating receptive syntax in on-line and off-line tasks. *Neuropsychologia*, **36**: 343–51.

Kataria, S., Goldstein, D.J. & Kushnick, T. (1984). Developmental delays in Williams ("elfin faces") syndrome. *Applied Research in Mental Retardation*, **5**: 419–23.

Klein, A.J., Armstrong, B.L., Greer, M.K. & Brown, F.R. (1990). Hyperacusis and otitis media in individuals with Williams syndrome. *Journal of Speech and Hearing Disorders*, **55**: 339–44.

Martin, N.D.T., Snodgrass, G.J.A.I. & Cohen, R.D. (1984). Idiopathic infantile hypercalcaemia – a continuing enigma. *Archives of Disease in Childhood*, **59**: 605–13.

Meyerson, M.D. & Frank, R.A. (1987). Annotation: language, speech and hearing in Williams syndrome: Intervention approaches and research needs. *Developmental Medicine and Child Neurology*, **29**: 258–70.

Moncla, A., Livet, M.O., Auger, M., Mattei, J.F., Mattei, M.G. & Firaud, F. (1991). Smith-Magenis syndrome: a new contiguous gene syndrome: report of three new cases. *Journal of Medical Genetics*, **28**: 627–32.

Morris, C.A., Demsey, S.A., Leonard, C.O., Dilts, C. & Blackburn, B.L. (1988). The natural history of Williams syndrome: physical characteristics. *Journal of Pediatrics*, **113**: 318–26.

Pober, B.P., Lacro, V.L., Rice, C., Mandell, V. & Teele, R.L. (1993). Renal findings in forty individuals with Williams syndrome. *American Journal of Medical Genetics*, **46**: 271–4.

Potocki, L., Reiter, R.J., Glaze, D. & Lupski, J.R. (1997). Twenty-four hour urinary excretion of 6-sulphatoxymelatonin in Smith-Magenis syndrome. *American College of Medical Genetics Conference*, A31.

Smith, A.C.M., Dykens, E. & Greenberg, F. (1998a). Behavioural phenotype of Smith-Magenis syndrome (del 17 p11.2). *American Journal of Medical Genetics*, **81**: 179–85.

Smith, A.C.M., Dykens, E. & Greenberg, F. (1998b). Sleep disturbance in Smith-Magenis syndrome (del 17 p11.2). *American Journal of Medical Genetics*, **81**: 186–91.

Smith, A.C.M., McGavran, L., Robinson, J. et al. (1986). Interstitial deletion of (17) (p11.2p11.2) in nine patients. *American Journal of Medical Genetics*, **24**: 393–414.

Smith, A.C.M., McGavran, L. & Waldstein, G. (1982). Deletion of the 17 short arm in two patients with facial clefts. *American Journal of Human Genetics*, **34**(Suppl.): A410.

Stratton, R.F., Dobyns, W.B., Greenberg, F. et al. (1986). Interstitial deletion of (17) (p11.2p11.2): report of six additional patients with a new chromosome deletion syndrome. *American Journal of Medical Genetics*, **24**: 421–32.

Turk, J. & Sales, J. (1996). Behavioural phenotypes and their relevance to child mental health professionals. *Child Psychology and Psychiatry Review*, **1**: 4–11.

Udwin, O. (1990). A survey of adults with Williams syndrome and idiopathic infantile hypercalcaemia. *Developmental Medicine and Child Neurology*, **32**: 129–41.

Udwin, O., Davies, M. & Howlin, P. (1996). A longitudinal study of cognitive abilities and educational attainment in Williams syndrome. *Developmental Medicine and Child Neurology*, **38**: 1020–9.

Udwin, O., Howlin, P. & Davies, M. (1996a). *Adults with Williams Syndrome: Guidelines for Families and Professionals*. Tonbridge Kent: The Williams Syndrome Foundation.

Udwin, O., Howlin, P. & Davies, M. (1996b). *Adults with Williams Syndrome: Guidelines for Employers*. Tonbridge Kent: The Williams Syndrome Foundation.

Udwin, O., Howlin, P., Davies, M. & Mannion, E. (1998). Community care for adults with Williams syndrome: How families cope and the availability of support networks. *Journal of Intellectual Disability Research*, **42**: 238–45.

Udwin, O., Webber, C. & Horn, I. (2001). Abilities and attainment in Smith-Magenis syndrome. *Developmental Medicine and Child Neurology*, **43**: 823–8.

Udwin, O. & Yule, W. (1990). Expressive language of children with Williams syndrome. *American Journal of Medical Genetics*, **6**(Suppl.): 108–14.

Udwin, O. & Yule, W. (1991). A cognitive and behavioural phenotype in Williams syndrome. *Journal of Clinical and Experimental Neuropsychology*, **13**: 232–344.

Udwin, O. & Yule, W. (1998a). *Williams Syndrome: Guidelines for Parents*. Tonbridge Kent: The Williams Syndrome Foundation.

Udwin, O. & Yule, W. (1998b). *Williams Syndrome: Guidelines for Teachers*. Tonbridge Kent: The Williams Syndrome Foundation.

Udwin, O., Yule, W. & Martin, N. (1987). Cognitive abilities and behavioural characteristics of children with idiopathic infantile hypercalcaemia. *Journal of Child Psychology and Psychiatry*, **28**: 297–309.

Vostanis, P., Harrington, R., Prendergast, M. & Farndon, P. (1994). Case reports of autism with interstitial deletion of chromosome 17 (p11.2p11.2) and monosomy of chromosome 5 (5pter → 5p15.3). *Psychiatric Genetics*, **4**: 109–11.

Webber, C. (1999). *Cognitive and Behavioural Phenotype of Children with Smith-Magenis Syndrome*. Unpublished Doctoral Dissertation, University of Leicester.

Wing, L. (1980). The MRC handicaps, behaviour and skills (HBS) schedule. *Acta Psychiatrica Scandinavica*, **62**: 241–8.

Wing, L. & Gould, J. (1994). *Diagnostic Interview for Social and Communication Disorders* (DISCO). London: National Autistic Society Centre for Social and Communication Disorders.

Zhao, Z., Lee, C.C., Jiralerspong, S. et al. (1995). The gene for human microfibril-associated glycoprotein is commonly deleted in Smith-Magenis syndrome patients. *Human Molecular Genetics*, **4**: 589–97.

Zori, R.T., Lupski, J.R., Heju, Z. et al. (1993). Clinical, cytogenetic and molecular evidence for an infant with Smith-Magenis syndrome born from a mother having a mosaic 17p11.2p12 deletion. *American Journal of Medical Genetics*, **47**: 504–11.

Index